Clinical Optics

Section 3

2012–2013

(Last major revision 2009–2010)

BASIC AND CLINICAL SCIENCE COURSE

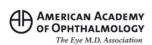

AMERICAN ACADEMY OF OPHTHALMOLOGY
The Eye M.D. Association

LEO

LIFELONG
EDUCATION FOR THE
OPHTHALMOLOGIST

The Basic and Clinical Science Course is one component of the Lifelong Education for the Ophthalmologist (LEO) framework, which assists members in planning their continuing medical education. LEO includes an array of clinical education products that members may select to form individualized, self-directed learning plans for updating their clinical knowledge. Active members or fellows who use LEO components may accumulate sufficient CME credits to earn the LEO Award. Contact the Academy's Clinical Education Division for further information on LEO.

The American Academy of Ophthalmology is accredited by the Accreditation Council for Continuing Medical Education to provide continuing medical education for physicians.

The American Academy of Ophthalmology designates this enduring material for a maximum of 15 *AMA PRA Category 1 Credits*™. Physicians should claim only the credit commensurate with the extent of their participation in the activity.

The Academy provides this material for educational purposes only. It is not intended to represent the only or best method or procedure in every case, nor to replace a physician's own judgment or give specific advice for case management. Including all indications, contraindications, side effects, and alternative agents for each drug or treatment is beyond the scope of this material. All information and recommendations should be verified, prior to use, with current information included in the manufacturers' package inserts or other independent sources, and considered in light of the patient's condition and history. Reference to certain drugs, instruments, and other products in this course is made for illustrative purposes only and is not intended to constitute an endorsement of such. Some material may include information on applications that are not considered community standard, that reflect indications not included in approved FDA labeling, or that are approved for use only in restricted research settings. **The FDA has stated that it is the responsibility of the physician to determine the FDA status of each drug or device he or she wishes to use, and to use them with appropriate, informed patient consent in compliance with applicable law.** The Academy specifically disclaims any and all liability for injury or other damages of any kind, from negligence or otherwise, for any and all claims that may arise from the use of any recommendations or other information contained herein.

Cover image courtesy of Perry Rosenthal, MD.

Basic and Clinical Science Course

Gregory L. Skuta, MD, Oklahoma City, Oklahoma, *Senior Secretary for Clinical Education*

Louis B. Cantor, MD, Indianapolis, Indiana, *Secretary for Ophthalmic Knowledge*

Jayne S. Weiss, MD, New Orleans, Louisiana, *BCSC Course Chair*

Section 3

Faculty Responsible for This Edition

Neal H. Atebara, MD, *Chair,* Honolulu, Hawaii
Penny A. Asbell, MD, New York, New York
Dimitri T. Azar, MD, Chicago, Illinois
Forrest J. Ellis, MD, Falls Church, Virginia
Eleanor E. Faye, MD, New York, New York
Kenneth J. Hoffer, MD, Santa Monica, California
Robert E. Wiggins, MD, Asheville, North Carolina
   Practicing Ophthalmologists Advisory Committee for Education

Financial Disclosures

Academy staff members who contributed to the development of this product state that they have no significant financial interest or other relationship with the manufacturer of any commercial product discussed in this course or with the manufacturer of any competing commercial product.

The authors state the following financial relationships:

Dr Asbell: Addition Technology, consultant, grant and lecture honoraria recipient; Alcon Laboratories, consultant, grant and lecture honoraria recipient; Allergan, consultant, grant and lecture honoraria recipient; Bausch & Lomb, consultant, grant and lecture honoraria recipient; Johnson & Johnson Medical, lecture honoraria recipient; Novartis Pharmaceuticals, consultant, grant and lecture honoraria recipient; Paragon Vision Sciences, consultant, grant and lecture honoraria recipient; Pfizer Ophthalmics, consultant, grant and lecture honoraria recipient; Santen, consultant, grant and lecture honoraria recipient; Vistakon, consultant, grant and lecture honoraria recipient.

Dr Azar: Advanced Medical Optics, lecture honoraria recipient; Alcon Laboratories, lecture honoraria recipient; Allergan, consultant, lecture honoraria recipient; Bausch & Lomb, consultant; Prism Ventures, consultant; Santen, lecture honoraria recipient; Sarentis, consultant.

Dr Hoffer: EyeLab, equity holder.

The other authors state that they have no significant financial interest or other relationship with the manufacturer of any commercial product discussed in the chapters that they contributed to this course or with the manufacturer of any competing commercial product.

Recent Past Faculty

Darren L. Albert, MD, Montreal, Quebec, Canada
Kevin M. Miller, MD, Los Angeles, California
Robert J. Schechter, MD, Los Angeles, California
Ming X. Wang, MD, PhD, Nashville, Tennessee

In addition, the Academy gratefully acknowledges the contributions of numerous past faculty and advisory committee members who have played an important role in the development of previous editions of the Basic and Clinical Science Course.

American Academy of Ophthalmology Staff

Richard A. Zorab, *Vice President, Ophthalmic Knowledge*
Hal Straus, *Director, Publications Department*
Christine Arturo, *Acquisitions Manager*
Stephanie Tanaka, *Publications Manager*
D. Jean Ray, *Production Manager*
Ann McGuire, *Medical Editor*
Steve Huebner, *Administrative Coordinator*

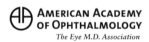

AMERICAN ACADEMY
OF OPHTHALMOLOGY
The Eye M.D. Association

655 Beach Street
Box 7424
San Francisco, CA 94120-7424

Contents

General Introduction

The Basic and Clinical Science Course (BCSC) is designed to meet the needs of residents and practitioners for a comprehensive yet concise curriculum of the field of ophthalmology. The BCSC has developed from its original brief outline format, which relied heavily on outside readings, to a more convenient and educationally useful self-contained text. The Academy updates and revises the course annually, with the goals of integrating the basic science and clinical practice of ophthalmology and of keeping ophthalmologists current with new developments in the various subspecialties.

The BCSC incorporates the effort and expertise of more than 80 ophthalmologists, organized into 13 Section faculties, working with Academy editorial staff. In addition, the course continues to benefit from many lasting contributions made by the faculties of previous editions. Members of the Academy's Practicing Ophthalmologists Advisory Committee for Education serve on each faculty and, as a group, review every volume before and after major revisions.

Organization of the Course

The Basic and Clinical Science Course comprises 13 volumes, incorporating fundamental ophthalmic knowledge, subspecialty areas, and special topics:

1 Update on General Medicine
2 Fundamentals and Principles of Ophthalmology
3 Clinical Optics
4 Ophthalmic Pathology and Intraocular Tumors
5 Neuro-Ophthalmology
6 Pediatric Ophthalmology and Strabismus
7 Orbit, Eyelids, and Lacrimal System
8 External Disease and Cornea
9 Intraocular Inflammation and Uveitis
10 Glaucoma
11 Lens and Cataract
12 Retina and Vitreous
13 Refractive Surgery

In addition, a comprehensive Master Index allows the reader to easily locate subjects throughout the entire series.

References

Readers who wish to explore specific topics in greater detail may consult the references cited within each chapter and listed in the Basic Texts section at the back of the book. These references are intended to be selective rather than exhaustive, chosen by the BCSC faculty as being important, current, and readily available to residents and practitioners.

Related Academy educational materials are also listed in the appropriate sections. They include books, online and audiovisual materials, self-assessment programs, clinical modules, and interactive programs.

Study Questions and CME Credit

Each volume of the BCSC is designed as an independent study activity for ophthalmology residents and practitioners. The learning objectives for this volume are given on page 1. The text, illustrations, and references provide the information necessary to achieve the objectives; the study questions allow readers to test their understanding of the material and their mastery of the objectives. Physicians who wish to claim CME credit for this educational activity may do so by mail, by fax, or online. The necessary forms and instructions are given at the end of the book.

Conclusion

The Basic and Clinical Science Course has expanded greatly over the years, with the addition of much new text and numerous illustrations. Recent editions have sought to place a greater emphasis on clinical applicability while maintaining a solid foundation in basic science. As with any educational program, it reflects the experience of its authors. As its faculties change and as medicine progresses, new viewpoints are always emerging on controversial subjects and techniques. Not all alternate approaches can be included in this series; as with any educational endeavor, the learner should seek additional sources, including such carefully balanced opinions as the Academy's Preferred Practice Patterns.

The BCSC faculty and staff are continuously striving to improve the educational usefulness of the course; you, the reader, can contribute to this ongoing process. If you have any suggestions or questions about the series, please do not hesitate to contact the faculty or the editors.

The authors, editors, and reviewers hope that your study of the BCSC will be of lasting value and that each Section will serve as a practical resource for quality patient care.

Objectives

Upon completion of BCSC Section 3, *Clinical Optics,* the reader should be able to

- compare and contrast physical and geometric optics

- discuss the clinical and technical relevance of such optical phenomena as interference, coherence, polarization, diffraction, and scattering

- review the basic properties of laser light and how they affect laser–tissue interaction

- outline the principles of light propagation and image formation and work through some of the fundamental equations that describe or measure such properties as refraction, reflection, magnification, and vergence

- explain how these principles can be applied diagnostically and therapeutically

- describe the clinical application of Snell's law and the lensmaker's equation

- identify optical models of the human eye and describe how to apply them

- define the various types of visual perception and function, including visual acuity, brightness sensitivity, color perception, and contrast sensitivity

- summarize the steps for performing streak retinoscopy

- summarize the steps for performing a manifest refraction using a phoropter or trial lenses

- describe the use of the Jackson cross cylinder

- describe the indications for prescribing bifocals and common difficulties encountered in their use

- review the materials and fitting parameters of both soft and rigid contact lenses

- explain the optical principles underlying various modalities of refractive correction: spectacles, contact lenses, intraocular lenses, and refractive surgery

- discern the differences among these types of refractive correction and describe how to apply them most appropriately to the individual patient

- discuss the basic methods of calculating intraocular lens powers and the advantages and disadvantages of the different methods

- describe the conceptual basis of multifocal IOLs and how the correction of presbyopia differs between these IOLs and spectacles

- recognize the visual needs of low vision patients and how to address these needs through optical and nonoptical devices and/or appropriate referral

- describe the operating principles of various optical instruments in order to use them more effectively

CHAPTER **1**

Physical Optics

What is light? This question has been the subject of vigorous debate for centuries. One school of thought supported the wave theory, originally stated by Christian Huygens and amplified by Young and Maxwell. Opposed to this school were those who championed the corpuscular theory, originated by Newton and supported by Planck. Ultimately, however, both theories are necessary to account for all the phenomena associated with light. The science of quantum mechanics, which evolved from the quantum theory of Planck, successfully addresses the dual nature of light by incorporating both the particle and the wave aspects of light.

The description of optical phenomena is currently divided into the areas of physical optics, geometric optics, and quantum optics. *Physical optics* describes those phenomena that are most readily understood in terms of wave properties of light. *Geometric optics* conceives of light as rays and deals with the imaging properties of lenses and mirrors. *Quantum optics* is concerned with the interaction of light and matter and considers light as having both wave and particle (photon) characteristics.

In brief, light behaves like a *wave* as it passes through air, a vacuum, or transparent materials. Light exhibits some characteristics of photons when it is being generated or absorbed. The *ray-tracing model* is a simplified method for describing the propagation of light. Although it ignores the effects of diffraction and other physical optics phenomena, it provides a convenient method for calculations involving lenses and images.

Because, in ophthalmology, our primary interest is in the propagation of light through media, including transparent ocular tissues, we concentrate on the wave and ray descriptions of light, with only occasional references to its photon characteristics.

Wave Theory

Water waves provide a good analogy for understanding light waves. When a wave travels along the water's surface, particles at the surface move up and down as the wave is propagated, but they do not move along with the wave. In the case of light, no material substance moves as the light wave propagates. Rather, at each point the electric field increases, decreases, and reverses direction in a sinusoidal manner as the wave passes (Fig 1-1). The electric field is always perpendicular to the direction of propagation.

Among the principal characteristics of a wave, as illustrated in Figure 1-1, are its wavelength (λ) and amplitude *(A). Wavelength* is determined by the distance between crests of the wave. *Amplitude* is the maximum value attained by the electric field as the

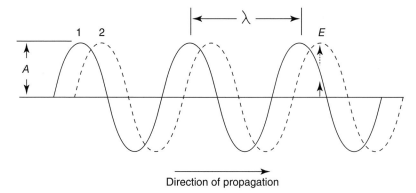

Figure 1-1 Instantaneous "snapshot" of a light wave. *1* represents the light at a particular instant; *2* represents the wave a short time later, after it has moved a fraction of 1 wavelength to the right. The wavelength, *λ,* is the distance between crests of the wave. The electric field, *E,* at a particular point, is represented by the *solid line* for wave 1 and by the *dashed line* for wave 2. The amplitude of the wave, *A,* is the maximum value of the electric field. The frequency is the number of wave crests that pass a fixed point per second and is dependent on the speed of the wave. *(Redrawn by C. H. Wooley.)*

wave propagates. It determines the intensity of the wave. A third characteristic of a wave, not shown in Figure 1-1, is the *frequency,* which is the number of wave crests that pass a fixed point per second. Finally, multiple waves of the same amplitude may be described as "in phase," which means the light intensity is doubled; "out of phase," meaning they cancel each other; or at some level in between, resulting in an intermediate level of intensity (Fig 1-2).

In addition to an electric field, a light wave has a magnetic field that increases and decreases with the electric field. As indicated in Figure 1-3, the magnetic field *(H)* is perpendicular both to the direction of propagation of the light and to the electric field. The magnetic field is less important than the electric field and is often omitted in descriptions of a light wave.

Figure 1-4 illustrates the electromagnetic wave spectrum, including the very small portion occupied by visible light. In common usage, the term *light* refers to the visible portion of the electromagnetic wave spectrum, but it can be applied to radiation in the infrared and near-UV portions of the spectrum as well. Although the region of visible light is normally defined as 400–700 nm, the boundaries are not precise, and under certain conditions the eye's sensitivity extends into the infrared and UV regions. For example, in aphakia, without the UV absorption of the natural lens, the retina is able to detect wavelengths well below 400 nm. X-rays also produce a response in the retina, but these waves are not focused by the optical components of the eye.

The speed of light in a vacuum *(c)* is one of the fundamental constants of nature, almost exactly 3×10^8 m/sec. The wavelength of light in a vacuum (λ.) is related to its frequency (ν) by the equation

$$\lambda.\nu = c$$

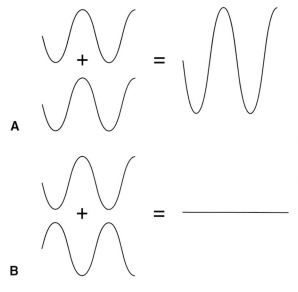

A

Figure 1-2 When light waves are fully "in phase" with one another, their superposition results in a doubling of the light intensity **(A).** When they are fully "out of phase," they cancel each other out, and the resulting light intensity is 0 **(B).** When they are in between these 2 extremes, the resulting light intensity is at an intermediate level **(C).** *(Illustration by C. H. Wooley.)*

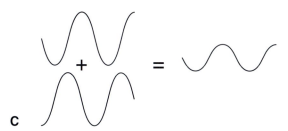

B

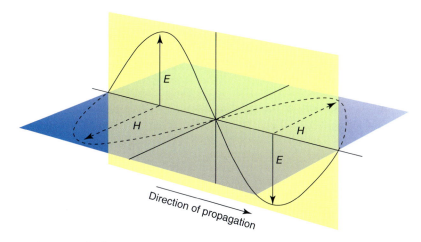

C

Figure 1-3 A magnetic field always accompanies the electric field in any electromagnetic wave. The magnetic field, represented by *H,* is always perpendicular to the electric field, *E.* *(Redrawn by Jonathan Clark.)*

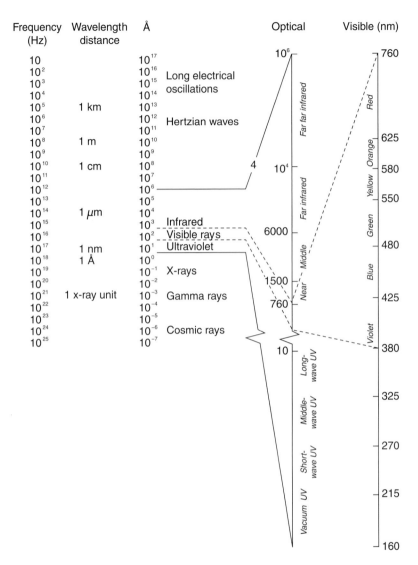

Figure 1-4 The electromagnetic spectrum. *(Modified with permission from Steinert RF, Puliafito CA. The Nd:YAG Laser in Ophthalmology: Principles and Clinical Applications of Photodisruption. Philadelphia: Saunders; 1985. Redrawn by C. H. Wooley.)*

When light travels through any transparent medium *(m)* other than a vacuum, its velocity *(V)* is reduced, but its frequency does not change. The index of refraction *(n)* of the medium is defined as the ratio of the speed of light in a vacuum to the speed of light in the given material and is written as

$$n_m = c/V$$

Lens materials have unique indices of refraction. The index of refraction of typical CR-39 plastic lenses is 1.50, whereas that of a typical high-index lens is 1.66. The higher the index of refraction, the thinner the lens. This is important for patients with higher refractive errors who prefer "thin lenses."

Given that the frequency of a wave does not change on traveling through a transparent medium, the wavelength (λ_m) becomes shorter, as governed by the relationship

$$n_m = c/V = \lambda_v/\lambda_m$$

where λ_v is the wavelength of light in a vacuum.

Photon Aspects of Light

When light interacts with matter, individual quanta of energy (photons) are emitted or absorbed. The amount of energy *(E)* per photon is equal to the Planck constant multiplied by the frequency and is written as

$$E = hv$$

where *v* is the frequency of the light wave and *h* is the *Planck constant:* 6.626×10^{-34} J/sec. Because the frequency of blue light is greater than that of red light (see Fig 1-4), a photon of blue light has greater energy than a photon of red light.

The diagnostic use of fluorescein demonstrates a practical application of this principle. For example, a photon of blue light is absorbed by an individual fluorescein molecule. When the molecule reemits light (fluoresces), the emitted photon has a lower energy, lying in the yellow-green portion of the spectrum. The remaining energy is converted into heat or chemical energy. As a rule, light emitted through fluorescence has a longer wavelength than the excitation light.

The particle–wave duality extends to other fundamental concepts as well. The electron, for example, behaves like a wave with a wavelength much shorter than that of light. Because diffraction effects are much reduced at shorter wavelengths (see the section Diffraction, later in this chapter), extremely high resolution can be obtained with the electron microscope.

Interference and Coherence

Interference occurs when 2 light waves originating from the same source are brought together. Interference occurs most readily when the light is monochromatic; that is, it lies within a narrow band of wavelengths. But interference can also be obtained with white light under optimum conditions.

In Figure 1-5, the curved lines represent the crests of the waves at a particular instant. Where the crests coincide (eg, at *A*), a maximum of intensity is produced because the energy of the electromagnetic fields is added together *(constructive interference)*. Where the crest of 1 wave coincides with the trough of the other wave *(B)*, the 2 electromagnetic fields cancel each other, and intensity is minimized *(destructive interference)*. If the 2 waves are exactly equal in amplitude, the destructive interference will be complete, and the light intensity will be zero. Thus, in Figure 1-5, the screen displays a series of light and dark bands corresponding to areas of constructive and destructive interference.

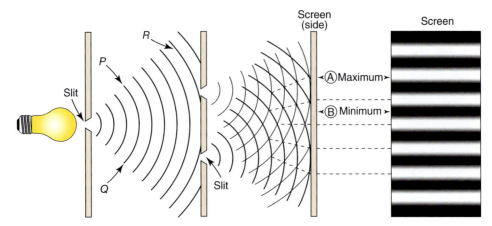

Figure 1-5 Interference. *A* represents constructive interference; *B* indicates destructive interference. *(Redrawn by Jonathan Clark.)*

The term *coherence* describes the ability of 2 light beams, or different parts of the same beam, to produce interference. *Spatial,* or lateral, coherence refers to the ability of 2 separated portions of the same wave (*P* and *Q* in Fig 1-5) to produce interference. *Temporal,* or longitudinal, coherence is the ability of 1 wave of a beam to interfere with a different wave within the same beam (*P* and *R*). A large, white light source has a coherence close to zero. However, if the light is passed through a narrow slit, as in Figure 1-5, the spatial coherence between *P* and *Q* improves, approaching unity as the slit approaches zero width. Temporal coherence is improved when a filter is used to select a narrow band of wavelengths, thereby making it highly monochromatic. Laser light is highly coherent. Most gas lasers approach perfect temporal coherence, meaning that a portion of the beam can be made to interfere with a much later portion of the beam.

Applications of Interference and Coherence

Interference resulting from the high degree of coherence in laser light can lead to serious problems in some laser applications. However, interference effects can also be put to practical use, as in *laser interferometry,* a technique for evaluating retinal function in the presence of a cataractous lens. In laser interferometry, a laser beam is split into 2 beams, which then pass through different parts of the pupil. Where the beams again overlap on the retina, interference fringes are formed, even if the beams have been diffused by the cataract.

One of the most important applications of interference is in *antireflection films* (Fig 1-6) and *interference filters* (Fig 1-7). If the 2 reflected beams in Figure 1-6 are equal in amplitude but exactly half a wavelength out of phase, the resulting destructive interference will cause the beams to cancel each other and thereby prevent reflection for a given wavelength. Modern low-reflection coatings consist of several thin layers of transparent materials designed to give a reflection of only a few tenths of a percent over the visible spectrum. Films are typically prepared by evaporation of the material in a vacuum chamber and deposition on the glass surface.

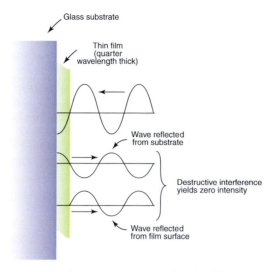

Figure 1-6 Destructive interference by an antireflection film. *(Redrawn by C. H. Wooley.)*

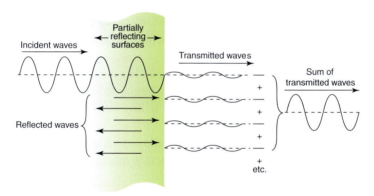

Figure 1-7 The interference filter transmits only that wavelength for which the internally reflected waves are in phase with one another. *(Redrawn by C. H. Wooley.)*

The *interference filter* (see Fig 1-7) is designed so that successive rays transmitted through the filter are exactly in phase and therefore interfere constructively. This condition applies exactly for only 1 wavelength; as a result, the filter transmits only that wavelength and a narrow band of wavelengths on either side. Other wavelengths are reflected by the interference filter. The reflecting layers can be thin films of metal such as silver or aluminum. More frequently they consist of multiple thin layers of transparent materials, with the thickness of each layer chosen to give the desired reflectance.

Thin layers can also be designed so that the transmission (or reflection) has the characteristic properties of a sharp cutoff filter. For example, a so-called *cold mirror* has a multilayer coating designed to reflect the visible (cold) light and transmit the infrared wavelengths. The excitation filter used in fluorescein angiography transmits short wavelengths, below about 500 nm, that cause fluorescein to fluoresce. The barrier filter used in the fundus camera transmits only the long wavelengths, above about 500 nm. Therefore, the fluorescent emission is received by the film, but all excitation light is excluded.

Optical coherence tomography (OCT), introduced into ophthalmology for in vivo imaging of the retina and optic nerve head, relies on low-coherence tomography, in which the signal carrying light returning from the eye is allowed to interfere with light that has traveled a path of known length. OCT is discussed in Chapter 8, Telescopes and Optical Instruments.

> van Velthoven ME, Faber DJ, Verbraak FD, van Leeuwen TG, de Smet MD. Recent developments in optical coherence tomography for imaging the retina. *Prog Retin Eye Res.* 2007;26(1): 57–77.

Polarization

In general, the human eye is not sensitive to polarization of light. Nevertheless, polarization has a number of applications in visual science and ophthalmology; these are discussed in the following section.

A good analogy for polarization is light waves moving through a picket fence. The fence lets through only waves of a certain direction, blocking the rest of the waves. *Plane-polarized,* or *linearly polarized,* light consists of waves that all have their electric fields in the same plane.

In a different analogy, we could turn one end of a rope in a circular motion. The wave would then travel along the rope as a circular oscillation. Similarly, in *circularly polarized light,* the electric field at any point rotates rapidly. In *elliptically polarized light,* the electric field both rotates and changes amplitude rapidly as the wave passes.

Unpolarized light consists of a random mixture of various plane-polarized beams. *Partial polarization,* as the name implies, produces a mixture of unpolarized light and polarized light (plane, circular, or elliptical).

One way to produce plane-polarized light is to pass a beam of unpolarized light through a polarizing filter (eg, sheet plastic). This is analogous to passing a vibrating rope through a picket fence so that only the vertical vibration is transmitted. Certain crystals, particularly calcite, can be used to polarize light. As will be seen later, reflection can also cause complete or partial polarization. Even the sky acts as a partial polarizer by means of the scattering properties of air molecules.

Applications of Polarization

One exception to the eye's lack of sensitivity to polarization is the Haidinger brush phenomenon, named after Austrian physicist Wilhelm Karl von Haidinger, who, in 1844, was the first to describe this entoptic phenomenon (Fig 1-8). The Haidinger brush can be demonstrated clinically when a polarizer is rotated continuously in front of a uniform blue field. A normal subject will see a rotating structure that looks like a double-ended brush or a propeller. This phenomenon is useful in localizing the fovea during sensory testing and in evaluating the status of the Henle fiber layer at the macula.

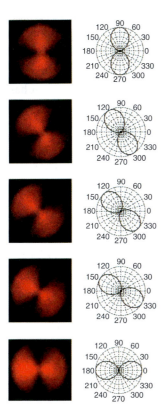

Figure 1-8 Sequence of experimentally generated photographs and polar intensity patterns showing the Haidinger brush pattern when linearly polarized light enters the eye at an orientation angle of 90°, 120°, 135°, 150°, and 180° with respect to the fast axis of the cornea. The dark brush is perpendicular to the incoming polarization. Panels progress from top to bottom; the phase shift of the cornea is $\Delta = 0\lambda$. The brush rotates uniformly with no loss in contrast. *(Adapted with permission from Rothmayer M, Dultz W, Frins E, Zhan Q, Tierney D, Schmitzer H. Nonlinearity in the rotational dynamics of Haidinger's brushes. Appl Opt. 2007;46(29):7244–7251.)*

Polarizing sunglasses are sometimes useful for reducing the glare from reflected sunlight. In boating, for example, sunlight reflected from the water surface is partially polarized. Because the predominant polarization is horizontal (see Fig 1-9), the sunglasses are constructed to pass only the vertical polarization. Similarly, when a person is driving, the light reflected from the road surface and from the painted or glass surfaces of other automobiles is also partially polarized, usually horizontally.

Certain materials such as glass or plastic, when stressed, will change the state of polarized light. A heat-treated ophthalmic lens, for example, will exhibit a distinctive pattern when placed between crossed polarizing sheets. People who wear polarizing sunglasses may be especially aware of stress patterns in glass doors and auto rear windows.

Polarized light is used in some ophthalmic instruments to eliminate the strong reflex from the cornea. The ophthalmologist looks through a polarizer that is placed 90° to the polarization of the light incident on the examined eye. The polarizer eliminates the light that is specularly reflected from the cornea, while partially transmitting the light diffusely reflected from the retina.

Polarizing projection charts are especially useful because they can be made to test 1 eye at a time while the patient is viewing binocularly through a pair of special polarizing glasses. For example, alternate letters on a Snellen chart can be polarized at 90° to each other and therefore are seen by each eye separately. Other charts provide sensitive

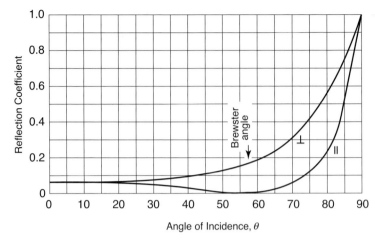

Figure 1-9 Reflection by a glass surface in air as a function of angle of incidence, θ. The symbol ⊥ indicates the polarization perpendicular to the plane of incidence; ‖ denotes the polarization parallel to the plane of incidence. At grazing incidence, 90°, the reflection coefficient approaches 100%. In this example, the glass has an index of refraction of 1.51; the Brewster angle for this index is 56.5°. At the Brewster angle, θ_B, the reflection of the parallel component is essentially 0. *(From Ditchburn RW. Light. 2nd ed. London: Blackie and Son; 1952:Fig 14.3. Redrawn by C. H. Wooley.)*

tests for binocular functions or abnormalities such as stereopsis, fixation disparity, and aniseikonia.

Reflection

The laws of reflection as they affect light rays and the formation of images are discussed in Chapter 2, Geometric Optics.

The magnitude of the reflection at an interface between 2 media depends primarily on the difference in index of refraction between the first and second media. An air–glass interface reflects approximately 4% (at normal incidence). The air–cornea interface reflects about 2%, whereas the cornea–aqueous interface reflects only about 0.02%.

Reflection from an interface also depends strongly on the angle of incidence. As illustrated in Figure 1-9, polarization becomes important for oblique incidence. At 1 particular angle (known as the *Brewster angle*) for every interface, only 1 polarization is reflected. The fact that 1 polarization is reflected more strongly than the other enables polarizing sunglasses to block reflected light, as explained in the earlier discussion of polarization and in the following paragraph.

Total reflection occurs when light from a medium with a high index of refraction encounters a medium with a lower index at oblique incidence (see Total Internal Reflection in Chapter 2). The basis for transmission of light in fiber optics is total reflection at the internal surface of the fiber. The fiber usually consists of a high-index core glass surrounded by a lower-index cladding glass.

Applications of Reflection

This topic is discussed in greater detail in Chapter 2, Geometric Optics.

As discussed in the previous section, total reflection occurs at the interface between a high-index glass and a lower-index glass. This interface must remain free of dirt, contamination, and contact with any other material that might degrade the total reflection. Reflection from metals such as silver or aluminum can be as high as 85%–95%. As with other materials, the reflectivity increases with the angle of incidence. Mirrors used in ophthalmic instruments usually consist of an aluminum layer that has been vacuum-evaporated on a glass substrate and then overcoated with a protective thin film of transparent material such as silicon monoxide to prevent oxidation and scratching of the aluminum surface.

Semitransparent mirrors, sometimes used as 1-way mirrors, often consist of a metallic layer thin enough to transmit a fraction of the incident light. They are not 100% efficient in that a substantial fraction of the light is also absorbed. In critical applications, partially reflecting mirrors can be made of other materials so that only a negligible fraction is lost to absorption.

Metallic reflection *partially* polarizes the reflected light. As with other materials, the perpendicular component is more strongly reflected than the parallel component. However, with metals there is no angle at which only 1 polarization is reflected; therefore, the polarization of the reflected light is never complete.

Transmission and Absorption

Transmission is the passing of radiant energy through a medium or space. It is measured in terms of transmittance, the percentage of energy that can pass through a particular medium. For absorbing materials, the transmittance is often a function of wavelength.

Absorption is usually expressed as an *optical density* (OD). An OD of 1 represents a transmittance of 10%; an OD of 2, a transmittance of 1% (0.01); and an OD of 3, a transmittance of 0.1% (0.001).

In general, the expression for optical density is OD = log $1/T$, where T is the transmittance. See also Chapter 4, Clinical Refraction, for a discussion of absorptive lenses.

Duke-Elder S, Abrams D, eds. *System of Ophthalmology.* Vol V, *Ophthalmic Optics and Refraction.* St Louis: Mosby; 1970:30–36.

Diffraction

Diffraction is the ability of light to bend around edges. All waves are subject to diffraction when they encounter an obstruction, an aperture, or another irregularity in the medium. Diffraction changes the direction of the wave; in the case of light, this corresponds to a bending of the light ray. The shorter the wavelength, the less the change of direction.

Diffraction is seldom seen alone; rather, it is usually combined with other effects, such as interference and refraction. One example in which diffraction dominates is in the light streaks seen through windshields that have been repeatedly rubbed by windshield wipers.

Each fine scratch diffracts the light into directions perpendicular to the scratch—that is, into a plane of rays normal to the diffracting groove. Another example is the pattern seen when a distant light is viewed through fine-woven curtain material. Again, the diffraction is in a direction perpendicular to the diffracting material—in this case, the threads. With cross-woven material, a 2-dimensional array of bright spots is seen. Here, diffraction is mixed with interference, producing discrete spots of light rather than continuous streaks.

Applications of Diffraction

Diffraction sets a limit on visual acuity when the pupil size is less than approximately 2.5 mm (for a person with emmetropia). The image formed on the retina from a distant small source takes the form of concentric light and dark rings surrounding a bright central disk, the *Airy disk* (Fig 1-10). The diameter, *d*, of the central disk increases as the pupil size decreases according to the equation

$$d = 2.44 f \lambda / a$$

where

λ = wavelength
a = diameter of the aperture (pupil)
f = focal length of the optical system (the eye)

This equation illustrates another property of diffraction: that longer wavelengths (red) diffract more than shorter wavelengths (blue) and therefore form a larger-diameter Airy disk. The best resolution obtainable from an optical instrument is limited by diffraction. The minimum resolvable distance is approximately equal to the radius of the Airy disk. Because of this, telescopes generally increase in resolution as the aperture of the objective lens is increased. However, ground-based astronomical telescopes larger than 10 inches in diameter are limited in resolution by atmospheric turbulence, the same phenomenon that gives rise to the familiar twinkling of stars. A space telescope operating in the relative vacuum high above the earth's atmosphere is unaffected by atmospheric conditions.

When no aberrations are present, an Airy pattern is formed in the image plane (Fig 1-11); hence, even when a small source is viewed through a small pupil, an Airy disk is

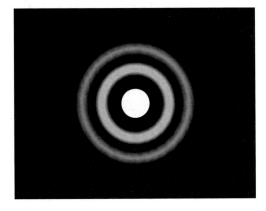

Figure 1-10 Diffraction pattern produced by a small circular aperture. The central bright spot is called an *Airy disk*. *(From Campbell CJ. Physiological Optics. Hagerstown, MD: Harper & Row; 1974:20.)*

seldom seen directly, usually because of aspherical irregularities in the cornea and the crystalline lens. In this way, diffraction combines with other aberrations to increase the blur circle size on the retina. (Blur circles are discussed in Chapter 2, under Image Quality.)

Because diffraction sets a limit on an optical system's resolution, there is a degree of precision in the fabrication of optical components beyond which any improvement in the

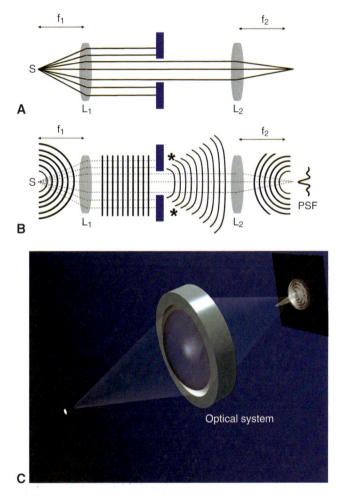

Figure 1-11 **A,** Geometric optics conceives of light as rays that propagate in a rectilinear fashion. This figure shows a light source *(S)* located at a distance f_1 (focal length) from lens L_1. The central rays are bent by lens L_2 to focus at a distance f_2 from L_2. **B,** Physical optics deals with light waves emanating from a point source *(S)*. Because of the diffraction caused by the edges of the aperture *(*)*, the transmitted wavefront is slightly distorted beyond the aperture. This causes the irradiance produced by an optical system with 1 or more lenses to take the form of a blurred spot over a finite area. This patch of light in the image plane is called the *point spread function (PSF)*. Diffraction thus decreases stigmatism. **C,** Schematic representation of the irradiance produced by an optical system free of aberrations, which corresponds to the diffraction figure of the input source; when no aberrations are present, an Airy pattern is formed in the image plane. *(Modified with permission from Gatinel D. Wavefront analysis. In: Azar DT, ed. Gatinel D, Hoang-Xuan T, associate eds. Refractive Surgery. 2nd ed. St Louis, MO: Elsevier-Mosby; 2007:117–145).*

image is negligible. This limit is given by the *Rayleigh criterion:* If the wavefront produced by the optical system is within one-quarter wavelength of being perfect, further improvement will not result in significantly better resolution. This tolerance has a practical application in setting standards for the fabrication of optical components.

Scattering

Scattering of light occurs at irregularities in the light path, such as particles or inclusions in an otherwise homogeneous medium. Scattering caused by very small particles, such as the molecules in the atmosphere, is called *Rayleigh scattering.* The effective size of a scattering particle is defined by the ratio *(x)* of its characteristic dimension $(2\pi r)$ and wavelength (λ):

$$x = \frac{2\pi r}{\lambda}$$

Although Rayleigh scattering is generally very weak, it varies according to the size of the particle and the wavelength of the light, with greater scattering at shorter wavelengths. In particular, the scattering coefficient, and therefore the scattered light's intensity, varies for small size parameter inversely with the fourth power of the wavelength. The sky appears blue because blue light from the sun is scattered more than sunlight of longer wavelengths. Scattered intensity is also proportional to r^6 (the sixth power of the radius). Therefore, larger particles, such as dust in the air, scatter light more intensely and with less dependence on wavelength.

Applications of Light Scattering

Scattering of light in ocular tissues can result from various pathologic conditions. Corneal haze is caused by excess water in the stroma, which disrupts the very regular, close-packed collagen structure of the stroma. In an early cataract, large molecules in the lens structure cause scattering. Anterior chamber flare is caused by protein in the aqueous humor (Tyndall effect).

Such scattering material interferes with vision in 2 ways. The primary effect is that of glare, starbursts, and halos. For example, when light from a source such as the sun or an oncoming headlight reaches the eye, a fraction of the light scattered within the ocular media falls on the retina. That which falls in the foveal area reduces the contrast and tends to obscure detail in the image of interest. The second effect, particularly important when the scattering is intense, is a reduction in the light available to form the image on the retina.

Illumination

The quantitative measurement of light is carried out in 2 different ways. *Radiometry* measures light in terms of power, the basic unit being the *watt.* For example, the *irradiance* on a surface is the number of watts per square meter incident on that surface.

Photometry measures light in units based on the response of the eye. The basic unit is the *candela,* a more precisely defined replacement for the old unit, the candle. A point source with output of 1 candela emits a total of 4π (ie, ≈ 12.6) *lumens.* The *illuminance* on a surface is the number of lumens per square meter incident on that surface. The *luminance* of a surface is the amount of light reflected or emitted by the surface.

If a source has a known output in watts, can we determine its output in lumens? Yes, provided we know the spectral properties of the lamp—that is, power at each wavelength. The output at each wavelength is multiplied by the sensitivity of the eye to that wavelength, and the results are summed to obtain the total response of the eye to light from that source. For example, if the source is monochromatic, with a wavelength at the peak of the eye's photopic sensitivity (555 nm), the conversion factor is 685 lumens per watt. At other wavelengths the factor is less, falling to approximately zero at 400 and 700 nm (Figs 1-12 and 1-13).

The *apostilb* is defined as the luminance of a perfectly diffusing surface that is emitting or reflecting 1 lumen per square meter. It is encountered in perimetry, where the luminance of the background and of the targets is often specified in apostilbs.

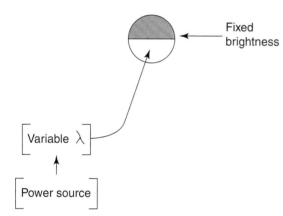

Fixed brightness

Variable λ

Power source

Figure 1-12 Schematic arrangement for measuring the spectral sensitivity of the eye. The subject is light-adapted. For λ_x, a certain amount of power (W_x) will be needed to match the standard brightness. A curve can then be constructed of W_x versus λ_x (see Fig 1-13). *(Redrawn by C. H. Wooley.)*

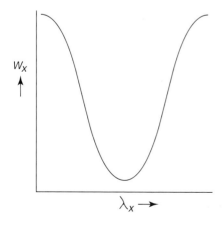

W_x

$\lambda_x \rightarrow$

Figure 1-13 The amount of power (W_x) at each wavelength (λ_x) needed to match a standard brightness in the arrangement of Figure 1-12. This curve is inverted with respect to the familiar photopic luminosity curve. The greatest energy efficiency is roughly in the middle of the visible spectrum, at a wavelength of 555 nm. *(Redrawn by C. H. Wooley.)*

Brightness is a subjective term referring to the sensation produced by a given illuminance on the retina. (Brightness and irradiance are discussed in the following section.)
The commonly used radiometric and photometric terms are summarized in Tables 1-1
and 1-2.

Michaels DD. *Visual Optics and Refraction: A Clinical Approach.* St Louis: Mosby; 1985:14–16.

Table 1-1 Principal Types of Photometric Light Measurement

	Description	Type	Units
	Quantity of light leaving a source or passing through a region of space	Luminous flux	Lumens (1 candle emits 4π lm)
	Light emitted per unit solid angle	Luminous intensity (candle power)	1 candela* = 1 lm/sr
	Quantity of light per unit area incident on a surface or at an image	Illuminance	1 lux = 1 lumen/square meter 1 foot-candle = 1 lumen/ square ft
	Light reflected or emitted by a surface, per unit area and per unit solid angle	Luminance	1 apostilb = $(1/\pi)$ lumen/ square meter/sr 1 foot-lambert = $(1/\pi)$ lumen/ square ft/sr
	Illuminance at the retina, adjusted for pupil size	Retinal illuminance	Trolands (luminance of 1 candle/square meter viewed through 1-square-mm pupil)

*A standard (new) candle is called a candela.

Modified from Armington JC. *The Electroretinogram.* New York: Academic Press; 1974:75.

Table 1-2 Radiometric Terminology for Medical Lasers

Term	Unit
Radiant energy	joule*
Radiant power	watt
Radiant energy density	joules/cm²
Irradiance	watts/cm²
Radiant intensity	watts/sr†
Radiance (brightness)	watts/sr cm²

*1 joule = 1 watt × 1 sec.
†Steradian is the unit of solid angle. There are 4π steradians in a sphere.

From Steinert RF, Puliafito CA. *The Nd:YAG Laser in Ophthalmology: Principles and Clinical Applications
of Photodisruption.* Philadelphia: Saunders; 1985.

Brightness and Irradiance

The word *brightness* is often used imprecisely. *Brightness* describes a visual perception: the response of the nervous system to light entering the eye. The individual's perception of brightness depends not only on the amount of light reaching the retina but also on many other factors such as the degree of dark adaptation and presence of pathology. *Irradiance* is a better term for discussing image characteristics. It is a purely physical measure of the amount of light per unit area of an image.

The relationship between irradiance and brightness is similar to the relationship between wavelength and color. If light of a given wavelength is observed by 2 people, one with normal color vision and the other with anomalous color perception, these 2 observers will "see" different colors. *Wavelength* is a physical property of the light itself, whereas *color* depends on the visual system. Likewise, *irradiance* depends only on light itself, whereas *brightness* is a perception.

Clinically, the most important use of irradiance is in the calibration of various testing apparatuses such as perimeters. Periodic calibration is essential to the reproducibility of visual tests.

Light Hazards

Although the eye requires light in order to function, it has long been recognized that light itself in excess, particularly at certain wavelengths, can be hazardous to various parts of the eye:

- The cornea and lens are particularly susceptible to UV injury in the wavelength range of 180–400 nm, from which photokeratitis and cataract can result.
- The retina is susceptible to photochemical injury from blue light in the wavelength range of 400–550 nm (310–550 nm for an aphakic eye). This is the basis for the incorporation of UV-blocking and blue-blocking chromophores in certain intraocular lenses.
- The retina is susceptible to thermal injury from optical radiation in the wavelength range of 400–1400 nm.
- The lens of the eye is susceptible to thermal injury from near-infrared radiation in the wavelength range of 800–3000 nm.
- The cornea and lens of the eye are susceptible to thermal injury from radiation in the wavelength range of 400–1200 nm.
- The cornea is susceptible to thermal injury from optical radiation in the wavelength range of 1400 nm–1 mm.

Laser Fundamentals

Laser is an acronym for *light amplification by stimulated emission of radiation*—a phrase that highlights the key events in producing laser light. In the most simplified sequence, an energy source excites the atoms in the *active medium* (a gas, solid, or liquid) to emit a particular wavelength of light. The light thus produced is amplified by an optical feedback system that reflects the beam back and forth through the active medium to increase its coherence, until the light is emitted as a laser beam. This process is described in greater detail in the following sections.

Although Einstein had developed the basic theory of laser emission more than 40 years earlier, it was not until 1960 that Theodore Maiman built the first successful laser with a ruby crystal medium.

Properties of Laser Light

Lasers are only one of many sources of light energy. The unique properties of laser light, however, make it particularly suitable for many medical applications. These properties are *monochromaticity, directionality, coherence, polarization,* and *intensity.*

Monochromaticity

Lasers emit light at only 1 wavelength or sometimes at a combination of several wavelengths that can be separated easily. Thus a "pure," or monochromatic, beam is obtained. Although the wavelength spread is not infinitesimally small, a gas laser emission line can be as narrow as 0.01 nm, compared with the 300-nm span of wavelengths found in white light. At best, a filter might reduce the transmission of white light to a color range (bandwidth) of 5 nm at the expense of most of the white light's energy. For medical purposes, the color of light can be used to enhance absorption or transmission by a target tissue with a certain absorption spectrum. The wavelength specificity of a laser greatly exceeds the absorption specificity of pigments in tissues. In addition, monochromatic light is not affected by chromatic aberration in lens systems. Thus, monochromatic light can be focused to a smaller spot than can white light.

Directionality

The second property of laser-emitted light is *directionality.* Lasers emit a narrow beam that spreads very slowly. As explained later in this chapter, lasers amplify only those photons that travel along a very narrow path between 2 mirrors. This process serves as a very efficient mechanism for collimating light. In a typical laser, the beam increases by approximately 1 mm in diameter for every meter traveled. Directionality makes it easy to collect all of the light energy in a simple lens system and focus this light to a small spot.

Coherence

Coherence, meaning that all the propagated energy from the source is in phase, is the term most often associated with lasers (see Fig 1-5 and the earlier discussion, Interference and Coherence). Laser light projected onto a rough surface produces a characteristic sparkling quality known as *laser speckle.* This phenomenon occurs because the irregular reflection of highly coherent light creates irregular interference patterns, or speckle. Coherence of laser light is utilized to create the interference fringes of the laser interferometer. In therapeutic ophthalmic lasers, coherence, like directionality, is important because it improves focusing characteristics.

Polarization

Many lasers emit linearly polarized light. *Polarization* is incorporated in the laser system to allow maximum transmission through the laser medium without loss caused by reflection.

Intensity

In most medical applications, the most important property of lasers is *intensity.* Intensity is the power in a beam of a given angular size, and the physical correlate of the perception of "brightness" is the intensity per unit area. In medical laser applications, the most important radiometric terms are *energy* (J), *power* (W), *radiant energy density* (J/cm^2), and *irradiance* (W/cm^2) (see Table 1-2). The laser output is fixed in either joules (J) or watts (W). Recall that energy is work, and power is the rate at which work is done. One joule = 1 watt × 1 second, or 1 W = 1 J/s. The tissue effect is then determined by the focal point spot size, which determines energy density and irradiance (or, less properly stated, "power density"). In ophthalmic lasers, spot size is conventionally given as the diameter. Thus, a 50-μm spot size has an area of π $(25 \times 10^{-4})^2$ cm^2, or about 2×10^{-5} cm^2.

Directionality, coherence, polarization, and, to some degree, monochromaticity enhance the most important characteristic of lasers, which is light intensity. The sun has a power of 10^{26} watts but emits energy in all directions at a great distance from the earth. Thus, a simple 1-mW helium neon laser has 100 times the radiance of the sun. Their intense radiance, combined with monochromaticity that can target selected tissues and avoid others on the basis of spectral absorption, makes lasers a unique tool in medicine. This is particularly true in ophthalmology, as the eye is designed to allow light transmission to most of its structures. Figure 1-14 summarizes the major properties of laser light in comparison with a conventional light source.

Elements of a Laser

All ophthalmic lasers currently in use require 3 basic elements: (1) an *active medium* to emit coherent radiation; (2) energy input, known as *pumping;* and (3) *optical feedback,* to reflect and amplify the appropriate wavelengths.

In 1917, Albert Einstein explained the mathematical relationships of 3 atomic transition processes: *absorption, spontaneous emission,* and *stimulated emission.* According to the fundamental principles of quantum physics, certain atomic energy transitions are highly probable, or "allowed." Light energy can readily induce such an allowed transition, causing the energy of the atom to move from its ground state (E_0) to an excited state (E_1). The atom absorbs a quantum of energy at a predictable frequency appropriate to cause the specific transition. If the source of illumination is white light, a discrete frequency (line spectrum) will be subtracted from the illuminating beam. Each atomic element has a characteristic line spectrum. This process is known as *absorption* (Fig 1-15A).

Because the lowest energy state is the most stable, the excited atom soon emits a quantum of energy at the same frequency in order to return to the ground state. This process can occur without external stimulation (*spontaneous emission;* Fig 1-15B) or as a result of

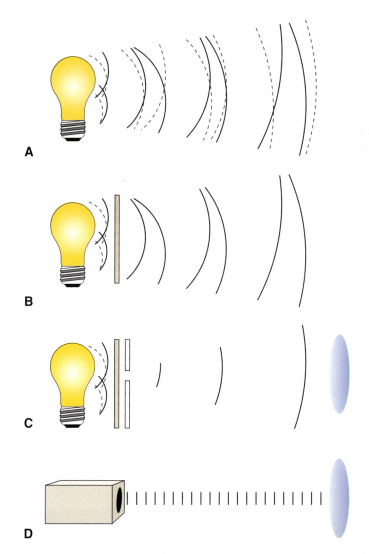

Figure 1-14 Comparison of properties of incandescent and laser light sources. **A,** The incandescent bulb emits incoherent, rapidly divergent light with a broad mixture of wavelengths *(solid and broken waves)*. **B,** A narrow-band pass filter absorbs all but a narrow portion of the spectrum *(solid waves)* but, in doing so, absorbs much of the light energy. **C,** Directionality and coherence are improved by the addition of a pinhole aperture, but still more energy is lost; a lens system collects some of the light and brings it to a focus. **D,** A laser emits monochromatic, directional, coherent light that is readily collected by a lens system and brought to a much smaller focal area. Compared with the incandescent source, the power and irradiance of the laser system are many orders of magnitude greater. *(Reproduced with permission from Steinert RF, Puliafito CA. The Nd:YAG Laser in Ophthalmology: Principles and Clinical Applications of Photodisruption. Philadelphia: Saunders; 1985. Redrawn by Jonathan Clark.)*

stimulation by a photon of light at the same frequency (*stimulated emission;* Fig 1-15C). Spontaneous emission occurs randomly in time, whereas stimulated emission is in phase with the stimulating wave. Therefore, stimulated emission is coherent. After absorption, the majority of energy release is through spontaneous emission occurring incoherently in

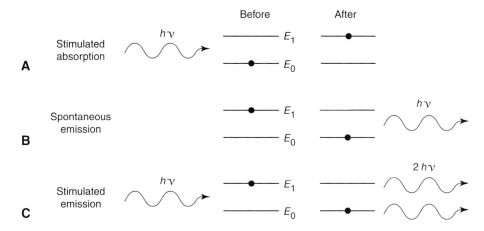

Figure 1-15 Schematic representation of an electron moving between the lowest energy (ground) state (E_0) and an allowed excited state (E_1) in conjunction with absorption of a quantum of light energy ($\Delta E = E_1 - E_0 = h\nu$). **A,** Stimulated absorption. **B,** Spontaneous emission. **C,** Stimulated emission. *(Reproduced with permission from Steinert RF, Puliafito CA.* The Nd:YAG Laser in Ophthalmology: Principles and Clinical Applications of Photodisruption. *Philadelphia: Saunders; 1985. Redrawn by C. H. Wooley.)*

all directions, and only a small fraction of the energy is normally released as coherent stimulated emission. The laser environment, however, amplifies only the stimulated emission.

As indicated in Figure 1-15C, stimulated emission occurs when an incident photon of the proper frequency interacts with an atom in the upper energy state. The result is the emission of a photon of the same wavelength and the return of the atom to its lower energy state. The emitted photon also has the same phase and direction of propagation as the incident photon.

The *active medium* is an atomic or molecular environment that supports stimulated emission. The active medium allows a large number of atoms to be energized above the ground state so that stimulated emission can occur. Recall that $\nu = c/\lambda$; hence, the particular atomic energy transition determines the wavelength of the emission ($E = h\nu = hc/\lambda$). Lasers are usually named for the active medium. The medium can be a gas (argon, krypton, carbon dioxide, argon-fluoride excimer, or helium with neon), a liquid (dye), a solid (an active element supported by a crystal, such as neodymium supported by yttrium-aluminum-garnet [Nd:YAG] and erbium supported by yttrium-lanthanum-fluoride [Er:YLF]), or a semiconductor (diode).

The second requirement for a laser is a means of imparting energy to the active medium so that a majority of the atoms are in an energy state higher than the ground state. This condition is known as a *population inversion* because it is the inverse of the usual condition in which the majority of atoms are in the ground energy state. The energy input that makes possible population inversion is known as *pumping*. Gas lasers are usually pumped by electrical discharge between electrodes in the gas. Dye lasers are often pumped by other lasers. Solid crystals are usually pumped by incoherent light such as the xenon arc flashlamp.

Once population inversion in an active medium has been achieved, *optical feedback* is required to promote stimulated emission and suppress spontaneous emission. The laser cavity acts as an optical resonator. Mirrors are placed at each end of a beam path to reflect light back and forth through the active medium, in which pumping maintains a population inversion (Fig 1-16). Each time the light wave resonates through the active medium, the total coherent light energy is increased through stimulated emission. Spontaneous emission, which occurs randomly in all directions, rarely strikes a mirror and therefore is not amplified.

The last element in this schematic laser design is a mechanism for releasing some of the oscillating laser light from the cavity. This is achieved by making one of the mirrors fully reflective and the other mirror only partially reflective. A portion of the light waves striking the second mirror is emitted from the cavity as the laser beam. The reflectivity of the mirror is selected to satisfy the requirements for efficient amplification in a particular system. For example, if a laser has a 98% reflective mirror, the light waves are coherently amplified by stimulated emission during an average of 50 round-trips through the active medium before they are emitted as the laser beam.

Laser Sources

Solid-state laser sources commonly used in medical applications are ruby and Nd:YAG. Refractive surgery uses excimer lasers (ablative procedures) and, less commonly, infrared holmium:YLF (IntraLase, Advanced Medical Optics, Santa Ana, CA) and holmium:YAG lasers (laser thermal keratoplasty [LTK], laser in situ keratomileusis [LASIK]). Argon, krypton, carbon dioxide, and argon-fluoride excimer are the most important gas laser sources used in medicine. The dye laser is the only liquid laser used in ophthalmology.

In 1975, it was shown that rare gas atoms in metastable excited states could react with halogens to form diatomic rare gas halides in a bound excited dimer *(excimer)* state.

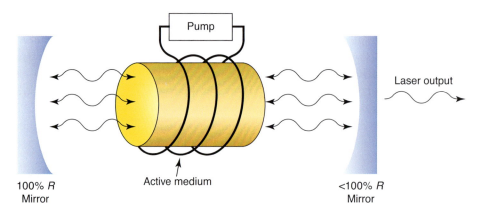

Figure 1-16 Elementary laser schematic illustrating the active medium within the optical resonance cavity formed by the mirrors and the pump, which creates a population inversion in the active medium. One mirror is fully reflective (100% *R*), whereas the other is partially transparent (<100% *R*). As drawn, the mirror is 66% reflective, and the average light wave makes 3 round-trips through the active medium before being emitted. *(Reproduced with permission from Steinert RF, Puliafito CA. The Nd:YAG Laser in Ophthalmology: Principles and Clinical Applications of Photodisruption. Philadelphia: Saunders; 1985. Redrawn by Jonathan Clark.)*

Decay of these excimer molecules to a weakly bound or unbound ground state is accompanied by emission of a photon with UV frequency. Excimer lasers efficiently produce high-power UV irradiation. A number of different excimer molecules can be created, and each is associated with a specific transition and emission wavelength: argon fluoride, or ArF (193 nm); krypton fluoride, or KrF (249 nm); and xenon fluoride, or XeF (351 nm).

Semiconductor diode lasers are solid-state lasers that are extremely compact and highly efficient. These laser sources are commonly used in communications applications and in digital information and audio systems. The increased power output of semiconductor diode lasers makes them feasible for retinal photocoagulation and for some glaucoma applications.

Laser–Tissue Interactions

Photocoagulation

Even before the invention of lasers, light energy had been employed therapeutically to heat and permanently alter target tissue. This early phototherapy had its origins in observations of solar retinitis and was used in the treatment of numerous retinal disorders and glaucoma. A laser could now achieve similar effects in a more controlled manner. The term *photocoagulation* refers to the selective absorption of light energy and conversion of that energy to heat, with a subsequent thermally induced structural change in the target. These processes and their therapeutic results depend on laser wavelength and laser pulse duration. A variety of photocoagulating lasers are currently in clinical use: argon, krypton, dye, holmium, and the solid-state gallium arsenide lasers.

Photodisruption

A second category of laser–tissue interaction uses high-peak-power pulsed lasers to ionize the target and rupture the surrounding tissue. In clinical practice, this process (known as *photodisruption*) uses laser light as a pair of virtual microsurgical scissors, reaching through the ocular media to open tissues such as lens capsule, iris, inflammatory membranes, and vitreous strands without damaging surrounding ocular structures. Currently, the Nd:YAG and Er:YAG lasers are the principal photodisruptive lasers used in clinical ophthalmology.

Photoablation

A third category of laser–tissue interaction, called *photoablation,* arose from the insight that high-powered UV laser pulses can precisely etch the cornea in the same manner that they etch synthetic polymers. The high energy of a single photon of 193-nm UV light exceeds the covalent bond strength of corneal protein. The high absorption of these laser pulses precisely removes a submicron layer of cornea without opacifying adjacent tissue, owing to the relative absence of thermal injury. Over a decade of laboratory and clinical investigation has brought excimer laser photoablation to clinical use in refractive surgery and corneal therapeutics. (See also BCSC Section 13, *Refractive Surgery.*)

Figure 1-17 shows some typical laser wavelengths.

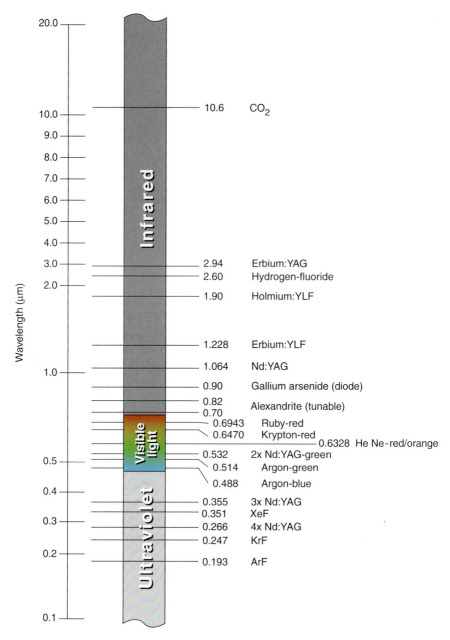

Figure 1-17 Typical laser wavelengths. *(Adapted from Steinert RF, Puliafito CA. The Nd:YAG Laser in Ophthalmology: Principles and Clinical Applications of Photodisruption. Philadelphia: Saunders; 1985. Redrawn by Jonathan Clark.)*

Azar DT, ed. Gatinel D, Hoang-Xuan T, associate eds. *Refractive Surgery*. 2nd ed. St Louis, MO: Elsevier-Mosby; 2007.

Campbell CJ. *Physiological Optics*. Hagerstown, MD: Harper & Row; 1974.

Rubin ML, Walls GL. *Fundamentals of Visual Science*. Springfield, IL: Charles C Thomas; 1969.

CHAPTER 2

Geometric Optics

Geometric optics is the study of light and images using geometric principles. In contrast, physical optics emphasizes the wave nature of light, and quantum optics (not covered in this text) emphasizes the particle nature of light and the interaction of light and matter. Geometric optics uses linear rays to represent the paths traveled by light.

Pinhole Imaging

The simplest imaging device is a pinhole aperture. Here's a simple experiment. Make a pinhole near the center of a large sheet of aluminum foil, light a candle, and extinguish all other illumination in the room. Hold a sheet of plain white or, better, waxed paper about 2 ft from the candle, and place the pinhole midway between the paper and the candle. Observe an inverted image of the candle flame on the paper (Fig 2-1).

The image is faint, but the object's features are faithfully duplicated. Moreover, the characteristics of the image are readily manipulated. For instance, moving the pinhole closer to the candle while keeping the paper stationary yields a larger image.

An object may be regarded as a collection of points. Geometric optics treats every point of an object as a *point source* of light. An object has an infinite number of point

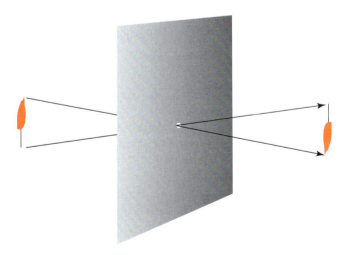

Figure 2-1 Pinhole imaging. *(Illustration developed by Edmond H. Thall, MD, and Kevin M. Miller, MD, and rendered by C. H. Wooley.)*

sources, and each point source is infinitesimally small. Light radiates in all directions from each point on an object. For practical purposes, an entire object may be treated as a single point source in certain instances. For example, stars other than our own sun, by virtue of their enormous distances from the earth, behave as point sources. The point source is mainly a conceptual tool: it is usually easier to understand an optical system by concentrating on the light radiating from a single object point or a few points.

For every object point, there is a specific image point. In optics, the term *conjugate* refers to these corresponding object and image points. An object point and its corresponding image point constitute a pair of *conjugate points* (Clinical Example 2-1). Light travels from an object point, passes through an optical system, and comes to a sharp focus at the corresponding image point. If the direction of travel were reversed, light would travel along the same path from the image point to the object point. It is common practice to use a letter to identify a specific point in the object and the same letter with a prime symbol to indicate the conjugate image point (eg, A and A').

A *ray* is a geometric construct indicating the path (or paths) of light as it travels from an object point to the corresponding image point. Rays represent only a path; they do not indicate the amount (ie, intensity) or wavelengths of the light traveling along the path. In illustrations, by convention, light is assumed to be traveling from left to right unless otherwise indicated. An arrowhead on the light ray is used as needed to indicate the direction of travel.

A *pencil of light* is a small collection (bundle) of light rays traveling in the same direction. The smaller the pencil, the more it behaves like a single ray of light.

Pinhole imaging has been known for millennia, but pinhole images are usually too faint to be useful. Only in rare situations is pinhole imaging practical. For instance, a solar eclipse can be safely observed when a pinhole is used to image the sun on a piece of paper. Of course, one should not look through the pinhole to directly view the sun!

Now what happens if we punch several pinholes in aluminum foil, separated by a few inches, and repeat the pinhole-imaging experiment? Several complete images of the flame

CLINICAL EXAMPLE 2-1

The concept of conjugate points is illustrated by retinoscopy. When performing retinoscopy, the examiner observes light emanating from the patient's retina and passing through the patient's pupil. Because the examiner is observing the light at the patient's pupil, the examiner's retina is conjugate to the patient's pupil (Fig 2-2A). At the point of neutrality in the refraction, the patient's retina is conjugate with the peephole of the retinoscope (Fig 2-2B). Adjustment for the distance between the examiner and the patient (working distance) makes the patient's retina conjugate with optical infinity (Fig 2-2C). (Retinoscopy is covered in detail in Chapter 4, Clinical Refraction.)

Another example of conjugacy is demonstrated by direct ophthalmoscopy. When the ophthalmoscope is focused to compensate for the

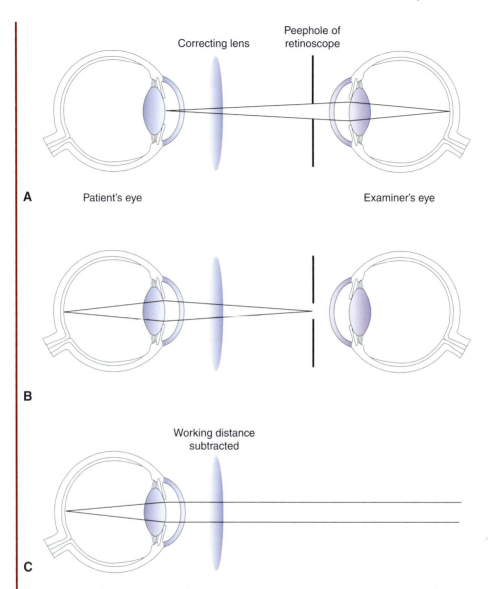

Figure 2-2 **A,** In retinoscopy, the examiner's eye is conjugate with the patient's pupil. **B,** At the point of neutrality, the patient's retina is conjugate with the retinoscope peephole. **C,** With the working distance subtracted, the patient's retina is conjugate with optical infinity. *(Illustration developed by Kevin M. Miller, MD, and rendered by C. H. Wooley.)*

refractive error of the examiner and that of the patient, the 2 retinas are conjugate (Fig 2-3). An image of the patient's retina is present on the examiner's retina and vice versa. However, the patient does not "see" the examiner's retina, because it is not illuminated by the ophthalmoscope light and because this light is so bright.

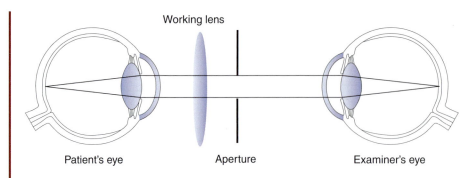

Figure 2-3 Conjugacy in direct ophthalmoscopy. *(Illustration developed by Kevin M. Miller, MD, and rendered by C. H. Wooley.)*

appear simultaneously (Fig 2-4). Each object point is a point source radiating light in all directions. Some light from each object point traverses every pinhole and produces an image. Note that only a small amount of light from each object point is necessary to yield a complete image. The pinhole restricts the brightness, not the size, of the image.

Imaging With Lenses and Mirrors

Repeat the pinhole-imaging demonstration, but replace the pinhole with a +6 D spherical trial lens, and note the improvement in the image. Vary the distances among the candle, lens, and paper, and observe the variety of different image characteristics that can be obtained from the same lens (Fig 2-5). Different lenses provide an even broader range of images.

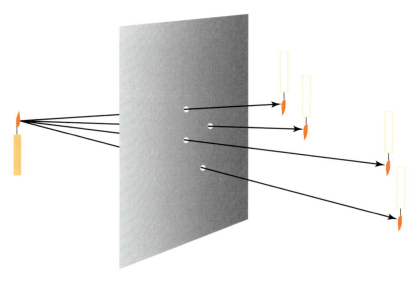

Figure 2-4 Multiple pinholes produce distinct, complete images. *(Illustration developed by Edmond H. Thall, MD, and Kevin M. Miller, MD, and rendered by C. H. Wooley.)*

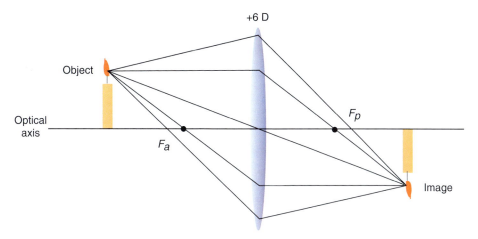

Figure 2-5 Basic imaging with a lens. The lens collects light from an object point and redirects the light to a small spot in the image. *(Illustration developed by Kevin M. Miller, MD, and rendered by C. H. Wooley.)*

Compared with the pinhole, the lens allows much more light from each object point to traverse the lens and ultimately contribute to the image. Generally, lenses produce better images than do pinholes. However, lenses do have some disadvantages. Place a lens at a fixed distance from the candle and note that the image appears in only 1 location. In pinhole imaging, an image appears at any location behind the aperture. Changing the distance between an object and a lens causes the distance between the image and the lens to change, but the image still forms in only one location.

Mirrors produce images in much the same way as lenses (Fig 2-6). The comments made in this section regarding lenses also apply to mirrors.

Most optical systems are rotationally symmetric about their long axis. This axis of symmetry is the *optical axis* (see Figs 2-5 and 2-6). Although the human eye is not truly rotationally symmetric, it is nearly symmetric, and theoretical models of the eye often approximate the eye as a rotationally symmetric system. (See the discussion of schematic eyes in Chapter 3, Optics of the Human Eye.)

Object Characteristics

Objects may be characterized by their location with respect to the imaging system and by whether they are luminous. If an object point produces its own light, such as the candle flame in the previous illustrations, it is called *luminous*. If it does not produce its own light, it can only be imaged if it is reflective and illuminated.

Image Characteristics

Images are described by characteristics such as magnification, location, quality, and brightness. Some of these features will be discussed briefly.

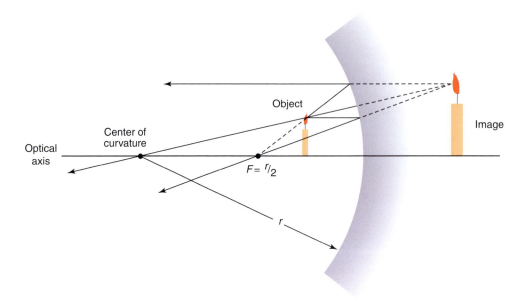

Figure 2-6 Basic imaging with a mirror. In this example, an upright, magnified, and virtual image is produced because the object is located inside the focal point, *F*. *(Illustration developed by Kevin M. Miller, MD, and rendered by C. H. Wooley.)*

Magnification

Three types of magnification are considered in geometric optics: transverse, angular, and axial.

The ratio of the height of an image to the height of the corresponding object is known as *transverse magnification* (Fig 2-7):

Transverse magnification = image height/object height

To calculate transverse magnification, we compare the height of an object (ie, the distance an object extends above or below the optical axis) to that of its conjugate image (ie, the distance its image extends above or below the axis). Object and image heights are measured perpendicular to the optical axis and, by convention, are considered positive when the object or image extends above the optical axis and negative, below the axis.

An image is a scale model of the object. If the object or image is upright (extending above the optical axis), a positive (+) sign is used; an inverted object or image (extending below the optical axis), is indicated by a minus (–) sign. The transverse magnification represents the size of the image in relation to that of the object. For instance, in Figure 2-7, the object height is +4 cm and the image height –2 cm; thus, the transverse magnification is –0.5, meaning that the image is inverted and half as large as the object. A magnification of +3 means the image is upright and 3 times larger than the object.

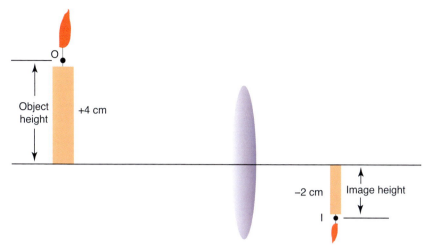

Figure 2-7 Object height and image height may be measured from any pair of off-axis conjugate points. In this illustration, an object point, *O*, on the wick, and its conjugate, *I*, are used to measure object and image height. *(Illustration developed by Edmond H. Thall, MD, and Kevin M. Miller, MD, and rendered by C. H. Wooley.)*

Transverse magnification applies to linear dimensions. For example, a 4 cm × 6 cm object imaged with a magnification of 2 produces an 8 cm × 12 cm image. Both width and length double, yielding a fourfold increase in image area.

The word *power* is sometimes used synonymously with transverse magnification. This is unfortunate because "power" has several different meanings, and confusion often arises. Other uses of the word include refracting power, resolving power, prism power, and light-gathering power. Generally, the multiplication sign, ×, is used to indicate magnification. The transverse magnification of microscope objectives, for example, is sometimes expressed by this convention.

Most optical systems have a pair of *nodal points* (Fig 2-8). Occasionally, the nodal points overlap, appearing as a single point, but technically they remain a pair of overlapping nodal points. The nodal points are always on the optical axis and have an important property. From any object point, a unique ray passes through the anterior nodal point. This ray emerges from the optical system along the line connecting the posterior nodal point to the conjugate image point (Fig 2-9). These rays form 2 angles with the optical axis. The essential property of the nodal points is that these 2 angles are equal for any selected object point. Because of this feature, nodal points are useful for establishing a relationship among transverse magnification, object distance, and image distance. (See Quick Review of Angles, Trigonometry, and the Pythagorean Theorem.)

Regardless of the location of an object, the object and the image subtend equal angles with respect to their nodal points. Therefore, the 2 triangles in Figure 2-9 are similar, and the lengths of corresponding sides of similar triangles are proportional. Therefore,

$$\text{Transverse magnification} = \frac{\text{image height}}{\text{object height}} = \frac{\text{image distance}}{\text{object distance}}$$

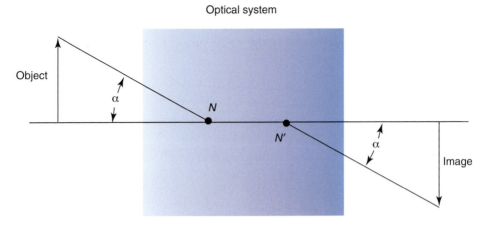

Figure 2-8 The anterior and posterior nodal points (*N* and *N'*, respectively) of an optical system. Any ray from an object point to the anterior nodal point will emerge along the line joining the posterior nodal point and the image point. The angles formed by these rays with the optical axis are identical. *(Illustration developed by Kevin M. Miller, MD, and rendered by C. H. Wooley.)*

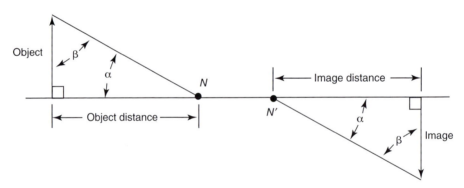

Figure 2-9 Lines perpendicular to the optical axis may be extended to the object points and image points. The triangles formed by these lines are similar. *(Illustration developed by Kevin M. Miller, MD, and rendered by C. H. Wooley.)*

QUICK REVIEW OF ANGLES, TRIGONOMETRY, AND THE PYTHAGOREAN THEOREM

It is useful to review a few basic principles of geometry and trigonometry. A circle is divided angularly into 360° or 2π radians. π is approximately 3.14, so 360° corresponds approximately to 6.28 radians. It is frequently necessary to convert between degrees and radians when optics problems are being solved. A degree is subdivided into 60' (minutes); each minute is subdivided into 60" (seconds).

The sum of the angles in a triangle equals 180° or π radians. For any right, or right-angled, triangle with sides a, b, and c (Fig 2-10) and angle θ between sides b and c, the trigonometric function is defined as follows:

$$\tan\theta = \frac{a}{b}$$

The Pythagorean theorem states that $c^2 = a^2 + b^2$; as a result, therefore, $c = \sqrt{a^2 + b^2}$. Triangles are said to be similar when their angles are equal. When 2 triangles have identical angles, their sides are proportional. The triangles in Figure 2-11 are similar.

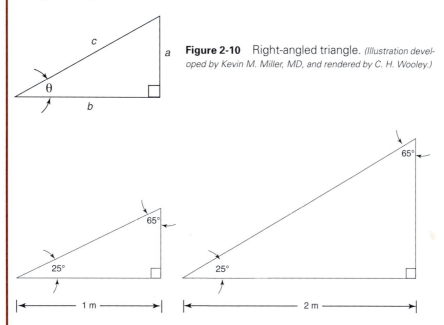

Figure 2-10   Right-angled triangle. *(Illustration developed by Kevin M. Miller, MD, and rendered by C. H. Wooley.)*

Figure 2-11   These 2 triangles are similar because their angles are equal. *(Illustration developed by Kevin M. Miller, MD, and rendered by C. H. Wooley.)*

As a practical matter, object and image distances must obey a sign convention consistent with the established convention for transverse magnification (ie, negative when the object or image is below the axis. Object and image distances are always measured along the optical axis. For the purpose of calculating transverse magnification, object distance is measured from the object to the anterior nodal point, and image distance is measured from the posterior nodal point to the image. For a simple thin lens immersed in a uniform medium such as air, the nodal points overlap in the center of the lens. Object and image distances are negative when they point to the left and positive when they point to the right (see Fig 2-9).

Here is a simple experiment. Use a pinhole to image the sun onto a piece of paper 50 cm behind the pinhole. What is the size of the image? Assume that the sun subtends an angle of 0.5° and that the nodal points for pinhole imaging overlap in the middle of the pinhole.

From trigonometry:

$$\tan(0.25°) = \frac{x}{50 \text{ cm}} = \frac{x}{500 \text{ mm}}$$

Thus,

$$x = (500 \text{ mm}) \tan(0.25°) = 2.2 \text{ mm}$$

The radius of the image is 2.2 mm, which is fairly small, and the diameter or overall height of the image is 4.4 mm.

Angular magnification is the ratio of the angular height subtended by an object seen by the eye through a magnifying lens, to the angular height subtended by the same object viewed without the magnifying lens. By convention, the standard viewing distance for this comparison is 25 cm. For small angles, the angular magnification provided by a simple magnifier *(P)* is independent of the actual object size:

$$M = (1/4) \, P \qquad \text{or} \qquad M = P/4$$

More will be said about simple magnifiers later.

Axial magnification, also known as *longitudinal magnification,* is measured along the optical axis. For small distances around the image plane, axial magnification is the square of the transverse magnification.

$$\text{Axial magnification} = (\text{transverse magnification})^2$$

Image Location

Another important characteristic of an image is its location. Refractive errors result when images formed by the eye's optical system are in front of or behind the retina. Image location is specified as the distance (measured along the optical axis) between a reference point associated with the optical system and the image.

The reference point depends on the situation. It is often convenient to use the back surface of a lens as a reference point. The back lens surface is usually not at the same location as the posterior nodal point, but it is easier to locate.

Frequently, image distance is measured from the posterior principal point to the image. The principal points (discussed later in the chapter), like the nodal points, are a pair of useful reference points on the optical axis. The nodal points and principal points often overlap.

Whatever reference point is used to measure image distance, the sign convention is always the same. When the image is to the right of the reference point, image distance is positive; when the image is to the left of the reference point, the distance is negative.

Depth of Focus

Perform the basic imaging demonstration with a lens as described in the earlier section Imaging With Lenses and Mirrors, and notice that if the paper is moved forward or backward within a range of a few millimeters, the image remains relatively focused. With the paper positioned outside this region, the image appears blurred. The size of this region represents the depth of focus, which may be small or large depending on several factors. (See Clinical Example 2-2.) In the past, depth of focus was of concern only in the management of presbyopia. However, it is an important concept in refractive surgery as well.

Depth of focus applies to the image. *Depth of field* is the same idea applied to objects. If a camera or other optical system is focused on an object, nearby objects are also in focus. Objects within the range of depth of field will be in focus, whereas objects outside the depth of field will be out of focus.

Image Quality

Careful examination reveals that some details in an object are not reproduced in the image. Images are imperfect facsimiles, not exact scaled duplicates of the original object.

Consider an object 50 cm in front of a pinhole 1 mm in diameter. Paper is placed 50 cm behind the pinhole, so the magnification is –1. A small pencil of rays from each object point traverses the pinhole aperture (Fig 2-12).

Each object point produces a 2-mm-diameter spot in the image. These spots are called *blur circles*. This term is somewhat misleading because off-axis object points technically produce elliptical spots in the image. In addition, this analysis ignores diffraction effects that make the spot larger and more irregular. Regardless, each object point is represented by a blur circle in the image, and the farther the image is from the pinhole, the larger the blur circle in the image. To the extent that these blur circles overlap, the image detail is reduced (blurred).

To some extent, the loss of detail is mitigated with the use of a smaller pinhole (Fig 2-13). A smaller pinhole gives a dimmer, but more detailed, image. However, the smaller the pinhole, the more that diffraction reduces image quality.

While a smaller blur circle preserves more detail, the only way to avoid any loss of detail is to produce a perfect point image of each object point. Theoretically, if a perfect point image could be produced for every point of an object, the image would be an exact duplicate of the object. A perfect point image of an object point is called a *stigmatic image*. "Stigmatic" is derived from the Greek word *stigma*, which refers to a sharply pointed stylus.

Loss of detail occurs in lens and mirror imaging as well, because light from an object point is distributed over a region of the image rather than being confined to a perfect image point (Fig 2-14). Generally, lenses focus light from a single object point to a spot

---

CLINICAL EXAMPLE 2-2

Pinholes are often placed in front of the naked eye to screen for uncorrected refractive error. Positioned over existing glasses and contact lenses, a pinhole screens for residual refractive errors. What is the depth of focus of a pinhole?

When an object is distant from a pinhole aperture, the image formed is relatively focused and remains so over a relatively long range. Thus, a pinhole creates a very long depth of focus.

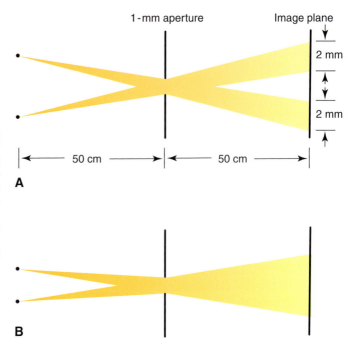

Figure 2-12 **A,** In pinhole imaging, a small pencil of rays from each object point traverses the aperture, producing a small spot in the image. **B,** If the object points are too close to each other, their images overlap. *(Illustration developed by Kevin M. Miller, MD, and rendered by C. H. Wooley.)*

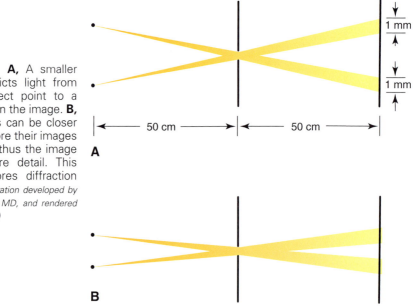

Figure 2-13 **A,** A smaller pinhole restricts light from a single object point to a smaller spot in the image. **B,** Object points can be closer together before their images overlap, and thus the image contains more detail. This analysis ignores diffraction effects. *(Illustration developed by Kevin M. Miller, MD, and rendered by C. H. Wooley.)*

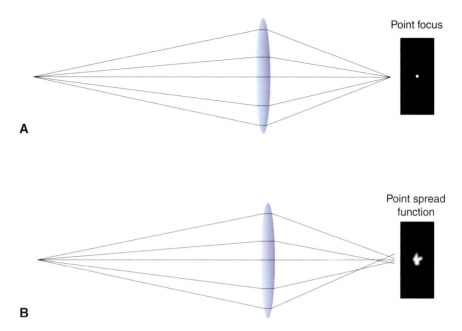

Figure 2-14 **A,** Textbooks often illustrate images produced by lenses as stigmatic. **B,** In most cases, however, the images are not stigmatic. The point spread function reveals how faithfully an imaging system reproduces each object point. *(Illustration developed by Kevin M. Miller, MD, and rendered by C. H. Wooley.)*

10–100 μm across. This is better than a typical pinhole, but the shape of the spot is very irregular. The term *blur circle* is especially misleading when applied to lenses and mirrors. A better term is *point spread function (PSF),* which describes the way light from a single object point is spread out in the image.

To summarize, a *stigmatic* image is a perfect point image of an object point. However, in most cases, images are not stigmatic. Instead, light from a single object point is distributed over a small region of the image known as a blur circle or, more generally, a PSF. The image formed by an optical system is the spatial summation of the PSF for every object point. The amount of detail in an image is related to the size of the blur circle or PSF for each object point. The smaller the PSF, the better the resemblance between object and image.

Light Propagation

An intensive investigation of light propagation was begun in the late 1500s. Numerous experiments measuring light deviation were carried out, and the data were collected and summarized as laws. These laws are summarized in the following sections.

Optical Media and Refractive Index

Light travels through a variety of materials, such as air, glass, plastics, liquids, crystals, some biological tissues, the vacuum of space, and even some metals. A *medium* is any material that transmits light.

Light travels at different speeds in different media. Light moves fastest in a vacuum and slower through any material. The *refractive index* of an optical medium is the ratio of the speed of light in a vacuum to the speed of light in the medium and is usually denoted in mathematical equations by the lowercase letter n. The speed of light in a vacuum is 299,792,458 m/s. This is approximately 300,000 km/s or 186,000 miles/s. In 1983 the Système International defined a meter as the distance light travels in a vacuum during 1/299,792,458 of a second. Refractive index is always greater than or equal to 1. In computations, it is often easier to work with the refractive index of a material than directly with the speed of light.

$$n = \frac{\text{speed of light in vacuum}}{\text{speed of light in medium}}$$

Refractive index is quite sensitive to a material's chemical composition. A small amount of salt or sugar dissolved in water changes its refractive index. Because refractive index is easy to measure accurately, chemists use it to identify compounds or determine their purity. Glass manufacturers alter the refractive index of glass by adding small amounts of rare earth elements. Until recently, clinical labs screened for diabetes by measuring the refractive index of urine. Table 2-1 lists the refractive indices of various tissues and materials of clinical interest.

Refractive index varies with temperature and barometric pressure, but these changes are usually small enough to be ignored. One exception is silicone polymer. The refractive index of polymerized silicone at room temperature (20°C) differs enough from its index at eye temperature (35°C) that manufacturers of silicone intraocular lenses (IOLs) have to account for the variation.

Refractive index also varies with wavelength. As discussed earlier in this text, physical optics regards light in the spectrum of electromagnetic waves. The visual system perceives different wavelengths of light as different colors. Long wavelengths appear red, intermediate wavelengths appear yellow or green, and short wavelengths appear blue. In a vacuum, all wavelengths travel at the same speed. In any other medium, short wavelengths usually travel more slowly than long wavelengths. This phenomenon is called *dispersion*.

In the human eye, chromatic dispersion leads to *chromatic aberration*. If yellow wavelengths are focused precisely on the retina, blue light will be focused in front of the retina and red light will be focused behind the retina. (See Clinical Example 2-3.)

Table 2-1 Refractive Index (Helium D Line) for Some Materials of Clinical Interest

Material	Refractive Index
Air	1.000
Water	1.333
Cornea	1.376
Aqueous and vitreous humor	1.336
Spectacle crown glass	1.523
Polymethylmethacrylate (PMMA)	1.492
Acrylic	1.460
Silicone	1.438

CLINICAL EXAMPLE 2-3

You may notice that red objects appear nearer than blue objects when they are displayed against a black background (Fig 2-15). This effect stands out in slide presentations that are rich in red and blue text and is known as *chromostereopsis.* It occurs because the human eye has approximately 0.5 D of chromatic aberration. Even individuals with red-green color blindness can observe the effect. To bring red print into focus, the eye must accommodate. To bring blue print into focus, the eye must relax accommodation. As a result, red print appears closer than blue print. The accommodative effort required to bring the various pieces of a chromatic image into focus imparts a 3-dimensional quality to the image.

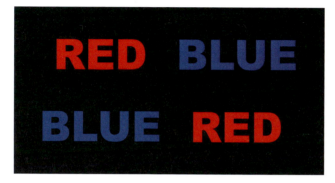

Figure 2-15 Chromostereopsis is demonstrated by this illustration of red and blue print on a black background. The illustration is not very dramatic unless rendered on a computer monitor or projected onto a screen. *(Illustration developed by Kevin M. Miller, MD, and rendered by C. H. Wooley.)*

Some media, such as quartz, are optically inhomogeneous. That is, the speed of light through the material depends on the direction of light propagation through the material.

Law of Rectilinear Propagation

The law of rectilinear propagation states that light in a homogeneous medium travels along straight-line paths called *rays* (Fig 2-16). The light ray is the most fundamental construct in geometric optics. Of particular note, rays traversing an aperture continue in straight lines in geometric optics. As stated earlier, a bundle of light rays traveling close to each other in the same direction is known as a *pencil* of light.

The law of rectilinear propagation is inaccurate insofar as it does not account for the effect of diffraction as light traverses an aperture (see Chapter 1, Physical Optics). The basic distinction between physical optics and geometric optics is that the latter, being based on the law of rectilinear propagation, ignores diffraction. For clinical purposes, diffraction effects are rarely important. However, in situations where diffraction effects are significant, geometric optics does not fully describe the image.

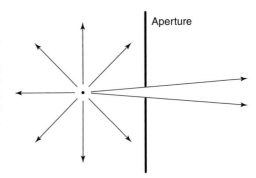

Figure 2-16 The law of rectilinear propagation. Light in a homogeneous medium propagates along straight-line paths originating from a point source. A ray is a geometric construct that represents a light path. Notice that rays traversing an aperture continue along a straight line. *(Illustration developed by Edmond H. Thall, MD, and Kevin M. Miller, MD, and rendered by C. H. Wooley.)*

Optical Interfaces

The boundary between 2 different optical media is called an *optical interface.* Typically, when light reaches an optical interface, some light is transmitted through the interface, some is reflected, and some is absorbed or converted to heat by the interface. The amount of light transmitted, reflected, and absorbed depends on several factors.

When light reaches smooth optical interfaces, it undergoes specular reflection and transmission (Fig 2-17); at rough optical interfaces, light undergoes diffuse reflection and transmission (Fig 2-18). If a pencil of light is reduced to a single ray, it is reflected and transmitted specularly by a rough interface.

Specular Reflection: Law of Reflection

In specular reflection, the direction of the reflected ray bears a definite relationship to the direction of the incident ray. To express a precise relationship between incident rays and reflected rays, it is necessary to construct an imaginary line perpendicular to the optical interface at the point where the incident ray meets the interface. This imaginary line is a *surface normal* (Fig 2-19). The surface normal and the incident ray together define an

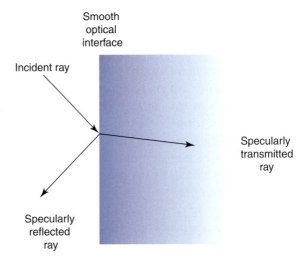

Figure 2-17 Light striking a smooth optical interface is specularly reflected and specularly transmitted. *(Illustration developed by Edmond H. Thall, MD, and Kevin M. Miller, MD, and rendered by C. H. Wooley.)*

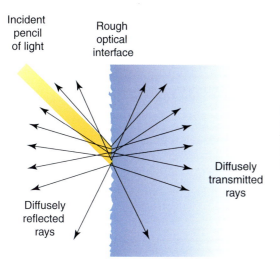

Figure 2-18 A pencil of light striking a rough optical interface is diffusely reflected and diffusely transmitted. *(Illustration developed by Kevin M. Miller, MD, and rendered by C. H. Wooley.)*

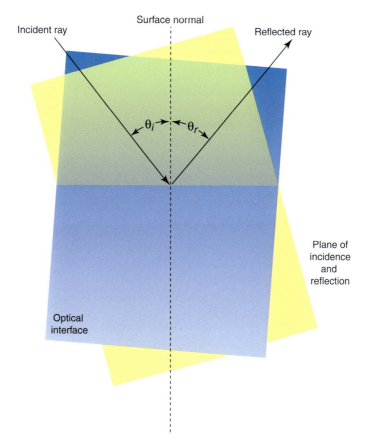

Figure 2-19 The angle of incidence, angle of reflection, surface normal, and the plane of incidence and reflection *(yellow). (Illustration developed by Edmond H. Thall, MD, and Kevin M. Miller, MD, and rendered by C. H. Wooley.)*

imaginary plane known as the *plane of incidence and reflection.* The angle formed by the incident ray and surface normal is the *angle of incidence* θ_i. This is not the angle between the incident ray and the optical interface. The reflected ray and the surface normal form the *angle of reflection* θ_r.

The *law of reflection* states that the reflected ray lies in the same plane as the incident ray and the surface normal (ie, the reflected ray lies in the plane of incidence) and that $\theta_i = \theta_r$ (Fig 2-20).

The amount of light reflected from a surface depends on θ_i and the plane of polarization of the light. The general expression for reflectivity is derived from the Fresnel equations, which are beyond the scope of this text. The reflectivity at normal incidence is simple and depends only on the optical media bounding the interface. The *reflection coefficient* for normal incidence is given by

$$R = \left(\frac{n_2 - n_i}{n_2 + n} \right)^2$$

The reflection coefficient is used to calculate the amount of light transmitted at an optical interface if absorption losses are minimal. (See Clinical Example 2-4.)

Specular Transmission: Law of Refraction

In specular transmission, the transmitted ray's direction bears a definite relation to the incident ray's direction. Again, a surface normal is constructed, and the angle of incidence and the plane of incidence and transmission are defined just as they were for reflection (Fig 2-21). The angle formed by the transmitted ray and the surface normal is the *angle of refraction,* also known as the *angle of transmission.* The angle of transmission θ_t is preferred in this text because the angle of refraction θ_r might otherwise be confused with the angle of reflection θ_r.

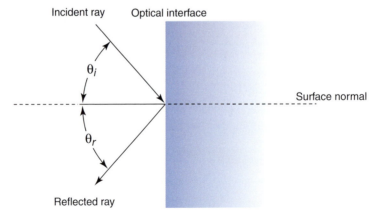

Figure 2-20 The law of reflection. Note that the optical interface is vertical instead of horizontal. The surface normal, incident ray, and reflected ray all lie in the same plane (in this case the plane of the paper). The angle of incidence equals the angle of reflection. *(Illustration developed by Edmond H. Thall, MD, and Kevin M. Miller, MD, and rendered by C. H. Wooley.)*

CLINICAL EXAMPLE 2-4

How much more reflective is a PMMA intraocular lens (IOL) than a silicone IOL? Assume that the index of refraction of a PMMA IOL is 1.492 and the index of refraction of silicone is 1.43.

An IOL is immersed in aqueous, which has an index of refraction of 1.33. The reflectivity coefficient of a PMMA IOL inside the eye is

$$R_{PMMA} = \left(\frac{1.492 - 1.330}{1.492 + 1.330}\right)^2 = 0.003295 = 0.329\%$$

The reflectivity coefficient of a silicone IOL inside the eye is

$$R_{silicone} = \left(\frac{1.430 - 1.330}{1.430 + 1.330}\right)^2 = 0.001313 = 0.131\%$$

Therefore, a PMMA IOL is 0.329/0.131 = 2.51 times more reflective than a silicone IOL.

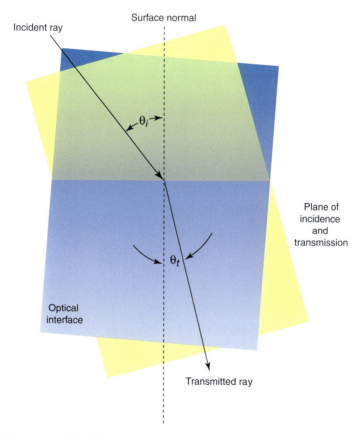

Figure 2-21 The angle of incidence, angle of transmission, surface normal, and the plane of incidence and transmission *(yellow)*. *(Illustration developed by Edmond H. Thall, MD, and Kevin M. Miller, MD, and rendered by C. H. Wooley.)*

At the optical interface, light undergoes an abrupt change in speed that, in turn, usually produces an abrupt change in direction. The *law of refraction,* also known as *Snell's law,* in honor of its discoverer, states that the refracted or transmitted ray lies in the same plane as the incident ray and the surface normal and that

$$n_i \sin \theta_i = n_t \sin \theta_t$$

where

n_i = refractive index of incident medium
n_t = refractive index of transmitted medium
θ_i = angle of incidence
θ_t = angle of transmission

When light travels from a medium of lower refractive index to a medium of higher refractive index, it bends toward the surface normal. Conversely, when light travels from a higher to a lower refractive index, it bends away from the surface normal (Fig 2-22; Clinical Example 2-5).

Normal Incidence

Normal incidence occurs when a light ray is perpendicular to the optical interface. In other words, the surface normal coincides with the ray. If the interface is a refracting surface, the ray is undeviated. Light changes speed as it crosses the interface but does not change direction. If the surface reflects specularly, rays and pencils of light will be reflected back along a 90° angle to the surface.

Total Internal Reflection

Total internal reflection (TIR) occurs when light travels from a high-index medium to a low-index medium and the angle of incidence exceeds a certain *critical angle.* Under these circumstances, the incident ray does not pass through the interface; all light is reflected

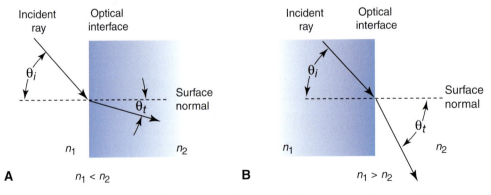

Figure 2-22   **A,** Light moving from a lower index to a higher one bends toward the surface normal. **B,** Conversely, light moving from higher to lower index bends away from the surface normal. *(Illustration developed by Edmond H. Thall, MD, and Kevin M. Miller, MD, and rendered by C. H. Wooley.)*

CLINICAL EXAMPLE 2-5

Imagine you are fishing from a pier and you spot a "big one" in front of you a short distance below the surface of the water. You don't have a fishing rod, but instead you are armed with a spear (Fig 2-23). How should you throw the spear to hit the fish?

From your knowledge of Snell's law, you know that the fish is not where it appears to be. If you throw the spear at the fish, you will certainly miss it. What you have to do is throw the spear in front of the virtual fish, the one you see, to hit the real fish.

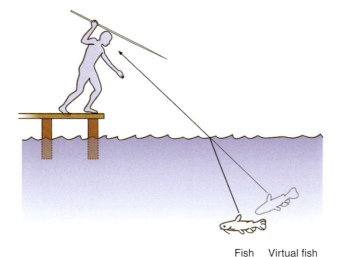

Fish   Virtual fish

Figure 2-23 The fisherman must throw the spear in front of the virtual fish to hit the actual fish. *(Illustration developed by Kevin M. Miller, MD, rendered by Jonathan Clark, and modified by Neal H. Atebara, MD.)*

back into the high-index medium. The law of reflection governs the direction of the reflected ray.

Figure 2-24A shows a light ray traveling from a high-index medium (spectacle crown glass) into a low-index medium (air). In this situation, the transmitted ray bends away from the surface normal, and thus the angle of transmission exceeds the angle of incidence. As the angle of incidence increases, the angle of transmission increases to a greater degree. Eventually, the angle of transmission equals 90°. At this point, the ray grazes along the optical interface and is no longer transmitted (Fig 2-24B).

The critical angle is the angle of incidence that produces a transmitted ray 90° to the surface normal. The critical angle θ_c is calculated from Snell's law:

$$n_i \sin \theta_c = n_t \sin 90°$$

The sine of 90° is 1; thus,

$$n_i \sin \theta_c = n_t$$

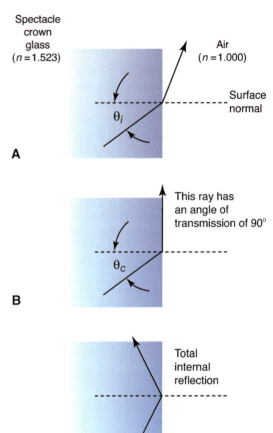

Figure 2-24 **A,** When light travels from a high-index medium to a low-index medium, it bends away from the surface normal. **B,** At the critical angle, θ_c, the refracted light travels in the optical interface. **C,** Beyond the critical angle, all light is reflected by the interface. In **A** and **B,** light is also reflected by the interface, but this is not drawn. *(Illustration developed by Kevin M. Miller, MD, and rendered by C. H. Wooley.)*

Rearranging gives

$$\sin\theta_c = \frac{n_t}{n_i}$$

So, the angle of transmission is 90° when the angle of incidence is

$$\theta_c = \arcsin\frac{n_t}{n_i}$$

In the current example, $n_i = 1.000$ and $n_t = 1.523$, so the critical angle is 41.0°.

What happens when the angle of incidence exceeds the critical angle? As Figure 2-24C shows, the angle of transmission increases as the angle of incidence increases, but the angle of transmission cannot exceed 90°. Consequently, refraction cannot occur. Indeed, Snell's law has no valid mathematical solution (in real numbers) when the critical angle is exceeded. Instead, the incident ray is 100% reflected.

TIR is a rather curious phenomenon. Consider light traveling from spectacle crown glass to air. If the angle of incidence is 10°, the light transmits easily as it crosses the interface. However, if the angle of refraction is 45°, the interface becomes an impenetrable barrier! The interface is transparent to some rays and opaque to others. Physicists have devoted a great deal of attention to this phenomenon.

TIR has great practical value. In the early 1600s, it was difficult to make a good mirror. The best surfaces could specularly reflect only about 80% of incident light, and the rest was diffusely reflected, which made these surfaces nearly useless as imaging devices. However, TIR is just that—total. When TIR occurs, 100% of the light is reflected. In the past, often the only way to make a practical mirror was to use internally reflecting prisms. Today, TIR is still used in prisms found in binoculars, slit lamps, and operating microscopes, to give just a few examples. Clinically, TIR is a nuisance when clinicians are trying to examine the anterior chamber angle (Clinical Example 2-6).

Dispersion

With the exception of a vacuum, which always has a refractive index of 1.000, refractive indices are not fixed values. They vary as a function of wavelength. In general, refractive

CLINICAL EXAMPLE 2-6

TIR makes it impossible to view the eye's anterior chamber angle without the use of a contact lens. Light from the angle undergoes TIR at the air–cornea interface (technically, the air–tear film interface) (Fig 2-25A). Light from the angle never escapes the eye. Using a contact lens to eliminate the air at the surface of the cornea (Fig 2-25B) overcomes the problem. Light travels from the cornea (or coupling gel) to the higher-index contact lens. TIR never occurs when light travels from a medium of lower index to one of higher index, so light enters the contact lens and is reflected from the mirror. TIR does not occur at the front surface of the contact lens because the angle of incidence is less than the critical angle.

Assuming the refractive index of the tear film on the front surface of the cornea is 1.333, the critical angle for the air–tear interface is

$$\theta_c = \arcsin\frac{1}{1.333} = 48.6°$$

From trigonometry, we can estimate the angle at which light rays from the trabecular meshwork strike the air–tear interface. The situation is illustrated in Figure 2-26 with average anatomical dimensions. We ignore the effect of the back surface of the cornea because this surface has relatively little power and we are performing only a rough calculation. From basic trigonometry,

$$\theta_i = \arctan\frac{5.5}{3.5} = 57.5°$$

Interestingly, this rough calculation shows that θ_c is exceeded by only a few degrees. When the cornea is ectatic (as in some cases of keratoconus), the angle of incidence is less than θ_c and the angle structures are visible without a goniolens.

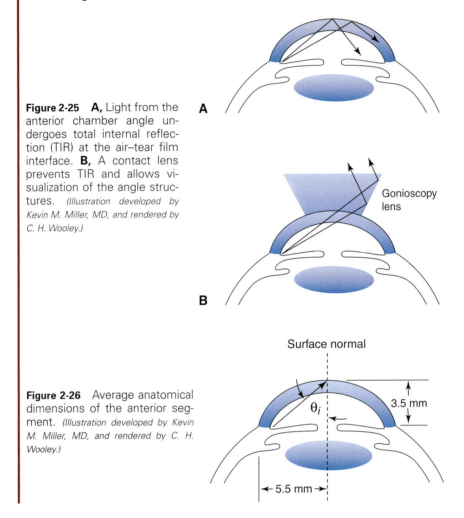

Figure 2-25 **A,** Light from the anterior chamber angle undergoes total internal reflection (TIR) at the air–tear film interface. **B,** A contact lens prevents TIR and allows visualization of the angle structures. *(Illustration developed by Kevin M. Miller, MD, and rendered by C. H. Wooley.)*

Figure 2-26 Average anatomical dimensions of the anterior segment. *(Illustration developed by Kevin M. Miller, MD, and rendered by C. H. Wooley.)*

indices are higher for short wavelengths and lower for long wavelengths. As a result, blue light travels more slowly than red light in most media, and Snell's law predicts a greater angle of refraction for blue light than for red light (Fig 2-27).

The *Abbe number,* also known as the V-number, is a measure of a material's dispersion. Named for the German physicist Ernst Abbe (1840–1905), the Abbe number V is defined as

$$V = \frac{n_{\mathrm{D}} - 1}{n_{\mathrm{F}} - n_{\mathrm{C}}}$$

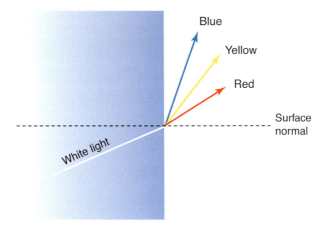

Figure 2-27 Chromatic dispersion. *(Illustration developed by Kevin M. Miller, MD, and rendered by C. H. Wooley.)*

where n_D, n_F, and n_C are the refractive indices of the Fraunhofer D, F, and C spectral lines (589.2 nm, 486.1 nm, and 656.3 nm, respectively). Low-dispersion materials, which demonstrate low chromatic aberration, have high values of V. High-dispersion materials have low values of V. Abbe numbers for common optical media typically range from 20 to 70.

Reflection and Refraction at Curved Surfaces

For the sake of simplicity, the laws of reflection and refraction were illustrated at flat optical interfaces. However, most optical elements have curved surfaces. To apply the law of reflection or refraction to curved surfaces, the position of the surface normal must be determined, because the angles of incidence, reflection, and refraction are defined with respect to the surface normal. Once the position of the surface normal is known, the laws of refraction and reflection define the relationship between the angle of incidence and the angles of refraction and reflection, respectively.

While there is a mathematical procedure for determining the position of the surface normal in any situation, the details of it are beyond the scope of this text. For selected geometric shapes, however, the position of the surface normal is easy to determine. In particular, the normal to a spherical surface always intersects the center of the sphere. For example, Figure 2-28 shows a ray incident on a spherical surface. The incident ray is 2 cm above, and parallel to, the optical axis. The surface normal is found with the extension of a line connecting the center of the sphere to the point where the incident ray strikes the surface. The angle of incidence and the sine of the angle of incidence are determined by simple trigonometry.

The Fermat Principle

The mathematician Pierre de Fermat believed that natural processes occur in the most economical way. The Fermat principle, as applied to optics, implies that light travels from one point to another along the path requiring the least time. Historically, the laws of reflection

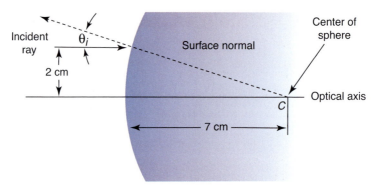

Figure 2-28 A ray 2 cm above and parallel to the optical axis is incident on a spherical surface. The surface normal is found by connecting the point where the ray strikes the surface to the center of the sphere (point *C*). The angle of incidence is found using similar triangles and trigonometry (arctan 2/7 = 16.6°). *(Illustration developed by Edmond H. Thall, MD, and Kevin M. Miller, MD, and rendered by C. H. Wooley.)*

and refraction were discovered by careful experimental measurements before Fermat's time. However, both the law of refraction and the law of reflection can be mathematically derived from the Fermat principle without the need for any measurements.

Suppose that the law of refraction were unknown, and consider light traveling from a point source in air, across an optical interface, to some point in glass (Fig 2-29). Unaware of Snell's law, we might consider various hypothetical paths that light might follow as it moves from point A to point B. Path 3 is a straight line from A to B and is the shortest total distance between the points. However, a large part of path 3 is inside glass, where light travels more slowly. Path 3 is not the fastest route. Path 1 is the longest route from A to B but has the shortest distance in glass. Nevertheless, the extreme length of the overall route makes this a fairly slow path. Path 2 is the best compromise between distance in glass and total path length, and this is the path light will actually follow.

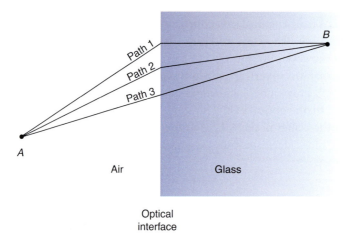

Figure 2-29 Light traveling from *A* to *B* follows only path 2 because it requires the least time. Light does not travel along either path 1 or 3. *(Illustration developed by Edmond H. Thall, MD, and Kevin M. Miller, MD, and rendered by C. H. Wooley.)*

Using mathematics beyond the scope of this text, it can be shown that the optimal path is the one predicted by Snell's law. Thus, Snell's law is a consequence of the Fermat principle.

The Fermat principle is an important conceptual and practical tool. The concept of *optical path length (OPL)* enhances the practical utility of this principle. OPL is the actual distance light travels in a given medium multiplied by the medium's refractive index. For instance, if light travels 5 cm in air ($n = 1.000$) and 10 cm in spectacle crown glass ($n = 1.523$), the OPL is 5 cm $\times$ 1.000 + 10 cm $\times$ 1.523 = 20.2 cm. According to the Fermat principle, light follows the path of minimum OPL.

Figure 2-30 shows light from an object point traveling along 2 different paths to the image point. According to the Fermat principle, for both paths to intersect at the image point, the time required to travel from object to image point (or alternatively, the OPL) must be absolutely identical for each path. If the time required for light to travel along each path is not exactly identical, the paths will not intersect at the image point.

Light traveling path 1 from object to image point traverses a relatively thick part of the lens. Light traveling the longer path 2 goes through less glass. If the lens is properly shaped, the greater distance in air is perfectly compensated for by the shorter distance in glass. So the time required to travel from object to image—and, thus, the OPL—is identical for both paths.

Stigmatic Imaging Using a Single Refracting Surface

By the early 1600s, the telescope and microscope had been invented. Although the images produced by these early devices were useful, their quality was not very high because the lenses did not focus stigmatically.

At the time, lensmakers were not very particular about the shape of the surfaces that were ground on the lens. It seemed that any curved surface produced an image, so lens surfaces were carefully polished but haphazardly shaped. However, as ideas such as stigmatic imaging and Snell's law developed, it became clear that the shape of the lens surfaces determined the quality of the image. In the 17th century, lensmakers began to carefully shape the lens surface in order to improve image quality.

The following question arose: what surface produces the best image? Descartes applied the Fermat principle to the simplest situation possible—a single refracting surface. Consider a single object point and a long glass rod (Fig 2-31). Descartes realized that if the

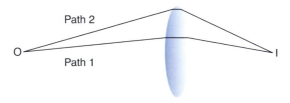

Figure 2-30 Light traveling the shorter distance from object to image point traverses a thick part of the lens. Light traveling the longer path 2 goes through less glass. If the lens is properly shaped, the greater distance in air is perfectly compensated for by the shorter distance in glass, and the time required to travel from object to image is identical for both paths. *(Illustration developed by Edmond H. Thall, MD, and Kevin M. Miller, MD, and rendered by C. H. Wooley.)*

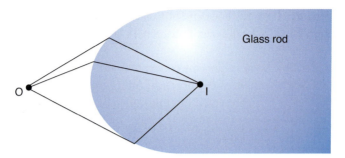

Figure 2-31 The Cartesian conoid is a single refracting surface that produces a stigmatic image for a single object point. *(Illustration developed by Edmond H. Thall, MD, and Kevin M. Miller, MD, and rendered by C. H. Wooley.)*

end of the rod were configured in a nearly elliptical shape, a stigmatic image would form in the glass. This shape became known as a Cartesian ellipsoid, or Cartesian conoid.

Some readers may be troubled by the fact that the image forms in glass instead of air, but this is not a problem. After all, in a myopic eye the image forms in the vitreous cavity, and in an emmetropic eye it forms on the retina. Once a stigmatic image is produced, the rod is cut and a second Cartesian ellipsoid placed on the back surface (Fig 2-32). The final image is also stigmatic. The Cartesian ellipsoid produces a stigmatic image of only 1 object point. All other object points image nonstigmatically.

Until about 1960, it was impossible to manufacture a Cartesian ellipsoid. The only surfaces that could be accurately figured were spheres, cylinders, spherocylinders, and flats. Now aspheric surfaces are relatively easy to manufacture.

Descartes established that a single refracting surface could, at best, produce a stigmatic image of only 1 object point. By means of mathematics, it has been demonstrated that an optical system can produce a stigmatic image for only as many object points as there are "degrees of freedom" in the optical system. A single lens has 3 degrees of freedom *(df)*: the front surface, the back surface, and the lens thickness. A combination of 2 lenses

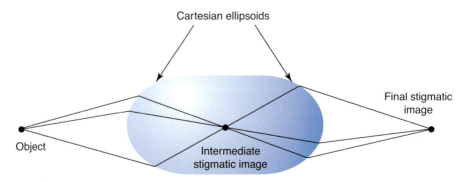

Figure 2-32 A combination of Cartesian ellipsoids also gives a stigmatic image. *(Illustration developed by Edmond H. Thall, MD, and Kevin M. Miller, MD, and rendered by C. H. Wooley.)*

has 7 *df*: the 4 lens surfaces, the 2 lens thicknesses, and the distance between the lenses. Optical systems utilizing multiple lenses improve image quality.

First-Order Optics

For centuries, the sphere was the only useful lens surface that could be manufactured. Descartes proved that lenses with spherical surfaces do not produce stigmatic images, but common experience shows that such lenses can produce useful images. Consequently, the properties of spherical refracting surfaces have been carefully studied.

Today, the accepted approach for studying the imaging properties of any lens is the method called *exact ray tracing*. In this technique, Snell's law is used to trace the paths of several rays, all originating from a single object point. A computer carries out the calculations to as high a degree of accuracy as necessary, usually between 6 and 8 significant figures.

Figure 2-33 shows an exact ray trace for a single spherical refracting surface. Because the image is not stigmatic, the rays do not converge to a single point. However, there is one location where the rays are confined to the smallest area, and this is the location of the image. The distribution of rays at the image location indicates the size of the blur circle or PSF. From the size of the blur circle, the image quality is determined. From the location of the image, other properties, such as magnification, are determined. Ultimately, all image properties may be determined with exact ray tracing.

Beginning in the 1600s, methods of analyzing optical systems were developed that either greatly reduced or eliminated the need for calculation. These methods are based on approximations—that is, these methods do not give exact answers. Nevertheless, carefully chosen approximations can yield results that are very close to the exact answer while greatly simplifying the mathematics.

The trick is to choose approximations that provide as much simplification as possible while retaining as much accuracy as possible. In this regard, the mathematician Carl Gauss (1777–1855) made many contributions to the analysis of optical systems. Gauss's

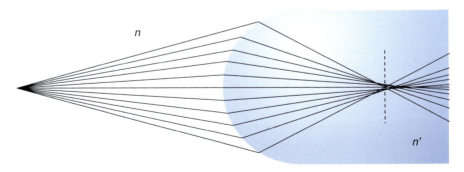

Figure 2-33 An exact ray trace for a single refracting surface. The image is not stigmatic. However, at one particular location, indicated by the *dotted line*, the rays are confined to the smallest area. This is the image location. *(Illustration developed by Edmond H. Thall, MD, and Kevin M. Miller, MD, and rendered by C. H. Wooley.)*

work, combined with that of others, developed into a system for analyzing optical systems that has become known as *first-order optics.*

Ignoring Image Quality

To determine image quality, it is necessary to know how light from a single object point is distributed in the image (ie, the PSF). To determine the PSF, hundreds of rays must be accurately traced. In Gauss's day, manufacturing techniques rather than optical system design limited image quality. Accordingly, there was little interest in theoretically analyzing image quality. Interest lay instead in analyzing other image features, such as magnification and location.

To determine all image characteristics except image quality requires tracing only a few rays. If image quality is ignored, analysis of optical systems is reduced from tracing hundreds of rays to tracing just 2 rays. In Gauss's time, exactly tracing even 2 rays was a daunting task, especially if the optical system consisted of several lenses.

Paraxial Approximation

To exactly trace a ray through a refracting surface, we need to establish a coordinate system. By convention, the origin of the coordinate system is located at the vertex, the point where the optical axis intersects the surface. Also by convention, the y-axis is vertical, the z-axis coincides with the optical axis, and the x-axis is perpendicular to the page (Fig 2-34). An object point is selected, and a ray is drawn from that object point to the refracting surface.

The first difficulty in making an exact ray trace is determining the precise coordinates (*y,z*) where the ray strikes the refracting surface. The formula for finding the intersection of a ray with a spherical surface requires fairly complicated calculations involving square roots.

Instead of tracing a ray through an optical system, it is easier to deal with rays extremely close to the optical axis, so-called *paraxial rays.* The portion of the refracting

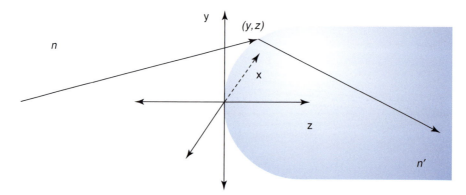

Figure 2-34 To exactly trace a ray through a refracting surface, it is necessary to establish a coordinate system (the x-, y-, and z-axes) and then find the precise coordinates (*y,z*) of the point where the ray intersects the surface. *(Illustration developed by Edmond H. Thall, MD, and Kevin M. Miller, MD, and rendered by C. H. Wooley.)*

surface near the optical axis may be treated as flat. Just as the earth's surface seems flat to a human observer, a refracting surface "seems" flat to a paraxial ray (Fig 2-35). For a ray to be paraxial, it must hug the optical axis over its entire course from object to image. A ray from an object point far off axis is not paraxial even if it strikes the refracting surface near the axis (Fig 2-36).

Treating a lens as a flat plane instead of a sphere eliminates the calculation necessary to find the intersection of the ray and the surface. The intersection of the ray with the surface is specified simply as a distance from the optical axis (h in Figure 2-37).

Small-Angle Approximation

To trace a paraxial ray, begin with an object point at or near the optical axis and extend a ray from the object point to the refracting surface, represented by a flat vertical plane (see Fig 2-37). The next step is to determine the direction of the ray after refraction.

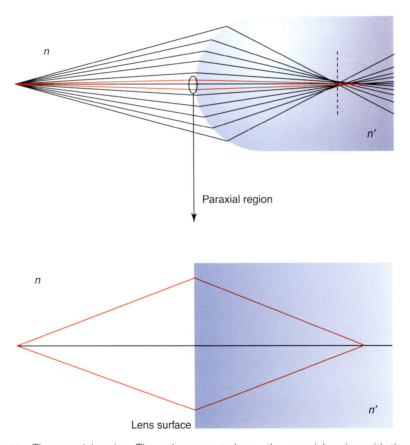

Figure 2-35 The paraxial region. The enlargement shows the paraxial region with the vertical scale greatly increased but the horizontal dimensions unchanged. Notice that in the paraxial region the lens is essentially flat. The paraxial rays are shown in *red*. *(Illustration developed by Edmond H. Thall, MD, and Kevin M. Miller, MD, and rendered by C. H. Wooley.)*

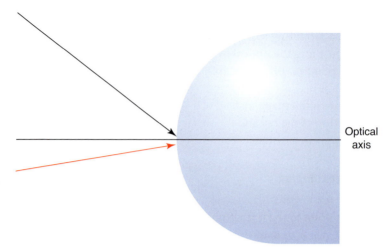

Figure 2-36 Both rays strike the refracting surface in the paraxial region. However, because the lower ray is close to the optical axis over its entire path, it is a paraxial ray. *(Illustration developed by Edmond H. Thall, MD, and Kevin M. Miller, MD, and rendered by C. H. Wooley.)*

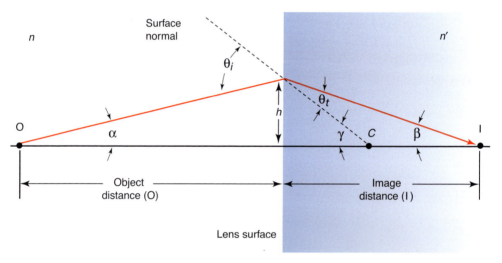

Figure 2-37 Detail of the paraxial region with the vertical scale greatly enlarged relative to the horizontal scale. The lens is spherical but appears flat in the paraxial region. The center of the lens is indicated by point *C*. The points *O* and *I* represent the object point and its image, respectively. θ_i and θ_t indicate the angles of incidence and transmission, respectively. *(Illustration developed by Edmond H. Thall, MD, and Kevin M. Miller, MD, and rendered by C. H. Wooley.)*

To determine the direction of the refracted ray, apply Snell's law. The angle of incidence is θ_i and the angle of transmission is θ_t. Thus,

$$n \sin \theta_i = n' \sin \theta_t$$

Now the polynomial expansion for the sine function is

$$\sin \theta = \theta - \frac{\theta^3}{3!} + \frac{\theta^5}{5!} - \frac{\theta^7}{7!} \cdots$$

where the angle θ is expressed in radians. If the angle θ is small, the third-order term $\theta^3/3!$ and every term after it become insignificant, and the sine function is approximated as

$$\sin\theta \approx \theta$$

This is the mathematical basis of the (essentially equivalent) terms *small-angle approximation, paraxial approximation,* and *first-order approximation.* Only the first-order term of the polynomial expansion needs to be used when the analysis is limited to paraxial rays, which have a small angle of entry into the optical system.

The angles appear large in the bottom part of Figure 2-35 because of the expanded vertical scale, but the upper part shows that in the paraxial region these angles are quite small.

Using the small-angle approximation, Snell's law becomes

$$n\theta_i = n'\theta_t$$

Now, using geometry and Figure 2-37, the angle of incidence θ_i is

$$\theta_i = \alpha + \gamma$$

and the angle of transmission θ_t is

$$\theta_t = \gamma - \beta$$

Thus, Snell's law becomes

$$n(\alpha + \gamma) = n'(\gamma - \beta)$$

or

$$n\alpha + n'\beta = \gamma(n' - n)$$

Now, the small-angle approximation also works for tangents:

$$\tan\alpha \approx \alpha \qquad \tan\beta \approx \beta \qquad \tan\gamma \approx \gamma$$

and

$$\tan\alpha = -\frac{h}{o}$$

The negative sign is used because the object distance (*o*), which extends backward from the lens to the object point, is considered a negative distance.

$$\tan\beta = -\frac{h}{i} \qquad \tan\gamma = \frac{h}{r}$$

Thus,

$$-\frac{nh}{o} + \frac{n'h}{i} = \frac{h(n' - n)}{r}$$

Canceling the common factor h gives

$$-\frac{n}{o} + \frac{n'}{i} = \frac{n'-n}{r}$$

Rearranging yields

$$\frac{n}{o} + \frac{(n'-n)}{r} = \frac{n'}{i}$$

Finally, we define the refractive power of the surface, $P = [(n'-n)/r]$. Thus,

$$\frac{n}{o} + P = \frac{n'}{i} \qquad \text{or} \qquad U + P = V$$

This is called the *lensmaker's equation*. The ratio n/o is the *reduced object vergence (U)* and the ratio n'/i is the *reduced image vergence (V)*. Vergence is discussed in detail in the section Ophthalmic Lenses.

The Lensmaker's Equation

The lensmaker's equation (LME) is one of the most important equations in ophthalmology. Unfortunately, it is also one of the most misused equations in all of ophthalmology.

Fundamentally, the LME says 2 things. First, the location of the image depends on the location of the object. Consider a specific example wherein the refractive index of a glass rod is 1.5 and the radius of curvature is 0.1 m. Suppose an object is in air with $n = 1.0$. The LME becomes

$$\frac{1}{o} + \frac{1.5-1.0}{0.1 \text{ m}} = \frac{1.5}{i}$$

or

$$\frac{1}{o} + 5\,\text{m}^{-1} = \frac{1.5}{i}$$

Note the units of reciprocal, or inverse, meters. Suppose the object is 1 m in front of the lens. Object distances are negative, so

$$\frac{1}{-1\,\text{m}} + 5\,\text{m}^{-1} = 4\,\text{m}^{-1} = \frac{1.5}{i}$$

$$i = \frac{1.5}{4\,\text{m}^{-1}} = 0.375\text{ m}$$

Thus, the image is 37.5 cm behind the refracting surface.

If the object moves closer to the lens—say to 50 cm—similar calculations yield an image distance of 0.5 m, or 50 cm. Thus, as the object moves closer to the lens, the image moves farther away. The object and image always move in the same direction (in this case, to the right) but not necessarily by the same distance (Fig 2-38).

Second, the LME establishes a relationship between the shape of the refracting surface and its optical function. The radius of the spherical refracting surface affects the image characteristics. The *refractive power* (or simply *power*) of a spherical refracting surface is

$$P = \frac{(n' - n)}{r}$$

To demonstrate the significance of power, consider 2 spherical refractive surfaces, both constructed from glass rods ($n = 1.5$). Suppose that 1 refracting surface has a radius of 10 cm, as in the previous example, and the other has a radius of 20 cm. If an object is 1 m in front of each surface, where is the image? As shown in the previous example, the first surface has a power of 5.0 D and produces an image 37.5 cm behind the surface. The second surface has a power of 2.5 D and forms an image 1 m behind the refracting surface. Notice that the second surface has half the power, but the image is more than twice as far behind the refracting surface.

Refractive power, strictly speaking, applies to spherical surfaces, but the cornea is not spherical. In general, every point on an aspheric surface is associated with infinitely many curvatures. There is no such thing as a single radius of curvature. The sphere is a very special case: a single radius of curvature characterizes the entire sphere. A single radius can characterize no other shape, and refractive power should not be applied to a nonspherical surface.

In addition, power is a paraxial concept; thus, it applies only to a small area near the optical axis. Power is not applicable to nonparaxial regions of the cornea. In the paraxial

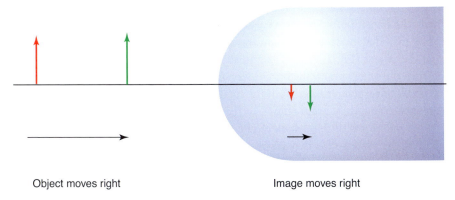

Object moves right   Image moves right

Figure 2-38 The object and the image always move in the same direction. When the object moves to the right, the image moves to the right and vice versa. *(Illustration developed by Edmond H. Thall, MD, and Kevin M. Miller, MD, and rendered by C. H. Wooley.)*

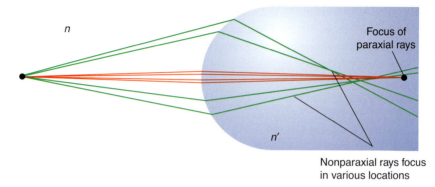

Focus of
paraxial rays

n

n'

Nonparaxial rays focus
in various locations

Figure 2-39 Rays in the paraxial region focus stigmatically. Rays outside the paraxial region do not focus at the image point, decreasing image quality. *(Illustration developed by Edmond H. Thall, MD, and Kevin M. Miller, MD, and rendered by C. H. Wooley.)*

region, imaging is stigmatic (ie, paraxial rays focus to a common point). Even for spherical surfaces, outside the paraxial region rays do not focus to a single point (Fig 2-39). That is, away from the paraxial region, rays do not focus as predicted when the LME is used.

Ophthalmic Lenses

In this section, we build upon the basic principles of first-order optics to show how both simple lenses and complex optical systems are modeled. We also demonstrate how imaging problems are solved.

We begin by considering the concept of vergence. Light rays emanating from a single object point spread apart and are referred to as *divergent.* Light rays traveling toward an image point, after passing through an optical lens, come together and are referred to as *convergent.* If rays are diverging, the vergence is negative; if rays are converging, the vergence is positive. Consider a lens placed close to an object point (Fig 2-40A). The lens collects a large fraction of the light radiating from the object point. When the lens is moved away from the object point, it collects a smaller portion of the light radiated by the object point. The rays that reach the lens are less divergent than they were when the lens was closer to the object (Fig 2-40B). Close to the object point, the light is more divergent; farther from the object point, the light is less divergent. Similarly, close to an image point, light is more convergent; farther from the image point, light is less convergent.

Vergence is inversely proportional to distance from the object or image point. Vergence is the reciprocal of the distance. The distances used most often in ophthalmology are 4 m, 2 m, 1 m, 0.5 m, 0.33 m, 0.25 m, and 0.2 m. The reciprocals of these distances are, respectively, 0.25 m^{-1}, 0.5 m^{-1}, 1 m^{-1}, 2 m^{-1}, 3 m^{-1}, 4 m^{-1}, and 5 m^{-1}. For convenience, the reciprocal meter (m^{-1}) is given another name, the *diopter (D)*.

As light travels away from an object point or toward an image point, its vergence constantly changes (Fig 2-41). To calculate the vergence of light at any point, one must know the location of the object or image point. Conversely, if one knows the vergence at a selected point, the position of the object or image point can be determined.

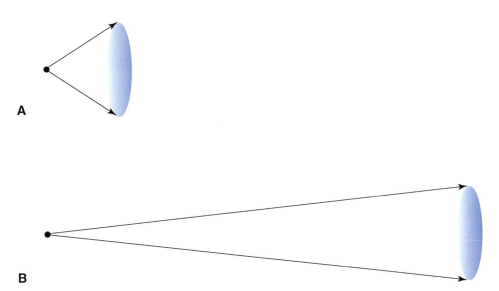

Figure 2-40 **A,** Close to an object point light is strongly divergent, so a lens placed close to the object point collects a large fraction of the light radiated from the point. **B,** Farther from an object point light is much less divergent, so a lens collects a much smaller portion of the light radiated by the object point. *(Illustration developed by Kevin M. Miller, MD, and rendered by C. H. Wooley.)*

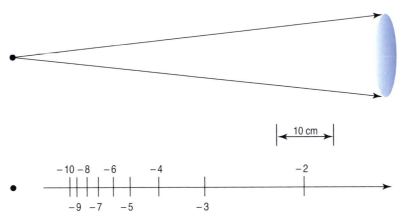

Figure 2-41 Every point on a ray has a different vergence. The numbers indicate vergence in diopters. The linear scale is shown for comparison. *(Illustration developed by Edmond H. Thall, MD, and Kevin M. Miller, MD, and rendered by C. H. Wooley.)*

Reduced vergence is vergence multiplied by the refractive index of the medium. This term is confusing because reduced vergence is numerically larger than vergence. For example, 1 m in front of an image point, light traveling in glass ($n = 1.5$) has a vergence of $+1.0$ D but a reduced vergence of $+1.5$ D. Confusing or not, however, the term *reduced vergence* is too well entrenched to be changed.

The LME can be interpreted in terms of reduced vergence. Light from an object point diverges, but the degree of divergence decreases as the light moves farther from the object point. Eventually, the light encounters the refracting surface, and just as it reaches the surface, it has a reduced vergence of n/o. The refracting surface suddenly changes the light's vergence by an amount equal to its power. As the light leaves the refracting surface, it has a reduced vergence of $(n/o) + P$, but because the light is converging to an image point, this must equal n'/i.

Calculations using the LME are inconvenient because they involve reciprocal distances. Vergence is a way to simplify the calculations. By means of reduced vergence, the LME

$$\frac{n}{o} + P = \frac{n'}{i}$$

can be written in a very simple form:

$$U + P = V$$

where U is reduced object vergence and V is reduced image vergence.

Consider an object in air 50 cm in front of a +5 D refracting surface with $n = 1.5$. Where is the image? Light diverging from the object has a negative vergence. When the light reaches the lens, it has a reduced vergence of –2 D. The lens adds +5 D, for a final reduced vergence at the lens of +3 D. The plus sign indicates that the light converges as it leaves the lens. Dividing the reduced vergence by the index of the glass gives a vergence of +2 D, so the image is 50 cm behind the refracting surface.

The most common mistake in working with vergence calculations is ignoring the negative sign for divergent light. One way to avoid this mistake is to deal with the signs first, rather than with the numbers. For example, to solve the previous problem, many people would begin by converting distance to diopters—that is, the object is 50 cm from the lens, so the vergence is 2 D. After this conversion has been performed, it is easy to forget about the minus sign. It is better to deal with the sign first. In this problem, begin by noting that light diverges from the object and has a negative value; then write down the negative sign and convert distance to vergence (–2). Always write the sign in front of the vergence, even when the sign is positive, as in the preceding example (+5 D and +3 D). If you encounter difficulties with a vergence calculation, check the signs first. The problem is most likely a dropped minus sign. (See Clinical Example 2-7.)

Transverse Magnification for a Single Spherical Refracting Surface

In the LME, object and image distances are measured from the vertex—that is, the point where the surface intersects the optical axis. To calculate transverse magnification using the equation given earlier, object and image distances should be measured from the nodal points. Rays intersecting the center of curvature strike the surface at normal incidence and travel undeviated through the nodal points (Fig 2-42).

If o and i are, respectively, the object and image distances for the LME, and r is the radius of curvature, then

$$\text{Transverse magnification} = \frac{i - r}{o - r}$$

CLINICAL EXAMPLE 2-7

Imagine you are having a difficult time outlining the borders of a sub-retinal neovascular membrane on a fluorescein angiogram. You pull out a 20 D indirect ophthalmoscopy lens and use it as a simple magnifier. If you hold the lens 2.5 cm in front of the angiogram, where is the image?

Light from the angiogram enters the 20 D lens with a reduced vergence of

$$U = -\frac{1}{0.025\,\text{m}} = -40\,\text{D}$$

It exits the lens with a reduced vergence of

$$-40\,\text{D} + 20\,\text{D} = -20\,\text{D}$$

The light is divergent as it exits the lens; thus, the virtual image you see is on the same side of the lens as the angiogram. It is located (1/20 D) = 0.05 m = 5 cm in front of the lens. Because the image is twice as far from the lens as the object, the transverse magnification is 2.

For calculating transverse magnification

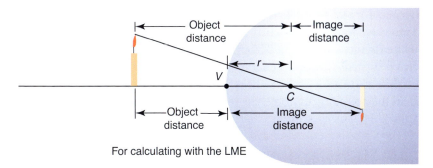

For calculating with the LME

Figure 2-42 For the lensmaker's equation (LME), object and image distances are measured from the vertex *(V)*. For the calculation of transverse magnification, object and image distances are measured from the nodal points, which are both located at the center of curvature *(C)*. The distance between the *C* and *V* is the radius of curvature, *r*. *(Illustration developed by Edmond H. Thall, MD, and Kevin M. Miller, MD, and rendered by C. H. Wooley.)*

It might appear that the denominator should be $o + r$ instead of $o - r$. However, $o - r$ is correct because the sign convention makes object distances negative. By algebraic manipulation, this is converted to a very simple equation involving reduced vergence:

$$\text{Transverse magnification} = \frac{U}{V}$$

Reduced vergence not only simplifies calculations with the LME but also simplifies calculation of magnification. Use of reduced vergence obviates the need for object or image distances, nodal points, or radius of curvature.

Thin-Lens Approximation

The LME deals with a single refracting surface, but, of course, lenses have 2 surfaces. According to the LME, when light from an object strikes the front surface of a lens, its (reduced) vergence changes by an amount equal to the power of the front surface P_f. The vergence continues to change as the light moves from the front to the back surface; this is known as the *vergence change on transfer* P_t. The back lens surface changes the vergence by an amount equal to the back-surface power P_b. Thus,

$$\frac{n}{o} + P_f + P_t + P_b = \frac{n'}{i}$$

The powers of the front and back lens surfaces are easily calculated, but the vergence change on transfer is difficult to calculate. However, because the vergence change on transfer is small in a thin lens, it is ignored to arrive at the *thin-lens approximation*. The total lens power is the sum of the front- and back-surface powers. Thus,

$$\frac{n}{o} + P = \frac{n'}{i}$$

This is the *thin-lens equation* (TLE). The TLE and LME appear to be the same. However, there is an important difference: in the LME, P is the power of a single surface; in the TLE, P is the combined power of the front and back surfaces.

For example, if a +5 D thin lens has water ($n = 1.33$) in front and air in back and an object is 33 cm in front of the lens, where is the image? Light from the object strikes the lens with a reduced vergence of $(-1.33/0.33 \text{ m}) = -4$ D. The lens changes the vergence by +5 D, so light leaves the lens with a vergence of +1 D, forming an image 1 m behind the lens.

The transverse magnification is the ratio of reduced object vergence to reduced image vergence. In the preceding example, the magnification is –4, indicating that the image is inverted and 4 times as large as the object.

Lens Combinations

Most optical systems consist of several lenses. For instance, consider an optical system consisting of 2 thin lenses in air. The first lens is +5 D, the second lens is +8 D, and they are separated by 45 cm. If an object is placed 1 m in front of the first lens, where is the final image and what is the transverse magnification?

In paraxial optics, the way to analyze a combination of lenses is to look at each lens individually. The TLE shows that the first lens produces an image 25 cm behind itself with a magnification of –0.25. Light converges to the image and then diverges again. The image formed by the first lens becomes the object for the second lens. The image is 20 cm in front of the second lens; thus, light strikes the second lens with a vergence of –5 D and forms an image 33 cm behind the second lens. The transverse magnification for the second lens alone is $(-5 \text{ D}/3 \text{ D}) = -1.66$. The total magnification is the product of the individual magnifications $-1.66 \times -0.25 = 0.42$.

It is absolutely essential to calculate the position of the image formed by the first lens. Only after locating the first image is it possible to calculate the vergence of light as it reaches the second lens.

Any number of lenses are analyzed in this way. Locate the image formed by the first lens and use it as the object for the second lens. Repeat the process for each subsequent lens. The overall transverse magnification is the product of the transverse magnifications produced by each individual lens.

Virtual Images and Objects

Many people find the subject of virtual images and virtual objects to be the most difficult aspect of geometric optics. Virtual images and objects can be understood with the use of a few simple rules. The trick is to not "overthink" the subject.

Consider an object 10 cm in front of a +5 D thin lens in air (Fig 2-43A). Light strikes the lens with a vergence of −10 D and leaves with a vergence of −5 D. In this case, unlike in all the previous examples, light emerges with a negative vergence, which means that light is still diverging after crossing the lens. No real image is produced. The reader can easily verify this by repeating the basic imaging demonstration with a +5 D spherical convex trial lens. Notice that an image does not appear, no matter where the paper is held.

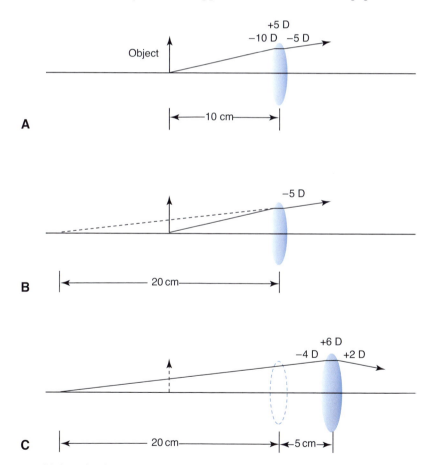

Figure 2-43 Light exits the +5 D lens with a vergence of −5 D **(A),** producing a virtual image 20 cm in front of the lens **(B).** The virtual image becomes the object for the +6 D lens, which in turn produces a real image 50 cm to the right of the lens **(C).** *(Illustration developed by Kevin M. Miller, MD, and rendered by C. H. Wooley.)*

Now, suppose a +6 D thin lens is placed 5 cm behind the first lens. Will an image form? If so, what are its characteristics? Light has a vergence of –5 D, but as the light crosses the 5 cm to the second lens, its vergence changes (the vergence change on transfer). In order to determine the vergence at the second lens, it is necessary to find the location of the image formed by the first lens. However, if the first lens does not form an image, how can the vergence at the second lens be calculated?

The solution is to use a mathematical trick. Light leaving the first lens has a vergence of –5 D. The same vergence would be produced by an object 20 cm away if the first lens were not present (Fig 2-43B).

So, light leaving the second lens appears to be coming from an object 20 cm away from the first lens and 25 cm away from the second lens. The virtual image formed by the first lens is a real object for the second lens. When this imaginary object is used as a reference point, it is easy to see that the vergence at the second lens is –4 D. When light leaves the second lens, it has a vergence of +2 D, forming a real image 50 cm behind the second lens (Fig 2-43C).

In this example, an imaginary reference point was used to determine the vergence at the second lens. In geometric optics, this reference point is commonly called the *virtual image* formed by the first lens. A virtual image is a mathematical convenience that allows all of the formulas developed so far (LME, TLE, transverse magnification) to be used even when a lens does not form a real image.

Mathematically, virtual images are used in exactly the same way as real images. In Figure 2-43, the first lens forms a virtual image 20 cm to the left. The transverse magnification for the first lens is (–10 D/–5 D) = 2. Thus, the virtual image is upright and twice as large as the original object. This virtual image now becomes the object for the second lens. The vergence at the second lens is –4 D, and after traversing the second lens, the vergence is +2 D. The image now formed is real and 50 cm to the right of the second lens. The transverse magnification for the second lens is –2 D. The total magnification is therefore 2 × –2 = –4. The final image is inverted and 4 times larger than the original. Again, this is verified with trial lenses.

Objects may also be virtual. Consider an object 50 cm in front of a +3 D thin lens in air. A +2 D thin lens in air is placed 50 cm behind the first lens. The first lens forms a real image 1 m to the right. However, before the light can reach this image, it strikes a second lens. The image formed by the first lens is the object for the second lens, but this object is on the wrong side of the lens. Thus, it is called a *virtual object* (Fig 2-44).

Here, unlike in all the previous examples, light is convergent when it strikes the second lens (vergence = +2 D). The second lens increases the vergence to +4 D, forming a real image 25 cm behind the second lens. The transverse magnification for the first lens is –2 and for the second lens +0.5, for a total magnification of –1.

A common misconception is that inverted images are real and upright images are virtual. This is not the case. The correct rule is very simple: For any individual lens, the object is virtual when light striking the lens is convergent, and the object is real when light striking the lens is divergent. When light emerging from the lens is convergent, the image is real, and when light emerging from a lens is divergent, the image is virtual.

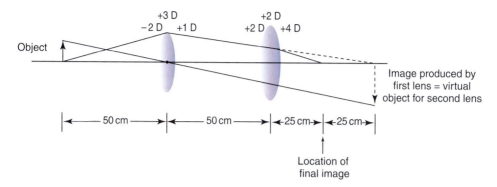

Figure 2-44 The real image formed by the +3 D lens is the virtual object for the +2 D lens. *(Illustration developed by Kevin M. Miller, MD, and rendered by C. H. Wooley.)*

Focal Points and Planes

The +5 D lens in Figure 2-45A has an *anterior (primary) focal point* F_a that is (1/5 D) = 0.2 m = 20 cm in front of the lens. By definition, light emanating from F_a exits the lens collimated and comes to a focus at plus optical infinity. The same is true of light emanating from any point in the *anterior focal plane* (Fig 2-45B). Collimated light entering a lens from minus optical infinity images to the *posterior (secondary) focal point* F_p (Fig 2-45C). Collimated off-axis rays from minus infinity focus to the *posterior focal plane* (Fig 2-45D). For a thin lens immersed in a uniform optical medium such as air or water, F_a and F_p are equidistant from the lens. For a convex (plus-power) spherical lens, F_a is located anterior to the lens and F_p is located posterior to the lens. For a concave (minus-power) spherical lens, the points are reversed: F_a is posterior to the lens; F_p, anterior to the lens. To avoid confusion, some authors prefer the terms F and F' instead of F_a and F_p.

Paraxial Ray Tracing Through Convex Spherical Lenses

From any object point, 3 simple rays are drawn through a thin lens to locate a corresponding point in the image. Only 2 rays are actually needed. The same rays are used to find corresponding points if a thick lens or a multi-element lens system is modeled by first-order optical principles. The first 2 rays traverse F_a and F_p. The final ray, known as the *central ray* or *chief ray*, traverses the nodal points. For a thin lens immersed in a medium with a uniform refractive index, the nodal points overlap at the optical center of the lens. The central ray traverses the nodal point undeviated; that is, it does not change direction with respect to the optical axis as it passes through the lens.

It is customary to represent objects as arrows to show size and orientation. The tip of an arrow represents a single object point. Suppose an object is placed 20 cm in front of a +10 D lens immersed in air (Fig 2-46).

A ray is drawn from the tip of the object through F_a. This ray emerges from the lens parallel to the optical axis and heads off to plus infinity. A second ray is drawn that parallels the optical axis until it enters the lens. It emerges from the lens and passes through

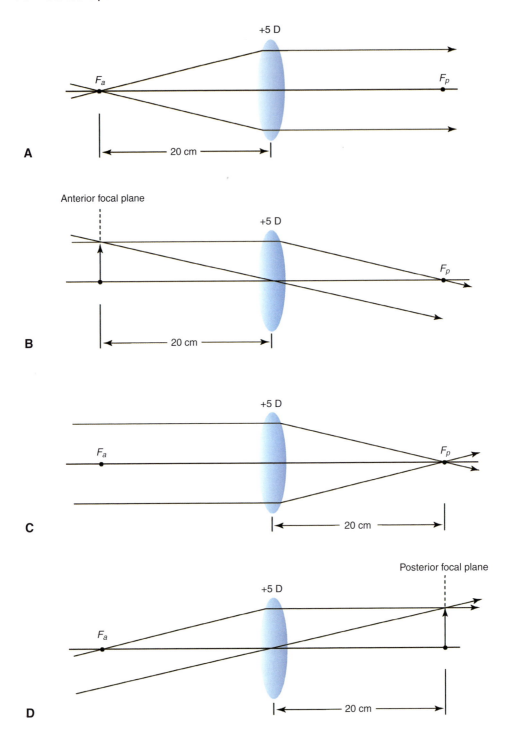

Figure 2-45 **A,** Light that emanates from the anterior focal point, F_a, leaves the lens collimated. **B,** All object points in the anterior focal plane focus to plus optical infinity. **C,** Collimated on-axis light from minus optical infinity focuses to the posterior focal point, F_p. **D,** Collimated off-axis rays focus to the posterior focal plane. *(Illustration developed by Kevin M. Miller, MD, and rendered by C. H. Wooley.)*

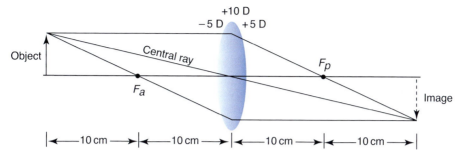

Figure 2-46 Ray tracing through a convex spherical lens. *(Illustration developed by Kevin M. Miller, MD, and rendered by C. H. Wooley.)*

F_p on its way to plus infinity. The intersection of these 2 rays defines the corresponding image point. Note that the image in this example is inverted. The location of the image is determined by vergence calculations. The vergence of light entering the lens is $(-1/0.2 \text{ m}) = -5$ D. By the LME, the vergence of light exiting the lens is -5 D $+ 10$ D $= +5$ D. The image is located $(1/5 \text{ D}) = 0.2 \text{ m} = 20$ cm to the right of the lens. Because the object and image are equidistant from the lens, the transverse magnification is -1. The central ray can also be drawn through the optical center of the lens to confirm the location of the image.

Now what if the object in the previous example is moved closer so that it is 5 cm in front of the lens instead of 20 cm in front (inside F_a), as shown in Figure 2-47A? The ray that leaves F_a and passes through the object point emerges from the lens parallel to the

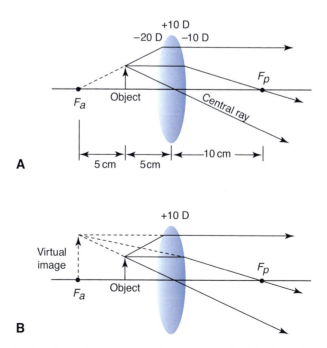

Figure 2-47 Ray tracing through a convex spherical lens. **A,** This time the object is located inside the anterior focal point. **B,** The image is magnified, upright, and virtual and is located to the left of the object. *(Illustration developed by Kevin M. Miller, MD, and rendered by C. H. Wooley.)*

optical axis. The ray that enters the lens parallel to the optical axis exits through F_p. Finally, the central ray traverses the optical center of the lens undeviated. On the back side of the lens, these 3 rays are divergent. So where is the image? If you are looking at the back side of the lens, you see the image point as the backward extension of all 3 rays (Fig 2-47B).

By the LME, the vergence of light exiting the lens is –10 D. The image is located (1/–10 D) = 10 cm to the left of the lens. The image is upright and virtual, and by similar triangles, its transverse magnification is +2. This is the optical basis of a simple, handheld plus-lens magnifier. An object positioned inside the focal point of a plus spherical lens will produce a magnified, upright, virtual image. Try this simple experiment with the lens you use for indirect ophthalmoscopy.

Concave Lenses

In the examples we have used thus far, the lenses have been convex, or positive. Light emerges from a convex lens more convergent—or at least less divergent—than it entered. By contrast, a concave, or negative, lens makes light more divergent.

A negative lens cannot produce a real image of a real object. Instead, a negative lens is usually used in combination with a positive lens to alter image characteristics. For instance, suppose that an object is 1 m in front of a +6 D thin lens in air. The image is 20 cm behind the lens and the magnification is –0.2 (Fig 2-48A). Suppose it is not convenient to have the image so close to the lens and that it would be better to have the image 50 cm behind the lens.

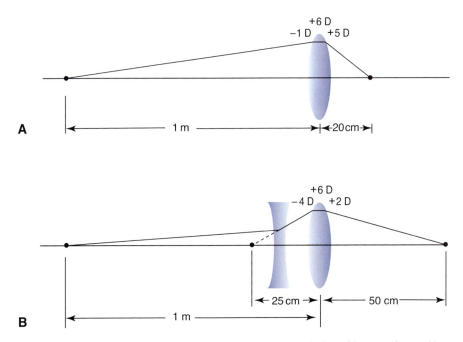

Figure 2-48 Negative lenses are used to change the characteristics of images formed by positive lenses. **A,** An object placed 1 m in front of a +6 D lens images 20 cm behind the lens. **B,** A concave (negative) spherical lens is placed in front of the +6 D lens to move the final image location to 50 cm. *(Illustration developed by Kevin M. Miller, MD, and rendered by C. H. Wooley.)*

For a +6 D lens to produce a real image 50 cm behind itself, the object must be 25 cm in front of the lens. As a practical matter, however, the position of the object usually cannot be changed. Instead, the problem is solved with placement of a negative thin lens between the +6 D lens and the object so the negative lens produces a virtual image 25 cm in front of the +6 D lens (Fig 2-48B).

As another example, a –5.55 D thin lens placed 10 cm in front of the +6 D thin lens (90 cm from the object) produces a virtual image 15 cm in front of the negative lens and 25 cm in front of the +6 D lens. The virtual image becomes a real object for the +6 D lens, which forms an image 50 cm behind itself. The overall magnification is –0.33.

Many different negative thin lenses could be used. Each different power of negative lens must be placed at a different distance from the +6 D lens. In particular, a –8.17 D lens placed 85.7 cm away from the object also produces a virtual image 25 cm in front of the +6 D lens, yielding a final real image in the desired location. Moreover, the final image has the same –0.25 magnification as the original image. So, in this case, it is possible to select a negative lens that changes the final image location without changing its size.

Paraxial Ray Tracing Through Concave Spherical Lenses

The principles of paraxial ray tracing are the same for concave spherical lenses as for convex spherical lenses. Consider a –2 D lens. Its F_a is (1/–2 D) = 50 cm behind the lens. By definition, a ray of light directed through F_a will exit the lens parallel to the optical axis (Fig 2-49A). Similarly, a virtual object in the anterior focal plane of a concave lens will image to plus infinity. A ray of light entering the lens parallel to the optical axis will pass through F_p after exiting the lens (Fig 2-49B). Similarly, a real object at minus

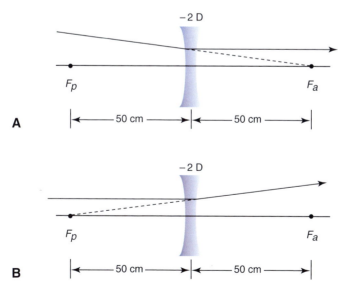

Figure 2-49 **A,** Incoming light directed through the anterior focal point, F_a, of a concave spherical lens exits the lens collimated. **B,** Collimated incoming light parallel to the optical axis leaves the lens as if it had come through the posterior focal point, F_p. *(Illustration developed by Kevin M. Miller, MD, and rendered by C. H. Wooley.)*

optical infinity will produce a virtual image in the posterior focal plane of a concave lens.

Now let's consider an object placed 100 cm in front of the lens. The 3 usual rays are drawn (Fig 2-50). A virtual image is formed 33 cm in front of the lens. By similar triangles, the transverse magnification is +0.33. No matter where a real object is placed in front of a minus lens, the resulting image is upright, minified, and virtual.

Objects and Images at Infinity

If an object is placed 50 cm in front of a +2 D thin lens in air, where is the image? Light emerges from the lens with a vergence of 0. A vergence of 0 means that light rays are neither convergent nor divergent but parallel, so the light is collimated. In this example, light rays emerge parallel to one another, neither converging to a real image nor diverging from a virtual image. In this case, the image is said to be at *infinity*.

Objects can be located at infinity as well. If a second lens is placed anywhere behind the first one, light striking the second lens has a vergence of 0; the object is at infinity. As a practical matter, a sufficiently distant object may be regarded as at infinity. Clearly, an object like the moon, which is 400 million meters away, has a vergence of essentially 0. For clinical work, objects more than 20 ft (6 m) distant may be regarded as being at optical infinity. An object 20 ft away has a vergence of about –0.17 D; clinically, this is small enough to be ignored. When a refractive correction is being determined, few patients can notice a change of less than 0.25 D.

Some people think that objects in the anterior focal plane are imaged in the posterior focal plane. This is not true. Objects in the anterior focal plane image at plus infinity; objects at minus infinity image in the posterior focal plane.

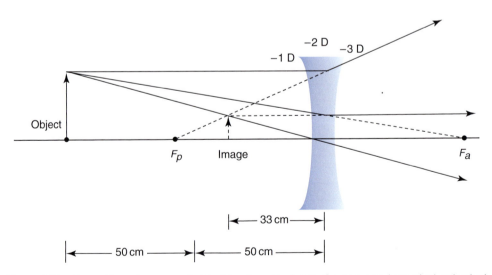

Figure 2-50 No matter where a real object is placed in front of a concave (negative) spherical lens, the image is upright, minified, and virtual. *(Illustration developed by Kevin M. Miller, MD, and rendered by C. H. Wooley.)*

Principal Planes and Points

If an object's position changes in front of a lens, both the location and magnification of the image change. Most optical systems have one particular object location that yields a magnification of 1. In other words, when an object is located in the correct position, the image will be upright and the same size as the object. The *principal planes* are perpendicular to the optical axis and identify the object and image locations that yield a magnification of 1. The principal planes are also called the *planes of unit magnification* and are geometric representations of where the bending of light rays occurs.

Consider an optical system consisting of 2 thin lenses in air (Fig 2-51). The first lens is +6 D, the second lens is +15 D, and the 2 lenses are separated by 35 cm. An object located 50 cm in front of the first lens is imaged 25 cm behind the first lens with a magnification of –0.5. The real image becomes a real object for the second lens, which produces a real image 20 cm behind the second lens with a magnification of –2. The *anterior principal plane* of this system is 50 cm in front of the first lens; the *posterior principal plane* is 20 cm behind the second lens. Often, both the anterior and posterior principal planes are virtual; in some cases, the posterior principal plane is in front of the anterior principal plane.

The intersection of the anterior and posterior principal planes with the optical axis defines the corresponding *anterior* and *posterior principal points.* Like the nodal points, the principal points are an important pair of reference points.

Collectively, the nodal points, focal points, and principal points are called the *cardinal points,* because these 3 pairs of points completely describe the first-order properties of an optical system. Notice that 2 pairs of cardinal points are conjugate. The posterior principal point is the image of the anterior principal point, and the same relationship holds for the nodal points. However, the focal points are not conjugate. Two pairs of cardinal points are associated with planes: the focal points and the principal points. However, there is no such thing as a nodal plane associated with a nodal point.

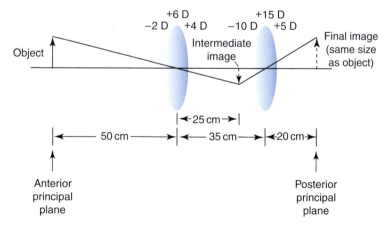

Figure 2-51 These 2 thin lenses in air produce an image that is upright, real, and the same size as the object. *(Illustration developed by Kevin M. Miller, MD, and rendered by C. H. Wooley.)*

Modeling an Unknown Optical System

In the previous examples, we showed how vergence calculations could be used to determine image location and magnification for a single lens or a combination of 2 lenses. However, most optical systems consist of many lenses. A typical 35-mm camera lens contains between 6 and 12 individual lenses. Vergence calculations become tedious for such systems; it is easier to analyze image characteristics graphically.

Thick lenses and complex optical systems are modeled using principal planes, nodal points, and focal points if the optical surfaces are spherical and we restrict the analysis to paraxial rays. The location of each point or plane is determined experimentally.

Consider an unknown optical system that contains any number of optical elements (Fig 2-52A). We will treat it as a "black box." A real object placed in front of the black box will image somewhere in space. If the image forms in front of the box, it is virtual. If it forms behind the box, it is real. Now consider a single ray of light that leaves a point on the object, such as the tip of the arrow in the drawing. A laser pointer is used to model the ray experimentally. At some angle of entry into the box with respect to the optical axis, the ray will exit the box parallel to the optical axis. The extension inside the box of the entering and exiting rays defines the location of the *anterior principal plane P* (Fig 2-52B). Similarly, a ray of light entering the black box parallel to the optical axis will exit the box at some angle to the optical axis. The intersection of these 2 rays inside the box defines the location of the *posterior principal plane P'* (Fig 2-52C). The intersection of the principal planes and the optical axis defines the principal points. If the indices of refraction of the media on either side of the black box are the same, the nodal points, N and N', correspond to the locations of the principal points (Fig 2-52D). The focal points, F_a and F_p, are determined the same way as for a thin lens. The result is an optical model that simplifies the complicated optical system (Fig 2-52E). If the media bounding the system are different (eg, the human eye has air on one side and vitreous gel on the other side), the nodal points "pull" in the direction of the medium with the higher refractive index. The anterior focal length of the system is the distance from F_a to the anterior principal point, not the distance to the first lens in the black box. The posterior focal length is the distance from F_p to the posterior principal point.

Thick Lenses

The thin-lens approximation is invalid in some clinical settings. For example, IOLs are treated as thick lenses. Consider a lens of arbitrary thickness (Fig 2-53).

The combined power of a thick lens P is not simply the sum of the individual surface powers; instead (as described under the section Thin-Lens Approximation), it includes the vergence change on transfer P_t:

$$P = P_f + P_b + P_t$$

where

P_f = power of the first lens surface
P_b = power of the second lens surface

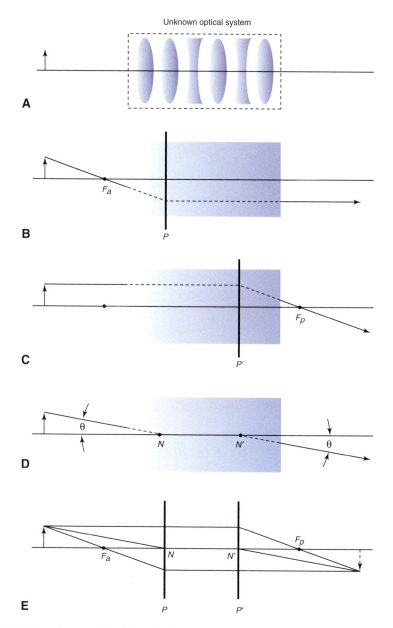

Figure 2-52 **A,** An unknown "black box" optical system may contain any number of optical elements. **B,** A ray of light from an object point is traced that leaves the system parallel to the optical axis. The intersection of this ray with the optical axis defines the anterior focal point, F_a. The intersection of rays entering and leaving the optical system defines the location of the anterior principal plane, P. **C,** Another ray of light from the same object point enters the optical system parallel to the optical axis and exits through the posterior focal point, F_p. The intersection of the 2 rays entering and leaving the system defines the posterior principal plane, P'. **D,** The nodal points are defined by entering and exiting rays that intersect the optical axis at the same angle. If the refractive indices of the media bounding the optical system are the same on both sides, the nodal points correspond to the principal points. **E,** The final model simplifies the complex unknown optical system. *(Illustration developed by Kevin M. Miller, MD, and rendered by C. H. Wooley.)*

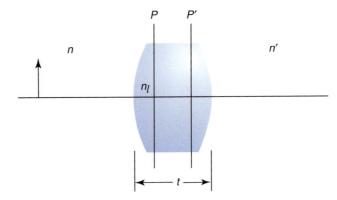

Figure 2-53 An example of a thick lens. *(Illustration developed by Kevin M. Miller, MD, and rendered by C. H. Wooley.)*

The vergence change on transfer is

$$P_t = -\frac{t}{n_l} P_f P_b$$

where

t = lens thickness
n_l = index of refraction of the lens

Thus, the power of a thick lens equals

$$P = P_f + P_b - \frac{t}{n_l} P_f P_b$$

When powers P, P_f, and P_b are in diopters, t is in meters. A lens with a front-surface power of +5.0 D, a back-surface power of +10.0 D, and a thickness of 1 cm, constructed from glass with an index of $n_l = 1.5$, has a total power of +14.7 D. In this case, the power of the thick lens is one-third of a diopter less than it would be if it were a thin lens. The difference is attributable to the vergence change that occurs as light travels from the front surface to the back surface.

Focal Lengths

For any optical system, the distance from the anterior principal point to the anterior focal point is the *anterior focal length (AFL)*. Similarly, the *posterior focal length (PFL)* is the distance from the posterior principal point to the posterior focal point.

Following the sign convention, focal lengths are negative when the focal point is to the left of the principal point and positive when the focal point is to the right of the principal point. For instance, a +5 D thin lens in air has an AFL of –20 cm and a PFL of +20 cm.

For any optical system, focal lengths and refractive power P are related by

$$\text{AFL} = \frac{n_o}{P} \qquad \text{PFL} = \frac{n_i}{P}$$

For any optical system, the distance from the anterior principal point to the anterior nodal point is always equal to the distance from the posterior principal point to the posterior nodal point. The distance between principal point and nodal point follows the sign convention and is given by

$$\text{Distance} = \text{AFL} + \text{PFL}$$

For instance, for a +5 D thin lens in air, AFL + PFL = –20 cm + 20 cm = 0. Thus, the nodal points and principal points overlap. For a +5 D thin lens with water ($n = 1.33$) in front and air in back, the AFL = –26.6 cm and the PFL = 20 cm. Thus, the nodal points are 6.6 cm to the left of the principal points.

Gaussian Reduction

Thus far, we have discussed the properties of a single optical system. The treatment of refractive errors usually involves adding a lens to an existing optical system, the patient's eye. Gaussian reduction describes what happens when 2 optical systems (such as a correcting lens and the eye) are combined.

When 2 optical systems—each with its own cardinal points—are combined, a totally new optical system is created that is described by a new set of cardinal points. The thick-lens equation is used to reduce the 2 individual systems to a single system with its own set of cardinal points. Typically, the combined system's cardinal points and power differ from those of either of the individual systems. Clinically, Gaussian reduction is most important in conjunction with the correction of ametropias (discussed in Chapter 4, Clinical Refraction) and in the calculation of IOL power (see Chapter 6, Intraocular Lenses).

Knapp's Law, the Badal Principle, and the Lensmeter

One problem in treating refractive errors is that the correcting lens often changes the size of the retinal image. If the retinal image in one eye differs in size from that in the other eye, the difference is usually tolerated by the patient unless this difference is large. The adult brain can fuse retinal images that differ in size by as much as 8%; the child's brain can handle an even greater disparity. According to Knapp's law, the size of the retinal image does not change when the center of the correcting lens (to be precise, the posterior nodal point of the correcting lens) coincides with the anterior focal point of the eye (Fig 2-54).

For example, if eyes have identical refractive power and differ only in axial length, then placing a lens at the anterior focal point of each eye will produce retinal images identical in size. However, it is rare that the difference between eyes is purely axial. In addition, the anterior focal point of the eye is approximately 17 mm in front of the cornea (see Chapter 3, Optics of the Human Eye). Although it is possible to wear glasses so the spectacle lens is 17 mm in front of the eye, most people prefer to wear them at a corneal

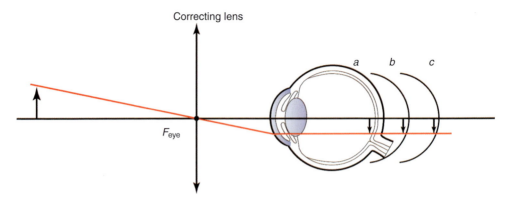

Figure 2-54 Illustration of Knapp's law. If the refractive power of eyes is the same but the axial length varies *(a, b, c)*, a correcting lens placed at the anterior focal point of each eye will produce an identical retinal image size regardless of the axial length. In this example, the power of the correcting lens will change depending on the axial length of the eye. However, the retinal image size will remain constant. *(Illustration by C. H. Wooley.)*

vertex distance of 10–15 mm. Because the clinician is rarely certain that any ametropia is purely axial, Knapp's law has limited clinical application.

Manual lensmeters make use of the same principle, although for an entirely different reason. When applied to lensmeters, Knapp's law is called the *Badal principle.* One type of optometer used for performing objective refraction is based on a variation of Knapp's law wherein the posterior focal plane of the correcting lens coincides with the anterior nodal point of the eye. The effect is the same. Retinal image size remains constant. In this application, the law is called the *optometer principle.* Optical engineers use a variation of Knapp's law called *telecentricity* to improve the performance of telescopes and microscopes. Regardless of the name, the principle remains the same.

Afocal Systems

Consider an optical system consisting of 2 thin lenses in air (Fig 2-55). The lens powers are +2 D and –5 D, respectively. Where is F_p for this system? The posterior focal point is where incoming parallel rays focus. However, as ray tracing demonstrates, rays entering the system parallel to the optical axis emerge parallel to the axis. This system has no focal points; in other words, it is an *afocal system.*

If an object is 2 m in front of the first lens, where is the image and what is the transverse magnification? Vergence calculations show that the image is virtual, 44 cm to the left of the second lens (14 cm to the left of the first lens), and that the transverse magnification is 0.4. If an object is 4 m in front of the first lens, vergence calculations show that the image is virtual, 76 cm to the left of the second lens, and that the transverse magnification is exactly 0.4. In afocal systems, the transverse magnification is the same for every object regardless of location.

Where are the principal planes for this system? Actually, it has no principal planes. Remember, the principal planes are the unique conjugates with a transverse magnification of 1. In this system, the transverse magnification is always 0.4 and never 1. If the transverse magnification were equal to 1, it would be 1 for every pair of conjugates. Consequently,

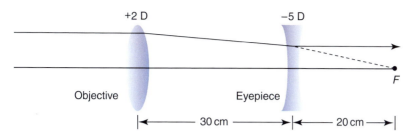

Figure 2-55 The Galilean telescope. The lenses are separated by the difference in focal lengths. *F* is simultaneously the posterior focal point of the plus lens and the anterior focal point of the minus lens. *(Illustration developed by Kevin M. Miller, MD, and rendered by C. H. Wooley.)*

there would be no unique set of planes that could be designated principal planes. In general, afocal systems do not have cardinal points.

Afocal systems are used clinically as telescopes or low vision aids. The 2 basic types of refracting telescopes are the *Galilean telescope* (named for, but not invented by, Galileo) and the *Keplerian,* or *astronomical telescope* (invented by Johannes Kepler). The Galilean telescope consists of 2 lenses. The first lens, the *objective lens,* is always positive and usually has a low power, whereas the second lens, the *eyepiece,* or *ocular,* is always negative and usually has a high power. The lenses are separated by the difference in their focal lengths. The afocal system depicted in Figure 2-55 is a Galilean telescope. The Galilean telescope is also used in some slit-lamp biomicroscopes (Fig 2-56).

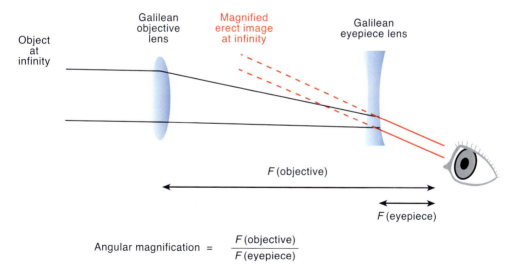

$$\text{Angular magnification} = \frac{F\,(\text{objective})}{F\,(\text{eyepiece})}$$

Figure 2-56 Slit-lamp biomicroscope, Galilean telescope. To produce even greater magnification than an astronomical telescope alone, an additional Galilean system is often used. A plus lens and a minus lens, separated by the difference in their focal lengths, produce an upright, virtual image. The angular magnification is equal to the focal length of the objective lens divided by the focal length of the eyepiece. If the positions of the plus and minus lenses are reversed, the image is minified. This optical property is used by the slit-lamp biomicroscope—a quick switch in lens positions allows 2 different magnification powers. *(Courtesy of Neal H. Atebara, MD. Redrawn by C. H. Wooley.)*

The Keplerian telescope also consists of 2 lenses, a low-power objective and a high-power ocular, but both are positive and separated by the sum of their focal lengths. The image is inverted (Fig 2-57). For comparison, construct a Keplerian telescope using +2 D and +5 D trial lenses.

For each telescope:

$$\text{Transverse magnification} = \frac{P_{eye}}{P_{obj}} = \frac{f_{obj}}{f_{eye}}$$

$$\text{Axial magnification} = m^2$$

where

P_{eye} = power of the eyepiece or ocular
P_{obj} = power of the objective lens
f_{obj} = focal length of the objective lens
f_{eye} = focal length of the eyepiece (negative for concave lenses)
m = transverse magnification

For afocal telescopes like the Galilean and the Keplerian telescope, the focal point of the objective lens and the focal point of the ocular lens are in the same position.

Each form of telescope has advantages and disadvantages. The advantage of a Galilean telescope is that it produces an upright image and is shorter than a Keplerian telescope. These features make the Galilean telescope popular as a spectacle-mounted visual aid or in surgical loupes.

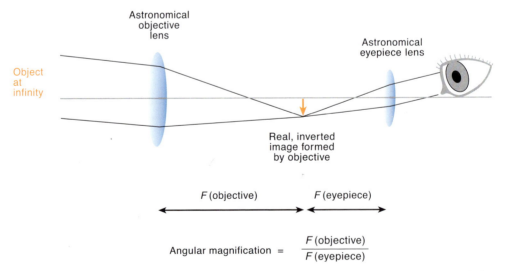

$$\text{Angular magnification} = \frac{F\,(\text{objective})}{F\,(\text{eyepiece})}$$

Figure 2-57 Slit-lamp biomicroscope, Keplerian telescope. One optical component of the slit-lamp biomicroscope is the astronomical telescope, which consists of 2 plus lenses separated by the sum of their focal lengths. This configuration produces a real, inverted image with an angular magnification equal to the focal length of the objective lens (the lens closer to the patient) divided by the focal length of the eyepiece (the lens closer to the observer). *(Courtesy of Neal H. Atebara, MD. Redrawn by C. H. Wooley.)*

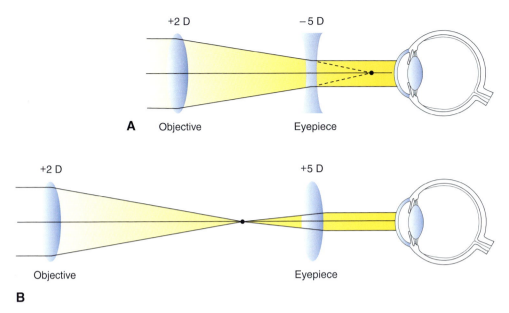

Figure 2-58 Comparison of Galilean and Keplerian telescopes. In the Galilean telescope **(A),** some of the light collected by the objective is lost. In the Keplerian telescope **(B),** all the light collected enters the eye. *(Illustration developed by Kevin M. Miller, MD, and rendered by C. H. Wooley.)*

Conversely, the Keplerian telescope uses light more efficiently, making faint objects easier to see (Fig 2-58). In the Keplerian design, all the light from an object point collected by the objective lens ultimately enters the eye. In the Galilean design, some of the light collected by the objective is lost. Because astronomical observation is largely a matter of making faint stars visible, all astronomical telescopes are of the Keplerian design. The inverted image is not a problem for astronomers, but inverting prisms are placed inside the telescope. Common binoculars and handheld visual aids are usually of the Keplerian design.

Ophthalmic Prisms

An ophthalmic prism is a wedge of transparent plastic or glass with a triangular cross section having an apex and a base (Fig 2-59). Low-power prisms with small apex angles may be incorporated into spectacle lenses and contact lenses. The doubled image viewed in keratometers is achieved with low-power prisms. High-power prisms with large apex angles are used to measure angles of strabismus, to produce the doubling in the measuring head of the Goldmann tonometer, and to apply laser treatment to the periphery of the fundus.

Plane Parallel Plate

The simplest prism has an apex angle of 0°; that is, the 2 faces are parallel. When a light ray traverses a plane parallel plate (such as a piece of window glass), it is refracted at both

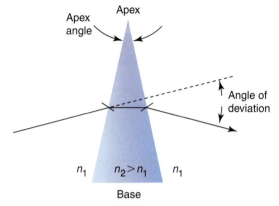

Figure 2-59 Cross section of a prism. Light rays are always bent toward the base of a prism. *(Illustration developed by Edmond H. Thall, MD, and Kevin M. Miller, MD, and rendered by C. H. Wooley.)*

surfaces; but because the bending is equal and opposite at the 2 surfaces, there is no net deviation. However, lateral displacement occurs for all incident rays that are not perpendicular to the surfaces (Fig 2-60).

When the surfaces of a wedge of glass are not parallel, light rays undergo a net deviation.

Angle of Deviation

In any prism with an apex angle greater than 0°, the total angle of deviation of light that passes through it is the sum of the deviations produced at each of the surfaces (see Fig 2-59). These 2 deviations may be in the same direction or in opposite directions, depending on the angle of incidence, but the total deviation is always toward the base of the prism (Fig 2-61).

Figure 2-60 Plane parallel plate. The light ray obeys the same laws at entry and exit; the result is lateral displacement without angular deviation. *(Illustration developed by Edmond H. Thall, MD, and Kevin M. Miller, MD, and rendered by C. H. Wooley.)*

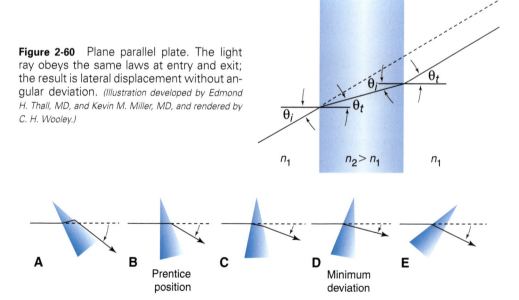

Figure 2-61 Variation of the angle of deviation depending on the angle of incidence. *(Illustration developed by Edmond H. Thall, MD, and Kevin M. Miller, MD, and rendered by C. H. Wooley.)*

The minimum angle of deviation produced by a prism occurs when the light ray undergoes equal bending at the 2 surfaces, as in Figure 2-61D. The angle of deviation is greater in any other situation.

Prism Diopter

Prism power defines the amount of light-ray deviation produced as the light ray traverses a prism. Prism power is the deviation, in centimeters, from the optical axis, measured 100 cm (1 m) from the prism (Fig 2-62). The amount is expressed in prism diopters (Δ).

The term *prism diopter* should never be shortened to "prisms" or "diopters" because the meanings of these terms are entirely different. For angles less than 100Δ ($45°$), each 2Δ is approximately equal to $1°$.

From Figure 2-62, it is apparent that the relationship between θ and Δ is

$$\tan\theta = \frac{\Delta}{100 \text{ cm}}$$

Therefore,

$$\Delta = 100\tan\theta$$

$$\theta = \arctan\frac{\Delta}{100}$$

Generally, the prisms that are used clinically to measure strabismus are plastic prisms. Prisms are calibrated for use in certain positions; if a prism is not used in the correct position, measurement errors may result. Plastic prisms and prism bars are calibrated according to the angle of minimum deviation. To approximate the angle of minimum deviation, the clinician should hold the plastic prism in the frontal plane position; in other words, the prism should be positioned so that its back surface is parallel to the facial plane of the patient (frontal plane) (Fig 2-63).

Prisms made of glass (not widely used) are calibrated according to the Prentice position—that is, with 1 face of the prism perpendicular to the direction in which the eye is directed. All of the bending occurs at the prism interfaces (see Fig 2-61B). If the rear surface of a 40Δ glass prism is erroneously held in the frontal plane, only 32Δ of effect will be achieved. This is the manner in which prism in spectacle lenses is measured on a lensmeter, with the back surface of the spectacle lens flat against the nose cone of the lensmeter.

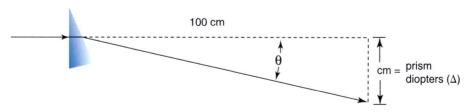

Figure 2-62 Definition of prism diopter. *(Illustration developed by Edmond H. Thall, MD, and Kevin M. Miller, MD, and rendered by C. H. Wooley.)*

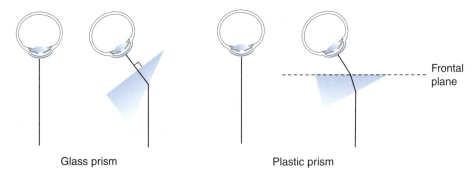

Glass prism   Plastic prism

Figure 2-63 Correct positions for holding glass and plastic orthoptic prisms. *(Illustration developed by Edmond H. Thall, MD, and Kevin M. Miller, MD, and rendered by C. H. Wooley.)*

Displacement of Images by Prisms

If a prism is introduced into the path of convergent light, all the light rays are bent toward the base of the prism, and the image is also displaced toward the base of the prism (Fig 2-64). In this case, the image is real, and real images are displaced toward the base of a prism.

If we turn the light around, making the image the object, and view the object through the prism, we will see a virtual image of the object. The object being viewed through the prism appears displaced toward the apex of the prism (Fig 2-65). In general, virtual images are displaced toward the apex of a prism, although the light rays themselves are

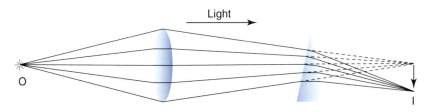

Figure 2-64 Real images displace toward the base of a prism. *(Illustration developed by Edmond H. Thall, MD, and Kevin M. Miller, MD, and rendered by C. H. Wooley.)*

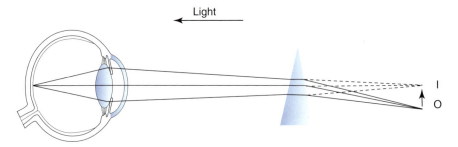

Figure 2-65 Virtual images displace toward the apex of a prism. *(Illustration developed by Edmond H. Thall, MD, and Kevin M. Miller, MD, and rendered by C. H. Wooley.)*

bent toward the base. The images we see when looking through prisms are always virtual images. This phenomenon is the source of the common teaching that a prism displaces images toward its apex.

Prismatic Effect of Lenses (the Prentice Rule)

A spherical lens behaves like a prism at every point on its surface except at its optical center. In plus lenses, the prism power bends light rays toward the optical axis. In minus lenses, the light bends away from the optical axis. Prism power increases as the distance from the optical center increases, in proportion to the dioptric power of the lens. This relationship is expressed mathematically by the Prentice rule (Fig 2-66). By similar triangles,

$$\frac{h}{\frac{100 \text{ cm}}{D}} = \frac{\Delta}{100 \text{ cm}}$$

$\Delta = hD$ (the Prentice rule)

where h is in centimeters.

The prismatic effect of lenses becomes clinically important in a patient with anisometropia. When the distance correction is different for the 2 eyes, prismatic effects occur. The patient usually notes these when in the reading position. With the eyes in downgaze, the prismatic effect of each lens differs and causes a different amount of image displacement in each eye. This leads to vertical diplopia if the image displacements are beyond the patient's fusion ability. Prismatic effects must be anticipated in the design of bifocal lenses to minimize image displacement and image jump (see Chapter 4, Clinical Refraction).

The clinician can induce prismatic effect in an ordinary spectacle lens simply by decentering the lens in the frame so that the visual axis in primary position does not pass through the optical center of the spectacle lens. The alternate method is grinding in prism. The power and size of the lens determine which method is used.

Remember that prism in a spectacle lens is read at the position of the visual axis in primary position. A washable felt-tip marker is helpful in marking this position before the glasses are transferred from the patient's face to the lensmeter.

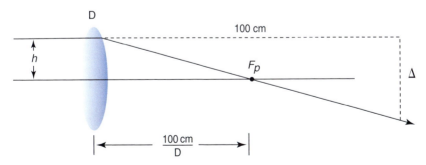

Figure 2-66 The Prentice rule. The prism power of a lens at any point on its surface, in prism diopters, Δ, is equal to the distance away from the optical center, h, in centimeters times the power of the lens in diopters. *(Illustration developed by Kevin M. Miller, MD, and rendered by C. H. Wooley.)*

Vector Addition of Prisms

Prismatic deviations in different directions are additive by straightforward vector addition. Vectors combine information about magnitude and direction. For instance, if 6Δ base up (BU) and 8Δ base out (BO) before the left eye are needed to correct a strabismic deviation, a single prism of 10Δ with base up and out in the 37° meridian accomplishes the same purpose (Fig 2-67).

When prescribing an oblique prism, remember to specify the direction of the base properly. A prism before the left eye cannot simply be specified as "base in, in the 37° meridian." It must be specified as either "base up and out in the 37° meridian" or "base down and in, in the 37° meridian."

A rotary prism (Risley prism), mounted on the front of most phoropters, consists of 2 prisms of equal power that are counter-rotated with respect to one another to produce prism power varying from 0 (prisms neutralize each other) to the sum of the 2 powers (prisms aligned in the same direction). Intermediate values may be determined by vector addition and are marked on the dial of the prism housing. The Risley prism is particularly useful in measuring phorias (often in conjunction with the Maddox rod) and fusional vergence amplitudes.

Prism Aberrations

Chromatic aberration produces colored fringes at the edges of objects viewed through prisms and can be bothersome to patients. Prisms have other aberrations, such as asymmetrical magnification and curvature of field. Although these aberrations are usually insignificant, they occasionally produce symptoms, even with low-power ophthalmic prisms.

Fresnel Prisms

A Fresnel (pronounced *fre-nell'*) prism is a series of small side-by-side prisms that act as a single large prism (Fig 2-68). It is typically used to avoid the weight and some of the aberrations of conventional prisms.

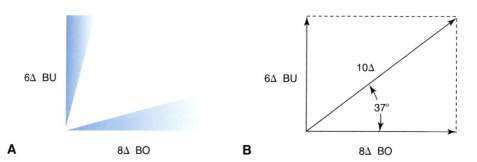

Figure 2-67   Vector addition of horizontal and vertical prisms. **A,** The magnitude of the sum vector is $\sqrt{8^2 + 6^2}$. **B,** The angle of the sum vector is arctan (6/8). *BU* = base up; *BO* = base out.

(Illustration developed by Kevin M. Miller, MD, and rendered by C. H. Wooley.)

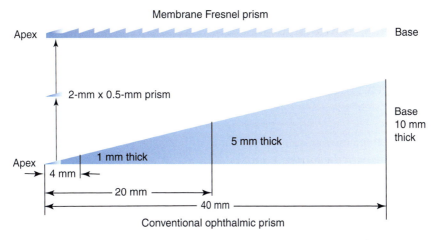

Figure 2-68 Cross-sectional construction of a Fresnel prism as compared to a conventional ophthalmic prism. *(Redrawn from Duane TD, ed.* Clinical Ophthalmology. *Hagerstown, MD: Harper & Row; 1976: vol 1, chap 52, fig 52-2.)*

The most popular form of Fresnel prism is a membrane molded from clear polyvinyl chloride. Known as a Press-On prism (3M, St Paul, MN), it is applied with water to the back surface of an ordinary spectacle lens. Press-On prisms are available in a variety of powers. Visual acuity is reduced because of light scattering at the groove edges, but the chromatic aberration of the prisms themselves produces most of the visual decrement. The advantages of these prisms far outweigh the disadvantages, and they are widely used in the fields of strabismus and orthoptics. Because of their ease of application and lower expense, Press-On prisms are especially useful for patients whose strabismus is changing (eg, patients with thyroid eye disease). Fresnel lenses are also available with concentric groove construction to approximate spherical lenses.

Mirrors

As discussed earlier in this chapter (under the section Imaging With Lenses and Mirrors), many of the vergence and ray-tracing concepts we developed for lenses also apply to mirrors. In the following pages, we consider some points specific to mirrors.

Reflecting Power

We can define the reflecting power of mirrors in the same way we define the refracting power of lenses: by the amount of vergence produced by the mirror.

- Convex mirrors add negative vergence (like minus lenses).
- Concave mirrors add positive vergence (like plus lenses).
- Plane mirrors add no vergence.

The focal length of a mirror in meters is equal to the reciprocal of the power of the mirror in diopters, and vice versa:

$$P_m = \frac{1}{f}$$

where

P_m = reflecting power of a mirror in diopters
f = focal length of the mirror in meters

Mirrors are often specified, however, not by focal length, but by radius of curvature. Because refractive index does not apply to reflective surfaces, the relationship between radius of curvature r and focal length is simple:

$$f = \frac{r}{2}$$

The focal length is half the radius of curvature. Therefore,

$$P_m = \frac{2}{r}$$

Reversal of Image Space

The basic vergence relationship, $U + P = V$, can be applied directly to mirrors if one remembers that the mirror reverses the image space. The incoming side of the mirror is the same as the outgoing side. If the incoming light rays are traveling from left to right, they will travel from right to left upon reflection. In this case, converging image rays (plus vergence) form a real image to the left of the mirror, and diverging image rays (minus vergence) appear to come from a virtual image to the right of the mirror.

Central Ray for Mirrors

The central ray for mirrors (Fig 2-69) is just as useful as the central ray for lenses, because if image location is determined by vergence calculation, the central ray immediately indicates the orientation and size of the image. Note that, in using the ratio of image distance to object distance to calculate the size of the image, the image and object distances are measured either from the center of curvature of the mirror or from the surface of the mirror.

Vergence Calculations

Because a *plane mirror* adds no vergence to light but simply reverses its direction, vergence does not change when light is reflected.

For example, light from an object 1 m to the left of a plane mirror has a vergence of –1 D at the mirror. On reflection, the vergence will still be –1 D; however, in tracing imaginary extensions of the reflected image rays to the far side of the mirror (into virtual image space), the virtual image is located 1 m to the right of the mirror.

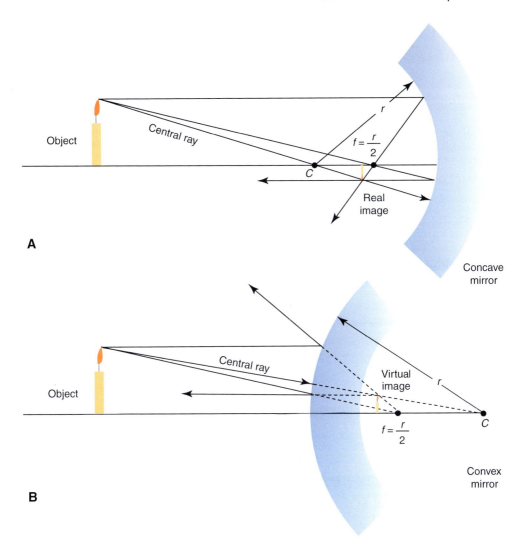

Figure 2-69 Ray tracing for concave **(A)** and convex **(B)** mirrors. The central ray for mirrors is different from the central ray for lenses in that it passes through the center of curvature of the mirror, not through the center of the mirror. *(Illustration developed by Kevin M. Miller, MD, and rendered by C. H. Wooley.)*

In general, plane mirrors create upright virtual images from real objects, with the virtual image located as far behind the mirror as the real image is in front. As illustrated in Figure 2-70, only half a full-length plane mirror is needed to see one's entire body.

A *concave mirror* (eg, makeup mirror, shaving mirror, or the internal limiting membrane of the fovea) adds positive vergence to incident light. It therefore has positive, or converging, power. If parallel rays strike the mirror, they reflect and converge toward a point halfway to the center of curvature. The focal point *F* of a concave mirror is not unique, for any central ray can serve as an optical axis. The anterior and posterior focal points of a concave mirror are in exactly the same place.

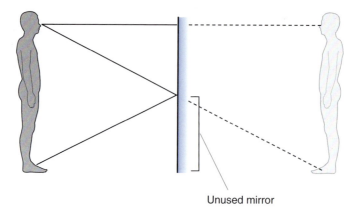

Figure 2-70 Using a half-length mirror for a full-length view. *(Illustration developed by Edmond H. Thall, MD, and Kevin M. Miller, MD, and rendered by C. H. Wooley.)*

As an example, consider an object 1 m to the left of a concave mirror with a radius of curvature of 50 cm. Where is the image?

The power of the mirror is equal to $1/f$, where $f = (r/2)$.

$$f = \frac{r}{2} = \frac{0.5}{2} = 0.25 \text{ m}$$

$$P_m = \frac{1}{f} = \frac{1}{0.25 \text{ m}} = +4 \text{ D}$$

$$U + P_m = V$$

$$-1 \text{ D} + (+4 \text{ D}) = +3 \text{ D}$$

$$\text{Transverse magnification} = \frac{U}{V} = \frac{-1 \text{ D}}{3 \text{ D}} = -0.33$$

Therefore, the image is located ⅓ m (33 cm) to the left of the mirror, in real image space. It is also minified and inverted.

A *convex mirror* adds negative vergence to incident light. It therefore has negative, or diverging, power. The anterior and posterior focal points, which coincide, are virtual focal points located halfway between the surface of the mirror and the center of curvature.

If the preceding example used a convex, rather than a concave, mirror with the same radius of curvature, the power of the mirror would be –4 D.

$$U + P_m = V$$

$$-1 \text{ D} + (-4 \text{ D}) = -5 \text{ D}$$

$$\text{Transverse magnification} = \frac{U}{V} = \frac{-1 \text{ D}}{-5 \text{ D}} = +0.20$$

In this case, the image rays are diverging, and a virtual image will appear to be located 20 cm to the right of the mirror. The image is minified and erect.

Optical Aberrations

In paraxial optics, the focus is essentially stigmatic. Peripheral or nonparaxial rays do not necessarily focus stigmatically. Deviations from stigmatic imaging are called *aberrations*. Aberrations are divided into monochromatic and chromatic forms. The 2 most common monochromatic aberrations are defocus (myopic and hyperopic spherical errors) and regular astigmatism. The clinical application of wavefront aberrometry makes it possible to measure *higher-order aberrations,* which were previously lumped into a catchall term—*irregular astigmatism.* Examples of higher-order aberrations include coma, spherical aberration, and trefoil. Spherical aberration is a particularly relevant higher-order aberration in keratorefractive surgery.

Regular Astigmatism

Unlike the spherical lens surface, the *astigmatic lens* surface does not have the same curvature and refracting power in all meridians. The curvature of an astigmatic lens varies from a minimum value to a maximum value, with the extreme values located in meridians 90° apart. Thus, the refracting power varies from one meridian to the next, and an astigmatic surface does not have a single point of focus. Instead, 2 focal lines are formed. The complicated geometric envelope of a pencil of light rays emanating from a single point source and refracted by a spherocylindrical lens is called the *conoid of Sturm* (Fig 2-71).

The conoid of Sturm has 2 focal lines, each parallel to one of the principal meridians of the spherocylindrical lens. All the rays in the pencil pass through each of the focal lines. The cross sections of the conoid of Sturm vary in shape and area along its length but are generally elliptical. At the dioptric mean of the focal lines, there is a cross section of the conoid of Sturm that is circular. This circular patch of light rays is called the *circle of least*

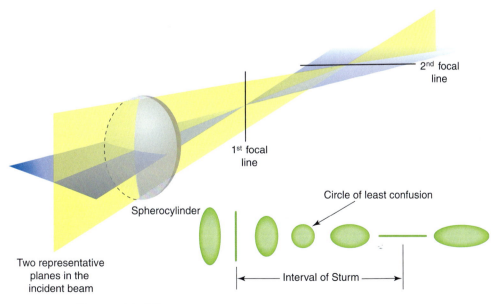

Figure 2-71 The conoid of Sturm. *(Illustration developed by Kevin M. Miller, MD, and rendered by Jonathan Clark.)*

confusion; it represents the best overall focus of the spherocylindrical lens. The circle of least confusion occupies the position where all the rays would be brought to focus if the lens had a spherical power equal to the average spherical power of all the meridians of the spherocylindrical lens. This average spherical power of a spherocylindrical lens is called the *spherical equivalent* of the lens. It is calculated by the following relationship:

$$\text{Spherical equivalent (D)} = \text{sphere (D)} + \frac{\text{cylinder (D)}}{2}$$

Although the cross section of each pencil of rays forming the conoid of Sturm is relatively easy to appreciate, the images produced by spherocylindrical lenses of extended objects, which are composed of an infinite number of pencils of light, are of somewhat different configuration (Fig 2-72).

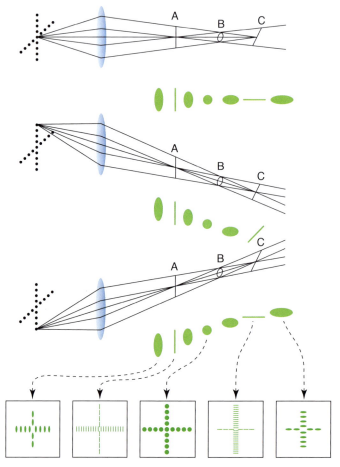

Figure 2-72 Images of an extended object (a cross) formed by a spherocylindrical lens at various distances from the lens. A line of the cross will appear clear only if the image is observed in the focal plane of one of the focal lines of the conoid of Sturm and, furthermore, only if the line is parallel with that particular focal line. *(Modified from Michaels DD.* Visual Optics and Refraction. *2nd ed. St Louis: Mosby; 1980: p 60; fig 2-37.)*

When calculating object and image relationships for spherocylindrical lenses, we must treat each principal meridian separately, applying the basic vergence relationship or graphical analysis. Once image positions are determined by these methods, we return to the 3-dimensional conoid of Sturm to understand the cross-sectional configurations of the pencils or beams of light that are intercepted (ie, by the retina of the eye) at various positions.

The simplest form of astigmatic lens is a *planocylindrical* lens, either plus or minus, as shown in Figure 2-73. The Maddox rod is an example of a high-power, clinically useful cylindrical lens (Fig 2-74).

The general form of an astigmatic surface is a *spherocylinder,* or torus, which might be likened to the surface of a curved barrel or American football (Fig 2-75). The meridians

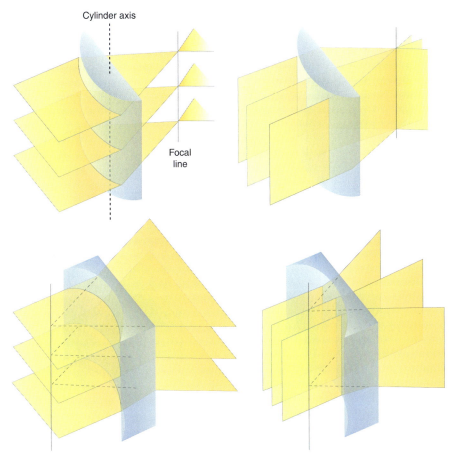

Figure 2-73 Image formation by plus and minus planocylinders. Each lens has maximum power in the horizontal meridian (perpendicular to the axis of the cylinder, which is in the vertical meridian) and no power in the vertical meridian. Light rays are bent only in the horizontal direction in passing through the lenses, forming vertical focal lines (a real focal line in the case of the plus cylinder and a virtual focal line in the case of the minus cylinder). The focal lines formed by planocylinders are always parallel to their axes. *(Illustration developed by Kevin M. Miller, MD, and rendered by Jonathan Clark.)*

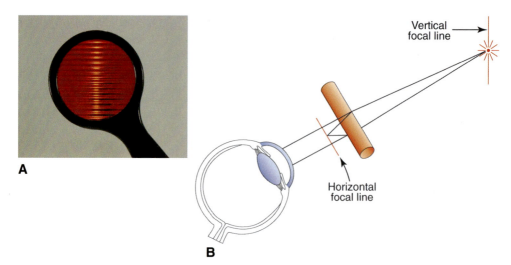

Figure 2-74 The Maddox rod. **A,** This high-power cylindrical lens is used clinically to form a line image from a point source of light. **B,** The real focal line produced by a Maddox rod is formed so close to the rod and so close to the patient's eye that the patient cannot focus on it. However, every astigmatic lens produces 2 focal lines perpendicular to each other; in the case of the Maddox rod, the second focal line is a virtual focal line passing through the point light source. *(Photograph courtesy of Kevin M. Miller, MD. Illustration developed by Kevin M. Miller, MD, and rendered by C. H. Wooley.)*

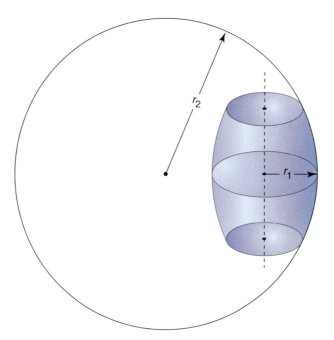

Figure 2-75 Toric surfaces having major and minor radii of curvature. *(Illustration developed by Kevin M. Miller, MD, and rendered by Jonathan Clark.)*

of greatest and least curvature—and therefore the meridians of greatest and least power of an astigmatic lens—are known as the *principal meridians* of that surface or lens. Although a spherocylindrical lens may be thought of as the combination of 2 planocylinders, it is more convenient to think of it as the combination of a spherical lens and a cylindrical lens. The orientation of the cylindrical lens is specified by the axis position according to conventional notation (Fig 2-76). The 0° meridian is the same as the 180° meridian, and the 180° notation is always used for this meridian.

The powers in the principal meridians and the cylinder axis of spherocylindrical lenses may be specified in several ways. The common graphical method is called the *power cross*. A cross is drawn oriented in the principal meridians, and each arm of the cross is labeled with the power acting in that meridian (Fig 2-77). The most common written notation specifies a sphere power, a cylinder power, and the axis of the cylinder. The following examples of spherocylindrical expression are entirely equivalent. Remember that the maximum power of a cylinder is in the meridian 90° away from the axis of the cylinder. To avoid errors in transcription and lens manufacture, it is helpful to notate the axis using all 3 digits and dropping the ° notation.

> Combined cylinder form: +1.00 × 180 +4.00 × 090
> Plus cylinder form: +1.00 +3.00 × 090
> Minus cylinder form: +4.00 –3.00 × 180

The spherical equivalent power of this lens is (+1 D + 4 D)/2 = +2.50 D. (See Clinical Example 2-8.)

Transposition

Sometimes we need to be able to transpose the notation for a spherocylindrical lens from plus cylinder form to minus cylinder form and vice versa. The 2 forms are different ways

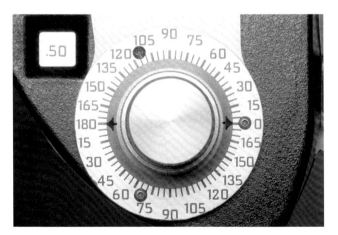

Figure 2-76 Meridian convention for specification of cylinder axis, the so-called *TABO* convention, named after the optical committee that adopted it in 1917. *(Courtesy of Kevin M. Miller, MD.)*

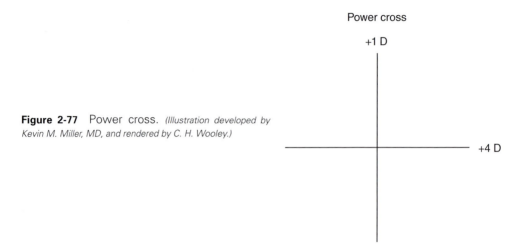

Figure 2-77 Power cross. *(Illustration developed by Kevin M. Miller, MD, and rendered by C. H. Wooley.)*

CLINICAL EXAMPLE 2-8

Imagine you have just performed streak retinoscopy on 1 eye of a child, using a rack of spherical lenses. The child was under general anesthesia and received cyclopentolate cycloplegia. When neutrality is achieved, the retinoscope neutralizes the power in the meridian that is perpendicular to the axis of the light streak. Stated differently, the axis of the light from the retinoscope is aligned with the plus axis of the required plus-power correcting cylinder. A +5 D sphere neutralizes the retinoscopic reflex when the axis of the streak is at the 175° meridian. A +3 D sphere neutralizes the reflex when the axis is at the 85° meridian. Assuming a working distance of 67 cm, what is the appropriate refractive correction for this child's eye?

Subtracting the working distance equivalent of 1.5 D from each measurement, we construct a power cross (Fig 2-78). The power cross may be separated into spherical and cylindrical components, if necessary. Remember that the +2.00 D power acting in the 85° meridian has its axis in the 175° meridian. The equivalent lens in spherocylindrical notation is +1.50 +2.00 × 175.

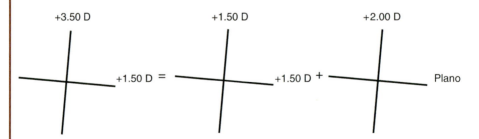

Figure 2-78 A power cross is separated into spherical and cylindrical components. *(Illustration developed by Kevin M. Miller, MD, and rendered by C. H. Wooley.)*

of specifying the same lens. One method of transposing is to convert the first cylinder form to the power cross notation and then convert the power cross notation to the second cylinder form. However, a simpler method is more frequently used. To convert a prescription from plus to minus cylinder form and vice versa:

- Add the sphere and cylinder powers together to obtain the new sphere.
- Change the sign of the cylinder to obtain the new cylinder.
- Rotate the axis 90° to obtain the new axis.

Combining Spherocylindrical Lenses

Spherocylindrical lenses can be added to one another to produce a single equivalent spherocylindrical lens. In fact, if any number of spherocylindrical lenses are combined, the result is always an equivalent spherocylindrical lens having principal meridians 90° apart. Similarly, a single spherocylindrical lens may be resolved into any number of component spherocylindrical lenses, provided that certain trigonometric rules are followed.

It is easy to add spherocylindrical lenses together if the principal meridians are aligned with one another. In this simple scenario, the principal meridians of the resultant lens are the same as those of the components. Combining 2 spherical lenses (placed close together) yields the algebraic sum of the lens powers. Combining cylinders at the same axis is just as simple and yields a resultant cylinder power that is just the algebraic sum of the cylinder powers; the axis remains unchanged. For cylinders separated by 90°, the situation is also straightforward. One of the cylinders is transformed into a cylinder with the opposite sign and located at the same axis as the other cylinder. Then the cylinders are added algebraically.

Combining Cylinders at Oblique Axes

It is more difficult to add spherocylindrical lenses when the principal meridians are not aligned with one another. A simple way of doing it is to read the power of the lens combination with a lensmeter.

Because cylinders have a power and axis, it might seem that cylinders could be treated as vectors and that the procedure for combining cylinders would be the procedure for combining vectors. Unfortunately, this is not entirely correct. Consider that a +1.00 cylinder at axis 180 is the same as a +1.00 cylinder at axis 0. If we add the vectors that correspond to these 2 angles, we get 0, and it is clear that if we add the 2 cylinders, we get +2.00 at either axis 0 or, equivalently, axis 180. Thus, cylinders cannot be treated as vectors for the purpose of combination. Calculating a combination of cylinders at oblique axes is complicated. Fortunately, computer programs are now available to facilitate these calculations.

Spherical Aberration

Spherical aberration causes night myopia and, in some cases, fluctuating vision following keratorefractive surgery. Although a spherical surface focuses rays stigmatically in the paraxial region (according to the LME), rays outside that region do not focus to a point.

For a positive spherical surface, the farther a ray is from the axis, the more anterior its focus (see Fig 2-33).

Spherical aberration has 2 effects. First, image quality (or visual acuity) decreases because the focus is not stigmatic. Second, the image location is changed from the position predicted by the LME and vergence equations. Roughly speaking, the best focus is achieved where the rays are confined to the smallest area. In the human eye, spherical aberration shifts the focus anteriorly, making the patient slightly more myopic than would be expected from vergence calculations.

Spherical aberration exacerbates myopia in low light (night myopia). In brighter conditions, the pupil constricts, blocking the more peripheral rays and minimizing the effect of spherical aberration. As the pupil enlarges, more peripheral rays enter the eye and the focus shifts anteriorly, making the patient slightly more myopic in low-light conditions. Typically, the amount of myopic shift is about 0.50 D. In addition, because of dark adaptation, the retinal rods become more sensitive to the shorter (blue) wavelengths of light, which are focused more anteriorly, contributing further to night myopia.

Spherical aberration accounts for some cases of fluctuating vision following keratorefractive surgery. Normally, the cornea is flatter peripherally than centrally, which decreases spherical aberration. Radial keratotomy makes the cornea more spherical, increasing spherical aberration. Laser in situ keratomileusis (LASIK) and photorefractive keratectomy (PRK) can make the central cornea flatter than the peripheral cornea. In general, the effect of spherical aberration increases as the fourth power of the pupil diameter. Doubling pupil diameter increases spherical aberration 16 times. Thus, a small change in pupil size can cause a significant change in refraction. This possibility should be considered in patients who have fluctuating vision despite stable K readings and well-healed corneas following keratorefractive surgery. (See Clinical Example 2-9.)

Chromatic Aberration

Thus far in our analysis of aberrations we have ignored the effect of wavelength. Ophthalmic lenses and the human eye are often treated as though they focus all wavelengths identically,

CLINICAL EXAMPLE 2-9

Following LASIK, what causes a patient to see halos when viewing distant lights at night?

This problem is typically encountered when a high correction is performed and a small optical zone results. If a pupil remains small enough to allow only light that has been refracted by the treated cornea to reach the fovea, the image will be relatively stigmatic (Fig 2-79A). If, however, the pupil opens widely under scotopic conditions, light refracted by the untreated peripheral cornea will enter the eye and form a myopic defocus on the retina. This defocused light, an effect of surgically induced spherical aberration, will be perceived as a halo (Fig 2-79B).

Small pupil

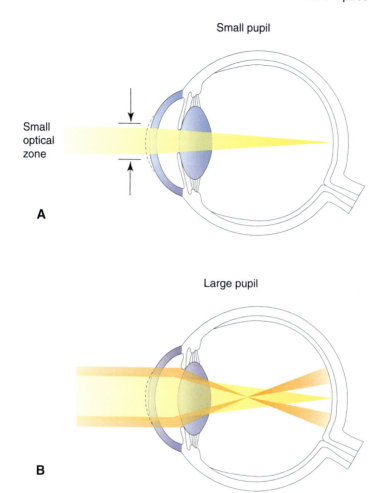

Large pupil

Figure 2-79 **A,** If the treated optical zone is larger than the entrance pupil, the image focuses stigmatically. **B,** If the optical zone is smaller than the entrance pupil, light refracting through the untreated peripheral cornea will cause spherical aberration. A patient viewing a distance point light source will see halos around the light. *(Illustration developed by Kevin M. Miller, MD, and rendered by C. H. Wooley.)*

but this is not true. Most lenses introduce dispersion. Dispersion in the human eye causes *chromatic aberration,* in which blue light focuses in front of red light (Fig 2-80).

The difference between the blue and red foci is about 0.5 D in the average eye, but may be much greater. Even if all monochromatic aberrations could be compensated for or eliminated by contact lenses or refractive surgery, chromatic aberration and diffraction would still limit the optical resolving power of the eye.

Chromatic compensation is common in microscope, telescope, and camera lenses but is not yet available in spectacle, contact, or intraocular lenses. Blue-blocking, red-blocking,

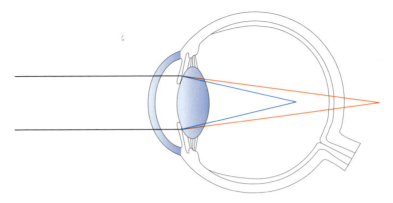

Figure 2-80 Chromatic aberration in the human eye. *(Illustration developed by Kevin M. Miller, MD, and rendered by C. H. Wooley.)*

and other colored sunglasses improve visual acuity by decreasing chromatic aberration. They do so, however, at the cost of reducing the color content of the perceived image.

CHAPTER 3

Optics of the Human Eye

The Human Eye as an Optical System

The eye obeys many of the same principles as optical instruments. This chapter presents conceptual tools ("schematic eyes") that were developed to help us understand the inner workings of the eye's optics. In addition, it covers the various methods used to measure the eye's ability to "see" and reviews the types of refractive errors of the eye. Treatment of refractive errors is covered in Chapter 4.

Schematic Eyes

The major challenges to understanding the optics of the human eye lie in the complexity of some of the eye's optical elements and in their "imperfections" as compared to mathematical ideals. Simplifications and approximations make models easier to understand but detract from their ability to explain all the complexities and subtleties of the inner workings of the eye's optical system. As an example, the anterior surface of the cornea is assumed to be spherical, but the actual anterior surface tends to flatten toward the limbus. Also, the center of the crystalline lens is usually decentered with respect to the cornea and the visual axis of the eye.

Many mathematical models of the eye's optical system are based on careful anatomical measurements and approximations. The model developed by Gullstrand (Fig 3-1, Table 3-1), a Swedish professor of ophthalmology, so closely approximated the human eye that he was awarded a Nobel Prize in 1911. As useful as this model is, it is cumbersome for certain clinical calculations and can be simplified further. Because the principal points of the cornea and lens are fairly close to each other, a single intermediate point can substitute for them. In a similar fashion, the nodal points of the cornea and lens can be combined into a single nodal point for the eye. Thus, we can treat the eye as if it were a single refracting element, an ideal spherical surface separating 2 media of different refractive indices: 1.000 for air and 1.333 for the eye (Fig 3-2). This is known as the *reduced schematic eye.*

Using this reduced schematic eye, we can calculate the retinal image size of an object in space (such as a Snellen letter). This calculation utilizes the simplified nodal point, through which light rays entering or leaving the eye pass undeviated. The geometric principle of similar triangles can be used for the calculation of retinal image size if the following information is given: (1) the actual height of a Snellen letter on the eye chart, (2) the

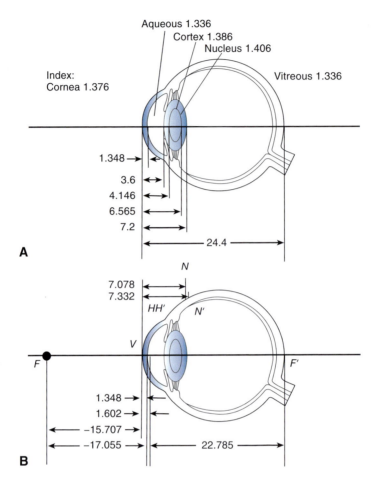

Figure 3-1 Optical constants of Gullstrand's schematic eye. All values in millimeters. **A,** Refractive indices of the media and positions of the refracting surfaces. **B,** Positions of the cardinal points, which are used for optical calculations. *(Illustration by C. H. Wooley.)*

distance from the eye chart to the eye, and (3) the distance from the nodal point to the retina (assumed to be 17 mm). The formula for this calculation is as follows:

$$\frac{\text{Retinal image height}}{\text{Snellen letter height}} = \frac{\text{nodal point to retina distance}}{\text{chart to eye distance}}$$

Although the distance from the eye chart to the nodal point should be measured, it is much easier to measure the distance to the surface of the cornea. The difference between these measurements is 5.6 mm, which is usually insignificant. As an example, if the distance between the nodal point and the retina is 17 mm, the distance between the eye chart and the eye is 20 ft (6000 mm), and the height of a Snellen letter is 60 mm, the resulting image size on the retina is 0.17 mm.

Katz M, Kruger PB. The human eye as an optical system. In: Tasman W, Jaeger EA, eds. *Duane's Clinical Ophthalmology.* Philadelphia: Lippincott Williams & Wilkins; 2003.

Table 3-1 The Schematic Eye

	Accommodation Relaxed	Maximum Accommodation
Refractive index		
Cornea	1.376	1.376
Aqueous humor and vitreous body	1.336	1.336
Lens	1.386	1.386
Equivalent core lens	1.406	1.406
Position		
Anterior surface of cornea	0	0
Posterior surface of cornea	0.5	0.5
Anterior surface of lens	3.6	3.2
Anterior surface of equiv. core lens	4.146	3.8725
Posterior surface of equiv. core lens	6.565	6.5275
Posterior surface of lens	7.2	7.2
Radius of curvature		
Anterior surface of cornea	7.7	7.7
Posterior surface of cornea	6.8	6.8
Equivalent surface of cornea		
Anterior surface of lens	10.0	5.33
Anterior surface of equiv. core lens	7.911	2.655
Posterior surface of equiv. core lens	−5.76	−2.655
Posterior surface of lens	−6.0	−5.33
Refracting power		
Anterior surface of cornea	48.83	48.83
Posterior surface of cornea	−5.88	−5.88
Equivalent surface of cornea		
Anterior surface of lens	5.0	9.375
Core lens	5.985	14.96
Posterior surface of lens	8.33	9.375
Corneal system		
Refracting power	43.05	43.05
Position of first principal point	−0.0496	−0.0496
Position of second principal point	−0.0506	−0.0506
First focal length	−23.227	−23.227
Second focal length	31.031	31.031
Lens system		
Refracting power	19.11	33.06
Position of first principal point	5.678	5.145
Position of second principal point	5.808	5.255
Focal length	69.908	40.416
Complete optical system of eye		
Refracting power	58.64	70.57
Position of first principal point, H	1.348	1.772
Position of second principal point, H'	1.602	2.086
Position of first focal point, F	−15.707	−12.397
Position of second focal point, F'	24.387	21.016
First focal length	−17.055	−14.169
Second focal length	22.785	18.930
Position of first nodal point, N	7.078	
Position of second nodal point, N'	7.332	
Position of fovea centralis	24.0	24.0
Axial refraction	−1.0	−9.6
Position of near point		−102.3

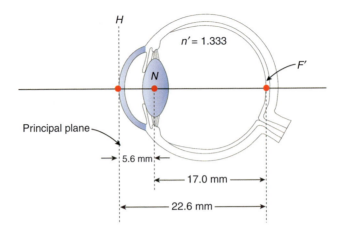

Figure 3-2 Dimensions of the reduced schematic eye, defined by the anterior corneal surface (H), the simplified nodal point of the eye (N), and the fovea (F'). The distance from the simplified nodal point to the fovea is 17.0 mm, and the distance from the anterior corneal surface to the nodal point is 5.6 mm. The refractive index for air is taken to be 1.000, and the simplified refractive index for the eye (n') is 1.333. The refractive power of this reduced schematic eye is 60 D, with its principal plane at the front surface of the cornea. *(Illustration by C. H. Wooley.)*

Important Axes of the Eye

Following are some important definitions of terms used to describe the axes of the eye:

Angle alpha (α)   The angle between the optical axis and the visual axis. This is considered positive when the visual axis in object space lies on the nasal side of the optical axis.

Angle kappa (κ)   The angle between the pupillary axis and the visual axis (Fig 3-3).

Optical axis   The line that best approximates the line passing through the optical centers of the cornea, lens, and fovea. Because the lens is usually decentered with respect to the cornea and the visual axis, no single line can precisely pass through each of these points. However, because the amount of decentration is small, the best approximation of this line is taken to be the optical axis.

Principal line of vision   The line passing through the fixation point, perpendicular to the corneal surface.

Pupillary axis   The imaginary line perpendicular to the corneal surface and passing through the midpoint of the entrance pupil.

Visual axis   The line connecting the fixation point and the fovea.

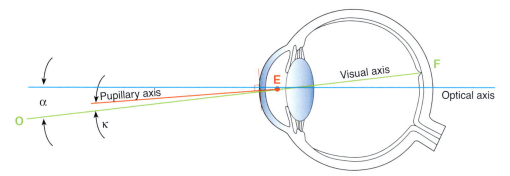

Figure 3-3 Angle kappa (κ). The pupillary axis *(red line)* is represented schematically as the line perpendicular to the corneal surface and passing through the midpoint of the entrance pupil *(E)*. The visual axis *(green line)* is defined as the line connecting the fixation point *(O)* and the fovea *(F)*. If all the optical elements of the human eye were in perfect alignment, these 2 lines would overlap. However, the fovea is normally displaced from its expected position. The angle between the pupillary axis and the visual axis is called *angle kappa (κ)* and is considered positive when the fovea is located temporally and downward from the expected position, as is the usual case. Angle alpha (α) is the angle between the optical axis and the visual axis of the eye and is considered positive when the visual axis in object space lies on the nasal side of the optical axis, as is normally the case. *(Courtesy of Neal H. Atebara, MD. Redrawn by C. H. Wooley.)*

Pupil Size and Its Effect on Visual Resolution

The size of the blur circle on the retina generally increases as the size of the pupil increases. If a pinhole aperture is placed immediately in front of an eye, it acts as an artificial pupil, and the size of the blur circle is reduced correspondingly (Fig 3-4; Clinical Problems 3-1).

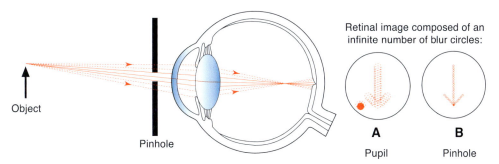

Figure 3-4 Light rays from each point on an object *(the upright arrow)* form a blur circle on the retina of a myopic eye. The retinal image is the composite of all blur circles, the size of each being proportional to the diameter of the pupil *(A)* and the amount of defocus. If a pinhole is held in front of the eye, the size of each blur circle is decreased; as a result, the overall retinal image is sharpened *(B)*. *(Courtesy of Neal H. Atebara, MD. Redrawn by C. H. Wooley.)*

CLINICAL PROBLEMS 3-1

Why do persons with uncorrected myopia squint?
To obtain a pinhole effect (or rather a stenopeic slit effect). Better visual acuity results from smaller blur circles (or even smaller blur "slits").

Does pupil size affect the measured near point of accommodation?
Yes. With smaller pupil size, the eye's depth of focus increases, and objects closer than the actual near point of the eye remain in better focus.

Why are patients less likely to need their glasses in bright light?
One reason is that the bright light causes the pupil to constrict, allowing the defocused image to be less blurred on the retina. Another is that bright light increases contrast.

The pinhole is used clinically to measure *pinhole visual acuity.* If visual acuity improves when measured through a pinhole aperture, a refractive error is usually present. The most useful pinhole diameter for general clinical purposes (refractive errors from –5 D to +5 D) is 1.2 mm. If the pinhole aperture is made smaller, the blurring effects of diffraction around the edges of the aperture overwhelm the image-sharpening effects of the small pupil. For errors greater than 5 D, one needs to use, in addition to the pinhole, a lens that corrects most of the refractive error.

The pinhole can also be used with a dilated pupil, after the best refractive correction has been determined. If visual acuity improves, optical irregularities such as corneal and lenticular light scattering or irregular astigmatism are likely to be present, with the pinhole restricting light to a relatively normal area of the eye's optics. (This technique also can be used to identify optical causes of *monocular diplopia.*) If visual acuity is worse, macular disease must be considered, as a diseased macula is often unable to adapt to the reduced amount of light entering through the pinhole.

Because of the refractive effects of the cornea, the image of the pupil, as viewed by the clinician, is about 13% larger than the actual pupil and is called the *entrance pupil.*

Visual Acuity

Clinicians often think of visual acuity primarily in terms of Snellen acuity, but visual perception is a far more complex process than is implied by this simple measuring system. Indeed, there are a multitude of ways to measure visual function. Following are definitions of terms used in the measurement of visual function:

- A patient's ability to recognize progressively smaller letters or forms is called the *minimum legible threshold,* of which Snellen acuity is the most common method.
- Measurement of the minimum brightness of a target so that the target may be distinguished from its background is called the *minimum visible threshold.*
- The smallest visual angle at which 2 separate objects can be discriminated is called the *minimum separable threshold.*

- The smallest detectable amount of misalignment of 2 line segments is called *Vernier acuity.*

Snellen acuity is measured with test letters (optotypes) constructed so that the letter as a whole subtends an angle of *5 minutes of arc,* whereas each stroke of the letter subtends 1 arc minute (arcmin). Letters of different sizes are designated by the distance at which the letter subtends an angle of 5 arcmin (Fig 3-5). The Snellen chart is designed to measure visual acuity in angular terms. However, the accepted convention does not specify acuity in angular measure but uses a notation in which the numerator is the *testing distance* (in feet or meters), and the denominator is the *distance at which a letter subtends the standard visual angle of 5 arcmin.* Thus, on the 20/20 line (6/6 in meters), the letters subtend an angle of 5 arcmin when viewed at 20 ft. On the 20/40 line (6/12), the letters subtend an angle of 10 arcmin when viewed at 20 ft or 5 arcmin when viewed at 40 ft. Conversions from the Snellen fraction to the *minimum angle of resolution* or *recognition* (MAR) and the *base-10 logarithm of the minimum angle of resolution* or *recognition* (logMAR) are shown in Table 3-2. For determining a mean of Snellen visual acuity in a series, logMAR is useful.

The standard Snellen eye chart, though widely accepted, is not perfect. The letters on different Snellen lines are not related to one another by size in any geometric or logarithmic sense. For example, the increase in letter size going from the 20/20 line to the 20/25 line is different from that going from the 20/25 line to the 20/30 line. In addition, certain

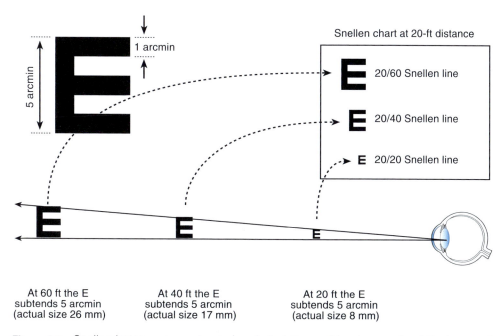

At 60 ft the E subtends 5 arcmin (actual size 26 mm)

At 40 ft the E subtends 5 arcmin (actual size 17 mm)

At 20 ft the E subtends 5 arcmin (actual size 8 mm)

Figure 3-5 Snellen letters are constructed such that they subtend an angle of 5 minutes of arc when located at the distance specified by the denominator. For example, if a Snellen E is 26 mm in height, it subtends 5 arcmin at 60 ft. Correspondingly, a 26-mm letter occupies the 20/60 line of the Snellen chart at the standard testing distance of 20 ft. *(Courtesy of Neal H. Atebara, MD. Redrawn by C. H. Wooley.)*

Table 3-2 Visual Acuity Conversion Chart

Feet	Snellen Fraction Meters	4-Meter Standard	Minimum Angle of Resolution	LogMAR	Decimal Notation
20/10	6/3	4/2	0.50	−0.30	2.00
20/15	6/4.5	4/3	0.75	−0.10	1.50
20/20	6/6	4/4	1.00	0.00	1.00
20/25	6/7.5	4/5	1.25	0.10	0.80
20/30	6/9	4/6	1.50	0.18	0.70
20/40	6/12	4/8	2.00	0.30	0.50
20/50	6/15	4/10	2.50	0.40	0.40
20/60	6/18	4/12	3.00	0.48	0.30
20/80	6/24	4/16	4.00	0.60	0.25
20/100	6/30	4/20	5.00	0.70	0.20
20/120	6/36	4/24	6.00	0.80	
20/150	6/45	4/32	7.50	0.88	0.13
20/200	6/60	4/40	10.00	1.00	0.10
20/400	6/120	4/80	20.00	1.30	0.05

letters (such as C, D, O, and G) are inherently harder to recognize than others (such as A and J) because there are more letters of the alphabet with which they can be confused. For these reasons, alternative visual acuity charts have been developed and popularized in clinical trials (eg, ETDRS, Bailey-Lovie) (Fig 3-6). Computer-based acuity devices that display optotypes on a monitor screen have also become popular because they allow presentation of a random assortment of optotypes and scrambling of letters and eliminate problems with memorization seen in patients who visit the office frequently.

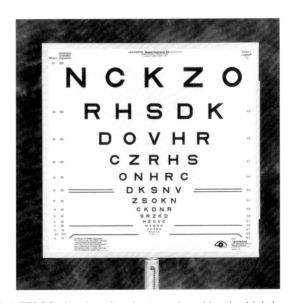

Figure 3-6 Modified ETDRS visual acuity chart produced by the Lighthouse. The chart is intended for use at 20 ft (6 m) but can also be used at 10 ft (3 m) or 5 ft (1.5 m) with appropriate scaling. *(Courtesy of Kevin M. Miller, MD.)*

Westheimer G. Visual acuity. In: Kaufman PL, Alm A, eds. *Adler's Physiology of the Eye.* 10th ed. St Louis: Mosby; 2003.

Contrast Sensitivity and the Contrast Sensitivity Function

An underappreciated variable in measuring visual function is the degree of contrast between the optotype and its background. In general, the higher the contrast, the easier the optotype is to decipher. One reason good illumination makes it easier to read a book is that more light creates a brighter background and therefore a higher contrast against the black letters on the page. If the brightness of an object (I_{min}) and the brightness of its background (I_{max}) are known, the following formula can be used to measure the degree of contrast between the object and its background:

$$\text{Contrast} = \frac{I_{max} - I_{min}}{I_{max} + I_{min}}$$

Thus, when letters are printed with perfectly black ink (ie, totally nonreflecting) on perfectly white paper (ie, 100% reflecting), the contrast will be 100%. Snellen acuity is commonly tested with targets, either illuminated or projected charts, that *approximate* 100% contrast. When we measure Snellen visual acuity, therefore, we are measuring the smallest optotype at approximately 100% contrast that can be resolved by the visual system. In everyday life, however, 100% contrast is rarely encountered, and most visual tasks must be performed in lower-contrast conditions.

To take contrast sensitivity into account when measuring visual function, we can use the *modulation transfer function (MTF)*. Consider a target in which the light intensity varies from some peak value to zero in a sinusoidal fashion. The contrast is 100%, but instead of looking like a bar graph, it looks like a bar graph with softened edges. The number of light bands per unit length or per unit angle is called the *spatial frequency* and is closely related to Snellen acuity. For example, the 20/20 E optotype is composed of bands of light and dark, where each band is 1 arcmin. Thus, 20/20 Snellen acuity corresponds (for a 100% contrast target) roughly to 30 cycles per degree of resolution when expressed in spatial frequency notation. If we take sine wave gratings with various spatial frequencies and describe how the optical system alters the contrast of each of them, we have a set of information that constitutes the MTF.

In clinical practice, the ophthalmologist presents a patient with targets of various spatial frequencies and peak contrasts. A plot is then made of the minimum resolvable contrast target that can be seen for each spatial frequency. The minimum resolvable contrast is the *contrast threshold.* The reciprocal of the contrast threshold is defined as the *contrast sensitivity,* and the manner in which contrast sensitivity changes as a function of the spatial frequency of the targets is called the *contrast sensitivity function (CSF)* (Fig 3-7). A typical contrast sensitivity curve obtained with sinusoidal gratings is shown in Figure 3-8. Contrast sensitivity can also be tested with optotypes of variable contrast (such as the Pelli-Robson or Regan charts), which may be easier for patients to use. Which of these approaches is more useful clinically remains controversial.

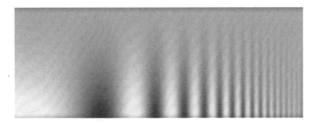

Figure 3-7 Contrast sensitivity grating. In this example, the contrast diminishes from bottom to top, and the spatial frequency of the pattern increases from left to right. The pattern appears to have a hump in the middle at the frequencies for which the human eye is most sensitive to contrasts. *(Courtesy of Brian Wandell, PhD.)*

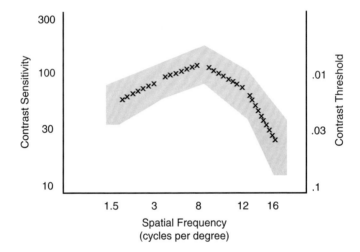

Figure 3-8 A typical contrast sensitivity curve is noted as x-x-x. The *shaded area* represents the range of normal values for 90% of the population. Expected deviations from the normal due to specific diagnoses are noted in the text discussion. *(Developed by Dr. Arthur P. Ginsburg. Courtesy of Stereo Optical Company, Inc, Chicago.)*

It is important to perform this test with the best possible optical correction in place. In addition, luminance must be kept constant when CSF is tested, because mean luminance has an effect on the shape of the normal CSF. In low luminance, the low spatial frequency falloff disappears and the peak shifts toward the lower frequencies. In brighter light, there is little change in the shape of the normal CSF through a range of luminance for the higher spatial frequencies. Generally, contrast sensitivity is measured at normal room illumination, which is approximately 30–70 foot-lamberts.

Contrast sensitivity is affected by various conditions of the eye, both physiologic and pathologic. Any corneal pathology that causes distortion or edema can affect contrast sensitivity. Lens changes, particularly incipient cataracts, may significantly decrease CSF, even with a normal Snellen acuity. Retinal pathology may affect contrast sensitivity more (as with retinitis pigmentosa or central serous retinopathy) or less (certain macular degenerations) than it does Snellen acuity. Glaucoma may produce a significant loss in the midrange. Retrobulbar optic neuritis may also be associated with a notch-type pattern loss. Amblyopia is associated with a generalized attenuation of the curve. Pupil size also has an effect on contrast sensitivity. With miotic pupils, diffraction reduces contrast sensitivity; with large pupils, optical aberrations may interfere with performance.

> Miller D. Glare and contrast sensitivity testing. In: Tasman W, Jaeger EA, eds. *Duane's Clinical Ophthalmology.* Philadelphia: Lippincott Williams & Wilkins; 1992.

Refractive States of the Eyes

In considering the refractive state of the eye, we can use either of the following concepts:

1. The *focal point* concept: The location of the image formed by an object at optical infinity through a nonaccommodating eye determines the eye's refractive state. Objects focusing anterior or posterior to the retina form a blurred image on the retina, whereas objects that focus on the retina form a sharp image.
2. The *far point* concept: The far point is the point in space that is conjugate to the fovea of the nonaccommodating eye; that is, the far point is where the fovea would be imaged if the optics were reversed and the fovea were made the object.

Emmetropia is the refractive state in which parallel rays of light from a distant object are brought to focus on the retina in the nonaccommodating eye (Fig 3-9A). The far point of the emmetropic eye is at infinity, and infinity is *conjugate* with the retina (Fig 3-9B). *Ametropia* refers to the absence of emmetropia and can be classified by presumptive etiology as *axial* or *refractive*. In *axial ametropia,* the eyeball is either unusually long *(myopia)* or short *(hyperopia)*. In *refractive ametropia,* the length of the eye is statistically normal, but the refractive power of the eye (cornea and/or lens) is abnormal, being either excessive (myopia) or deficient (hyperopia). *Aphakia* is an example of extreme refractive hyperopia unless the eye was highly myopic (>20 D) before lens removal. An ametropic eye requires either a diverging or a converging lens to image a distant object on the retina.

Ametropias may also be classified by the nature of the mismatch between the optical power and length of the eye. In myopia, the eye possesses too much optical power for its axial length, and (with accommodation relaxed) light rays from an object at infinity

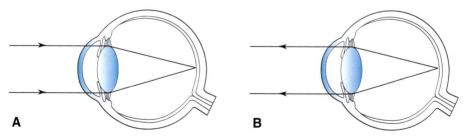

A   **B**

Figure 3-9   Emmetropia with accommodation relaxed. **A,** Parallel light rays from infinity focus to a point on the retina. **B,** Similarly, light rays emanating from a point on the retina focus at the far point of the eye at optical infinity. *(Illustration by C. H. Wooley.)*

converge too soon and thus focus in front of the retina (Fig 3-10A). This results in a defocused image on the retina. Similarly, the far point of the eye images in front of the eye, between the cornea and optical infinity (Fig 3-10B). In hyperopia, the eye does not possess enough optical power for its axial length, and (with accommodation relaxed) an object at infinity attempts to focus light behind the retina, again producing a defocused image on the retina (Fig 3-11A); the far point of the eye (actually a virtual point rather than a real point in space) is located behind the retina (Fig 3-11B).

Astigmatism [A = without, *stigmos* = point] is an optical condition of the eye in which light rays from an object do not focus to a single point, because of variations in the curvature of the cornea or lens at different meridians. Instead, there is a set of 2 *focal lines*. Each astigmatic eye can be classified by the orientations and relative positions of these focal lines (Fig 3-12). If 1 focal line lies in front of the retina and the other is on the retina, the condition is classified as *simple myopic astigmatism*. If both focal lines lie in front of the retina, the condition is classified as *compound myopic astigmatism*. If 1 focal line lies behind the retina and the other is on the retina, the astigmatism is classified as *simple hyperopic*. If both focal lines lie behind the retina, the astigmatism is classified as *compound hyperopic*. If 1 focal line lies in front of and the other behind the retina, the condition is classified as *mixed astigmatism*.

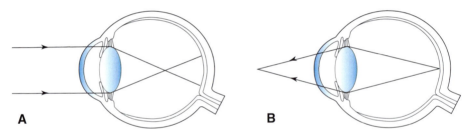

Figure 3-10 Myopia with accommodation relaxed. **A,** Parallel light rays from infinity focus to a point anterior to the retina, forming a blurred image on the retina. **B,** Light rays emanating from a point on the retina focus to a far point in front of the eye, between optical infinity and the cornea. *(Illustration by C. H. Wooley.)*

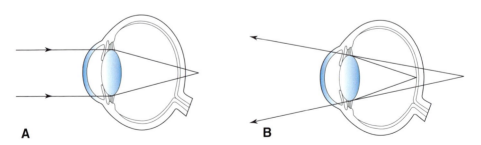

Figure 3-11 Hyperopia with accommodation relaxed. **A,** Parallel light rays from infinity focus to a point posterior to the retina, forming a blurred image on the retina. **B,** Light rays emanating from a point on the retina are divergent as they exit the eye, appearing to have come from a virtual far point behind the eye. *(Illustration by C. H. Wooley.)*

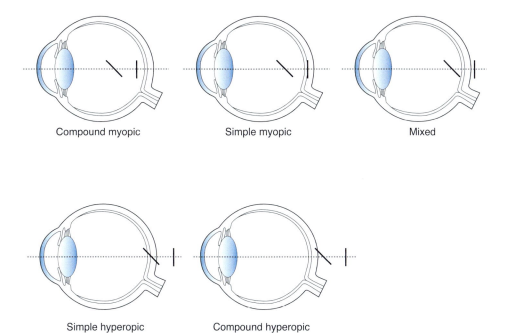

Compound myopic   Simple myopic   Mixed

Simple hyperopic   Compound hyperopic

Figure 3-12 Types of astigmatism. The locations of the focal lines with respect to the retina define the type of astigmatism. The main difference between the types of astigmatism depicted in the illustration is the spherical equivalent refractive error. All of the astigmatisms depicted are with-the-rule astigmatisms—that is, they are corrected with a plus cylinder whose axis is vertical. If they were against-the-rule astigmatisms, the positions of the vertical and horizontal focal lines would be reversed.

If the principal meridians (or *axes*) of astigmatism have constant orientation at every point across the pupil, and if the amount of astigmatism is the same at every point, the refractive condition is known as *regular astigmatism* and is correctable by cylindrical spectacle lenses. Regular astigmatism may itself be classified into *with-the-rule* and *against-the-rule astigmatism.* In *with-the-rule* astigmatism (the more common type in children), the vertical meridian is steepest (resembling an American football lying on its side), and a correcting plus cylinder should be used at or near axis 90°. In *against-the-rule* astigmatism (the more common type in older adults), the horizontal meridian is steepest (resembling a football standing on its end), and a correcting plus cylinder should be used at or near axis 180°. The term *oblique astigmatism* is used to describe regular astigmatism in which the principal meridians do not lie at, or close to, 90° or 180° but lie near 45° and 135°.

In *irregular astigmatism,* the orientation of the principal meridians or the amount of astigmatism changes from point to point across the pupil. Although the principal meridians are 90° apart at every point, it may sometimes appear by retinoscopy or keratometry that the principal meridians of the cornea, as a whole, are not perpendicular to one another. All eyes have at least a small amount of irregular astigmatism, and instruments such as corneal topographers and wavefront aberrometers can be used to detect this condition clinically. These *higher-order* aberrations in the refractive properties of the cornea and lens have been characterized by Zernike polynomials, which are mathematical shapes that approximate various types of irregular astigmatism more closely than the simple "football" model. They include such shapes as spherical aberration, coma, and trefoil. See BCSC Section 13, *Refractive Surgery*, for further discussion.

Binocular States of the Eyes

The spherical equivalent of a refractive state is defined as the algebraic sum of the spherical component and half of the astigmatic component. *Anisometropia* refers to any difference in the spherical equivalents between the 2 eyes. Uncorrected anisometropia in children may lead to amblyopia, especially if 1 eye is hyperopic. Although adults may be annoyed by uncorrected anisometropia, they may be intolerant of initial spectacle correction. Unequal image size, or *aniseikonia,* may occur, and the prismatic effect of the glasses will vary in different directions of gaze, inducing *anisophoria.* Anisophoria is usually more bothersome than aniseikonia for patients with spectacle-corrected anisometropias.

Aniseikonia can also be due to a difference in the shape of the images formed in the 2 eyes. The most common cause is the differential magnification inherent in the spectacle correction of anisometropia. Even though aniseikonia is difficult to measure, anisometropic spectacle correction can be prescribed in such a manner as to reduce aniseikonia. Making the front surface power of a lens less positive can reduce magnification. Decreasing center thickness also reduces magnification. Decreasing vertex distance diminishes both the magnifying effect of plus lenses and the minifying effect of minus lenses (these effects become increasingly noticeable as lens power increases). Contact lenses may provide a better solution than spectacles in most patients with anisometropia, particularly in children (in whom fusion may be possible).

Unilateral aphakia is an extreme example of hyperopic anisometropia arising from refractive ametropia. Spectacle correction produces an intolerable aniseikonia of about 25%; contact lens correction produces aniseikonia of about 7%, which is usually tolerated. By adjusting the powers of contact lenses and simultaneously worn spectacle lenses to provide the appropriate minifying or magnifying effect by the Galilean telescope principle, the clinician may reduce aniseikonia still further, if necessary. For further information on correcting aphakia, see Chapter 4, Clinical Refraction; Chapter 5, Contact Lenses; and Chapter 6, Intraocular Lenses.

Accommodation and Presbyopia

Accommodation is the mechanism by which the eye changes refractive power by altering the shape of its crystalline lens. The mechanisms that achieve this alteration have been described by Helmholtz. The posterior focal point is moved forward in the eye during accommodation (Fig 3-13A). Correspondingly, the far point moves closer to the eye (Fig 3-13B). *Accommodative effort* occurs when the ciliary muscle contracts in response to parasympathetic stimulation, thus allowing the zonular fibers to relax. The outward-directed tension on the lens capsule is decreased, and the lens becomes more convex. The movement of the equatorial edge of the lens is thus away from the sclera during accommodation

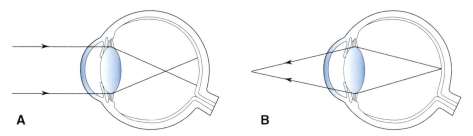

Figure 3-13 Emmetropia with accommodation stimulated. **A,** Parallel light rays now come to a point locus in front of the retina, forming a blurred image on the retina. **B,** Light rays emanating from a point on the retina focus to a near point in front of the eye, between optical infinity and the cornea. *(Illustration by C. H. Wooley.)*

and toward the sclera again when accommodation is relaxed. *Accommodative response* results from the increase in lens convexity (primarily the anterior surface), and it may be expressed as the *amplitude of accommodation* (in diopters) or as the *range of accommodation*, the distance between the far point of the eye and the nearest point at which the eye can maintain focus *(near point)*. It is evident that as the lens loses elasticity from the aging process, the accommodative response wanes (a condition called *presbyopia*), even though the amount of ciliary muscle contraction or accommodative effort is virtually unchanged. For calculation of the additional spectacle lens power requirement for an eye with this condition, the amplitude is a more useful measurement. For appraising an individual's ability to perform a specific visual task, the range is more informative.

Glasser A, Kaufman PL. The mechanism of accommodation in primates. *Ophthalmology*. 1999; 106(5):863–872.

Epidemiology of Refractive Errors

An interplay among corneal power, lens power, anterior chamber depth, and axial length determines an individual's refractive status. All 4 elements change continuously as the eye grows. On average, babies are born with about 3.0 D of hyperopia. In the first few months of life, this hyperopia may increase slightly, but it then declines to an average of about 1.0 D of hyperopia by age 1, because of marked changes in corneal and lenticular powers, as well as axial length growth. By the end of the second year, the anterior segment attains adult proportions; however, the curvatures of the refracting surfaces continue to change measurably. One study found that average corneal power decreased 0.1–0.2 D, and lens power decreased about 1.8 D, between ages 3 and 14 years.

From birth to age 6 years, the axial length of the eye grows by approximately 5 mm, and one might expect from this a high prevalence of myopia in infants. However, most children are actually emmetropic, with only a 2% incidence of myopia at 6 years. This phenomenon is due to a still undetermined mechanism called *emmetropization*. During the first 6 years of life, as the eye grows by 5 mm, a compensatory loss of 4 D of corneal power and 2 D of lens power keeps most eyes close to emmetropia. It appears that the immature human eye develops so as to reduce refractive errors.

Lawrence MS, Azar DT. Myopia and models and mechanisms of refractive error control. *Ophthalmol Clin North Am.* 2002;15(1):127–133.

Preferred Practice Patterns Committee, Refractive Management/Intervention Panel. *Refractive Errors.* San Francisco: American Academy of Ophthalmology; 2002.

Prevent Blindness America and the National Eye Institute. *Vision Problems in the U.S.: Prevalence of Adult Vision Impairment and Age-Related Eye Disease in America.* Schaumburg, IL: Prevent Blindness America; 2002.

Zadnik K, Mutti DO. Biology of the eye as an optical system. In: *Duane's Clinical Ophthalmology* (vol 1, ch 34). Philadelphia: Lippincott Williams & Wilkins; 2003.

Developmental Myopia

Myopia increases steadily with increasing age. In the United States, the prevalence of myopia has been estimated at 3% among children aged 5 to 7 years, 8% among those aged 8 to 10 years, 14% among those aged 11 to 12 years, and 25% among adolescents aged 12 to 17 years. In particular ethnic groups, a similar trend has been demonstrated, although the percentages in each age group may differ. Ethnic Chinese children have much higher rates of myopia at all ages. A national study in Taiwan found the prevalence was 12% among 6-year-olds and 84% among those aged 16 to 18 years. Similar rates have been found in Singapore and Japan.

Different subsets of myopia have been characterized. *Juvenile-onset myopia,* defined as myopia with an onset between 7 and 16 years of age, is due primarily to growth in axial length. Risk factors include *esophoria,* against-the-rule astigmatism, premature birth, family history, and intensive near work. In general, the earlier the onset of myopia, the greater the degree of progression. In the United States, the mean rate of childhood myopia progression is reported at about 0.5 D per year. In approximately 75% of teenagers, refractive errors stabilize at about age 15 or 16. In those whose errors do not stabilize, progression often continues into the 20s or 30s.

Adult-onset myopia begins at about 20 years of age, and extensive near work is a risk factor. A study of West Point cadets found myopia requiring corrective lenses in 46% at entrance, 54% after 1 year, and 65% after 2 years. The probability of myopic progression was related to the degree of initial refractive error. It is estimated that as many as 20%–40% of patients with low hyperopia or emmetropia who have extensive near-work requirements become myopic before age 25, as compared to less than 10% of persons without such demands. Older Naval Academy recruits have a lower rate of myopia development than younger recruits over a 4-year curriculum (15% for 21-year-olds versus 77% for 18-year-olds). Some young adults are at risk for myopic progression even after a period of refractive stability. It has been theorized that persons who regularly perform considerable near work undergo a process similar to emmetropization for the customary close working distance, and this results in a myopic shift.

The etiologic factors concerning myopia are complex, involving both genetic and environmental factors. Regarding a genetic role, identical twins are more likely to have a similar degree of myopia than are fraternal twins, siblings, or parent and child. Identical twins separated at birth and having different work habits do not show significant differences in refractive error. Some forms of severe myopia suggest dominant, recessive, and even sex-linked inheritance patterns. However, studies of ethnic Chinese in Taiwan show an increase in the prevalence and severity of myopia over the span of 2 generations, a finding that implies that genetics alone are not entirely responsible for myopia. Some studies have reported that near work is not associated with a higher prevalence and progression of myopia, especially with respect to middle-distance activities, such as those involving video display terminals. Higher educational achievement has been strongly associated with a higher prevalence of myopia. Poor nutrition has been implicated in the development of some refractive errors. Studies from Africa have found that children suffering malnutrition have an increased prevalence of high ametropia, astigmatism, and anisometropia.

Feldkamper M, Schaeffel F. Interactions of genes and environment in myopia. *Dev Ophthalmol.* 2003;37:34–49.

Fischer AJ, McGuire JJ, Schaeffel F, Stell WK. Light- and focus-dependent expression of the transcription factor ZENK in the chick retina. *Nat Neurosci.* 1999;2(8):706–712.

Hoffer KJ. Biometry of 7,500 cataractous eyes. *Am J Ophthalmol.* 1980;90(3):360–368. [Published correction appears in *Am J Ophthalmol.* 1980;90(3):890.]

Lin LL, Shih YF, Tsai CB, et al. Epidemiologic study of ocular refraction among schoolchildren in Taiwan in 1995. *Optom Vis Sci.* 1999;76(5):275–281.

McCarty CA, Taylor HR. Myopia and vision 2020. *Am J Ophthalmol.* 2000;129(4):525–527.

Winawer J, Wallman J, Kee C. Differential responses of ocular length and choroidal thickness in chick eyes to brief periods of plus and minus lens-wear. *Invest Ophthalmol Vis Sci Suppl.* 1999;40:S963.

Developmental Hyperopia

Less is known about the epidemiology of hyperopia than of myopia. There appears to be an increase in the prevalence of adult hyperopia with age apart from those who develop nuclear sclerotic cataracts. Nuclear sclerosis is usually associated with a myopic shift. In Caucasians, the prevalence of hyperopia increases from about 20% among those in their 40s to about 60% among those in their 70s and 80s. In contrast to myopia, hyperopia was associated with lower educational achievement.

Attebo K, Ivers RQ, Mitchell P. Refractive errors in an older population: the Blue Mountains Eye Study. *Ophthalmology.* 1999;106(6):1066–1072.

Lee KE, Klein BE, Klein R. Changes in refractive error over a 5-year interval in the Beaver Dam Eye Study. *Invest Ophthalmol Vis Sci.* 1999;40(8):1645–1649.

Prevention of Refractive Errors

Over the years, many treatments have been proposed to prevent or slow the progression of myopia. Optical correction in the form of bifocal spectacles, multifocal spectacles, or removal of distance spectacles when performing close work has been recommended to reduce accommodation, because accommodation is a postulated mechanism for the progression of myopia. Administration of atropine eyedrops has long been proposed to prevent progression of myopia because it inhibits accommodation, which may exert forces on the eye that result in axial elongation. Use of an agent that lowers intraocular pressure has been suggested as an alternative pharmacologic intervention; this agent works presumably by reducing internal pressure on the eye wall. It has also been postulated that use of rigid contact lenses could slow the progression of myopia in children. Visual training purported to reduce myopia includes exercises such as near–far focusing change activities and convergence exercises. Evidence reported in the peer-reviewed literature, including from randomized clinical trials, is currently insufficient to support a recommendation for intervention using any of these proposed treatments.

Saw SM, Shih-Yen EC, Koh A, Tan D. Interventions to retard myopia progression in children: an evidence-based update. *Ophthalmology.* 2002;109(3):415–421.

Treatment of Refractive Errors

The need to correct refractive errors depends on the patient's symptoms and visual needs. Patients with low refractive errors may not require correction, and small changes in refractive corrections in asymptomatic patients are not generally recommended. Correction options include spectacles, contact lenses, or surgery. Various occupational and recreational requirements as well as personal preferences affect the specific choices for any individual patient.

CHAPTER **4**

Clinical Refraction

Objective Refraction: Retinoscopy

The *retinoscope* allows the physician to objectively determine the spherocylindrical refractive error, as well as observe optical aberrations, irregularities, and opacities.

Most retinoscopes in use today employ the streak projection system developed by Copeland. The illumination of the retinoscope is provided by a bulb with a straight filament that forms a streak in its projection. The light is reflected from a mirror that is either half silvered (Welch-Allyn model) or totally silvered around a small circular aperture (Copeland instrument) (Fig 4-1).

The filament can be moved in relation to a convex lens in the system. If the light is slightly divergent, it appears to come from a point behind the retinoscope, as if the light had been reflected off a plano mirror ("plano mirror setting," Fig 4-2).

Alternatively, when the distance between the convex lens and the filament is increased by moving the sleeve on the handle, convergent light is emitted. In this situation, the image

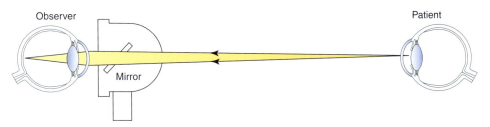

Figure 4-1   Observation system: light path from patient's pupil, through mirror, to observer's retina. *(Modified from Corboy JM.* The Retinoscopy Book: A Manual for Beginners. *Thorofare, NJ: Slack; 1979:13.)*

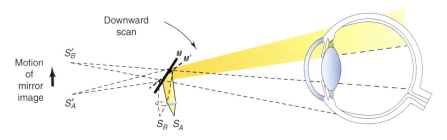

Figure 4-2   Illumination system: position of source with plano mirror effect.

of the filament is between the examiner and the patient, as if the light had been reflected off a concave mirror (Fig 4-3).

Retinoscopy is usually performed using the plano mirror setting. Not all retinoscopes employ the same sleeve position for this mirror setting. For example, the original Cope-land retinoscope is in plano position with the sleeve up; the Welch-Allyn is in plano posi-tion with the sleeve down. The axis of the streak is rotated by rotating the sleeve.

Positioning and Alignment

Ordinarily, the examiner uses the right eye to perform retinoscopy on the patient's right eye, and the left eye for the patient's left eye. If the examiner looks directly through the optical centers of the trial lenses while performing retinoscopy, the reflections from lenses may interfere. In general, if the examiner is too far off-axis, unwanted spherical and cylin-drical errors occur. The optimal alignment is just off-center, where the lens reflections can still be seen between the center of the pupil and the lateral edge of the lens.

Fixation and Fogging

Retinoscopy should be performed with the patient's accommodation relaxed. The patient should fixate at a distance on a nonaccommodative target. For example, the target may be a dim light at the end of the room or a large Snellen letter (20/200 or 20/400 size). (Chil-dren typically require pharmacologic cycloplegia.)

The Retinal Reflex

The projected streak illuminates an area of the patient's retina, and this light returns to the examiner. By observing characteristics of this reflex, one determines the refractive status of the eye. If the patient's eye is emmetropic, the light rays emerging from the patient's pupil are parallel to one another. If the patient's eye is myopic, the rays are convergent

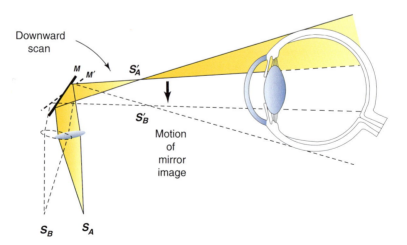

Figure 4-3 Illumination system: position of source with concave mirror effect.

(Fig 4-4); if the eye is hyperopic, they are divergent. Through the peephole in the retinoscope, these emerging rays are seen as a red reflex in the patient's pupil. If the examiner (specifically, the peephole of the retinoscope) is at the patient's far point, all the light leaving the patient's pupil enters the peephole and illumination is uniform (Fig 4-5). However, if the far point of the patient's eye is not at the peephole of the retinoscope, only some of the rays emanating from the patient's pupil enter the peephole, and illumination of the pupil appears incomplete.

    If the far point is between the examiner and the patient, the emerging rays will have focused and then diverged. The lighted portion of the pupil will move in a direction opposite to the motion (sweep) of the retinoscope streak (known as *against* motion; Fig 4-6)

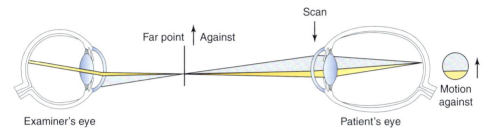

Figure 4-4   Observation system for myopia.

Neutralization

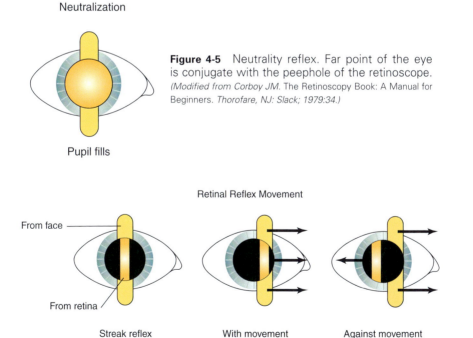

Figure 4-5   Neutrality reflex. Far point of the eye is conjugate with the peephole of the retinoscope. *(Modified from Corboy JM.* The Retinoscopy Book: A Manual for Beginners. *Thorofare, NJ: Slack; 1979:34.)*

Figure 4-6   Retinal reflex movement. Note movement of the streak from face and from retina in *with* versus *against* motion. *(Modified from Corboy JM.* The Retinoscopy Book. A Manual for Beginners. *Thorofare, NJ: Slack; 1979:32.)*

as it is moved across the patient's pupil. If the far point is behind the examiner, the light will move in the same direction as the sweep (*with* motion; see Fig 4-6).

When the light fills the pupil and does not move, the condition is known as *neutrality* (see Fig 4-5). The far point is moved with placement of a correcting lens in front of the patient's eye. At neutrality, if the examiner moves forward (in front of the far point), *with* motion is seen; if the examiner moves back and away from the far point, *against* motion is seen.

Characteristics of the reflex

The moving retinoscopic reflex has 3 main characteristics (Fig 4-7):

- *Speed.* The reflex seen in the pupil moves slowest when the far point is distant from the examiner (peephole of the retinoscope). As the far point is moved toward the peephole, the speed of the reflex increases. In other words, large refractive errors have a slow-moving reflex, whereas small errors have a fast reflex.
- *Brilliance.* The reflex is dull when the far point is distant from the examiner; it becomes brighter as neutrality is approached. *Against* reflexes are usually dimmer than *with* reflexes.
- *Width.* When the far point is distant from the examiner, the streak is narrow. As the far point is moved closer to the examiner, the streak broadens and, at neutrality, fills the entire pupil.

The Correcting Lens

When the examiner uses the appropriate correcting lenses (either with loose lenses or a phoropter), the retinoscopic reflex is neutralized. In other words, when the examiner brings the patient's far point to the peephole, the reflex fills the patient's entire pupil (Fig 4-8). The power of the correcting lens (or lenses) neutralizing the reflex helps determine the patient's refractive error.

The examiner determines the refractive error at the distance from which he or she is working. The dioptric equivalent of the working distance (ie, the inverse of the distance)

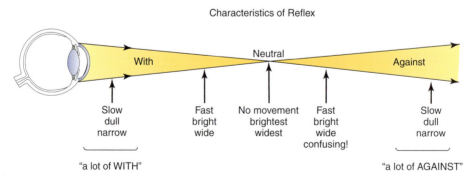

Figure 4-7 Characteristics of the moving retinal reflex on both sides of neutrality. The vertical arrows indicate the position of the retinoscope with regard to the point of neutrality. *(Modified from Corboy JM.* The Retinoscopy Book: A Manual for Beginners. *Thorofare, NJ: Slack; 1979:38.)*

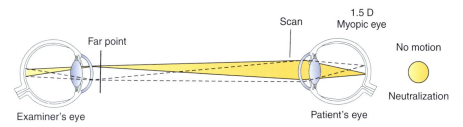

Figure 4-8 Observation system at neutralization.

should be subtracted from the power of the correcting lens to determine the actual refractive error of the patient's eye. Because a common working distance is 67 cm, many phoropters have a 1.50 D (1.00/0.67 m) "working-distance" lens for use during retinoscopy. However, this added lens can produce bothersome reflexes. Any working distance may be used. If the examiner prefers to move closer to the patient for a brighter reflex, the working-distance correction is adjusted accordingly.

For example, suppose that the examiner obtained neutralization with a total of +4.00 D over the eye (gross retinoscopy) at a working distance of 67 cm. Subtracting 1.50 D for the working distance yields a refractive correction of +2.50 D.

Finding Neutrality

In *against* movement, the far point is between the examiner and the patient. Therefore, to bring the far point to the peephole of the retinoscope, minus lenses are placed in front of the patient's eye. Similarly, in the case of *with* movement, plus lenses are placed in front of the patient's eye. This leads to the simple clinical rule: If you see *with* motion, add plus power (or subtract *minus*); if you see *against* motion, add minus power (or subtract *plus*) (Fig 4-9).

Because it is easier to work with the brighter, sharper *with motion* image, overminus the eye and obtain a *with* reflex; then reduce the minus (add plus) until neutrality is reached. Be aware that the slow, dull reflexes of high refractive errors may be confused with the neutrality reflex. Media opacities may also produce dull reflexes.

Retinoscopy of Regular Astigmatism

Most eyes have some regular astigmatism. In these cases, light is refracted differently by the 2 principal astigmatic meridians. Let us consider how the retinoscope works in greater detail.

As we sweep the retinoscope back and forth, we are really measuring the power along only a single axis. If we move the retinoscope from side to side (with the streak oriented at 90°), we are measuring the optical power in the 180° meridian. Power in this meridian is provided by a cylinder at axis 90°. The convenient result is that the streak of the retinoscope is aligned at the same axis as the axis of the correcting cylinder being tested. In a patient with regular astigmatism, we want to neutralize 2 reflexes, 1 from each of the principal meridians.

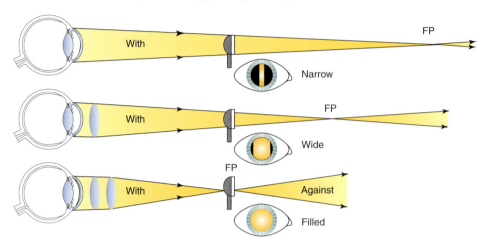

Approaching Neutrality

Figure 4-9 Approaching neutrality. Change in width of the reflex as neutrality is approached. Note that working distance remains constant, and the far point *(FP)* is pulled in with plus lenses. *(Modified from Corboy JM. The Retinoscopy Book: A Manual for Beginners. Thorofare, NJ: Slack; 1979:41.)*

Finding the cylinder axis

Before the powers in each of the principal meridians are determined, the axes of the meridians must be determined. Four characteristics of the streak reflex aid in this determination:

- *Break.* A break is seen when the streak is not oriented parallel to one of the principal meridians. The reflex streak in the pupil is not aligned with the streak projected on the iris and surface of the eye, and the line appears *broken* (Fig 4-10). The break disappears (ie, the line appears continuous) when the projected streak is rotated to the correct axis.
- *Width.* The width of the reflex in the pupil varies as it is rotated around the correct axis. The reflex appears narrowest when the streak, or intercept, aligns with the axis (Fig 4-11).
- *Intensity.* The intensity of the line is brighter when the streak is on the correct axis.
- *Skew.* Skew (oblique motion of the streak reflex) may be used to refine the axis in small cylinders. If the retinoscope streak is off-axis, it will move in a slightly different

Figure 4-10 Break. The retinal reflex is discontinuous with the intercept when the streak is off the correct axis. *(Modified from Corboy JM. The Retinoscopy Book: A Manual for Beginners. Thorofare, NJ: Slack; 1979:90.)*

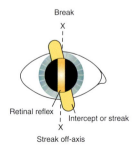

Thickness

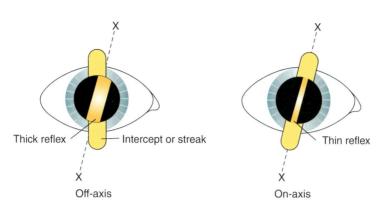

Thick reflex — Intercept or streak — Thin reflex

Off-axis — On-axis

Figure 4-11 Width, or thickness, of the retinal reflex. We locate the axis where the reflex is thinnest. *(Modified from Corboy JM. The Retinoscopy Book: A Manual for Beginners. Thorofare, NJ: Slack; 1979:90.)*

direction from the pupillary reflex (Fig 4-12). The reflex and streak move in the same direction when the streak is aligned with one of the principal meridians.

When the streak is aligned at the correct axis, the sleeve may be lowered (Copeland instrument) or raised (Welch-Allyn instrument) to narrow the streak, allowing the axis to be more easily determined (Fig 4-13).

This axis can be confirmed through a technique known as *straddling,* which is performed with the estimated correcting cylinder in place (Fig 4-14). The retinoscope streak is turned 45° off-axis in both directions, and if the axis is correct, the width of the reflex should be equal in both off-axis positions. If the axis is not correct, the widths will be unequal in these 2 positions. The axis of the correcting cylinder should be moved toward the narrower reflex and the straddling repeated until the widths are equal.

Finding the cylinder power

After the 2 principal meridians are identified, the previously explained spherical techniques are applied to each axis.

Skew

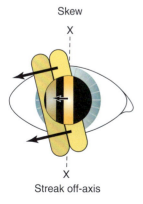

Streak off-axis

Figure 4-12 Skew. The *arrows* indicate that movements of the reflex and intercept are not parallel. The reflex and intercept do not move in the same direction but are skewed when the streak is off-axis. *(Modified from Corboy JM. The Retinoscopy Book: A Manual for Beginners. Thorofare, NJ: Slack; 1979:91.)*

Pinpointing Axis

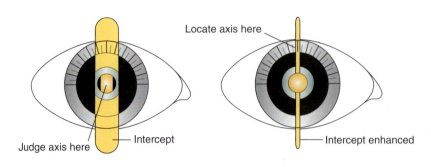

A Axis Determination   **B** Axis Location

Figure 4-13 Locating axis on the protractor. **A,** First determine the astigmatic axis. **B,** Then lower the sleeve to enhance the intercept until the filament is seen as a fine line pinpointing the axis. *(Modified from Corboy JM.* The Retinoscopy Book: A Manual for Beginners. *Thorofare, NJ: Slack; 1979:92.)*

Straddling

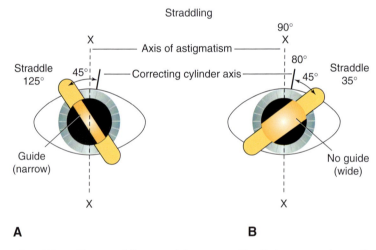

A   **B**

Figure 4-14 Straddling. The straddling meridians are 45° off the correcting cylinder axis, at roughly 35° and 125°. As you move back from the eye while comparing meridians, the reflex at 125° remains narrow **(A)** at the same distance that the reflex at 35° has become wide **(B)**. This dissimilarity indicates an axis error; the narrow reflex **(A)** is the guide toward which we must turn the correcting cylinder axis. *(Modified from Corboy JM.* The Retinoscopy Book: A Manual for Beginners. *Thorofare, NJ: Slack; 1979:95.)*

With 2 spheres: Neutralize 1 axis with a spherical lens; then neutralize the axis 90° away. The difference between these readings is the cylinder power. For example, if the 90° axis is neutralized with a +1.50 sphere and the 180° axis is neutralized with a +2.25 sphere, the gross retinoscopy is +1.50 +0.75 × 180. The examiner's working distance (ie, +1.50) is subtracted from the sphere to obtain the final refractive correction, plano +0.75 × 180.

With a sphere and cylinder: Neutralize 1 axis with a spherical lens. To enable the use of *with* reflexes, neutralize the *less plus* axis first. Then, with this spherical lens in place, neutralize the axis 90° away by adding a plus cylindrical lens. The spherocylindrical gross retinoscopy is read directly from the trial lens apparatus.

It is also possible to use 2 cylinders at right angles to each other for this gross retinoscopy.

Aberrations of the Retinoscopic Reflex

With irregular astigmatism, almost any type of aberration may appear in the reflex. Spherical aberrations tend to increase the brightness at the center or periphery of the pupil, depending on whether they are positive or negative.

As neutrality is approached, one part of the reflex may be myopic, whereas the other is hyperopic relative to the position of the retinoscope. This will produce the *scissors reflex*.

Occasionally, marked irregular astigmatism or optical opacity produces confusing, distorted shadows that reduce the precision of the retinoscopy. In such instances, other techniques such as subjective refraction may be used.

All of these aberrant reflexes are more noticeable with larger pupillary diameters. When a large pupil is encountered during retinoscopy, the examiner should neutralize the central portion of the light reflex.

Summary of Retinoscopy

The performance of streak retinoscopy using a plus-cylinder phoropter is summarized in the following steps:

1. Set the phoropter to 0 D sphere and 0 D cylinder. Use cycloplegia if necessary. Otherwise, fog the eyes or use a nonaccommodative target.
2. Hold the sleeve of the retinoscope in the position that produces a divergent beam of light. (If the examiner can focus the linear filament of the retinoscope on a wall, the sleeve is in the wrong position.)
3. Sweep the streak of light (the intercept) across the pupil perpendicular to the long axis of the streak. Observe the pupillary light reflex. Sweep in several different meridians.
4. Add minus sphere until the retinoscopic reflex shows *with* motion in all meridians. Add a little extra minus sphere if uncertain. If the reflexes are dim or indistinct, consider high refractive errors and make large changes in sphere (–3 D, –6 D, –9 D, and so on).
5. Continue examining multiple meridians while adding plus sphere until the retinoscopic reflex neutralizes in 1 meridian. (If all meridians neutralize simultaneously, the patient's refractive error is spherical; subtract the working distance to obtain the net retinoscopy).
6. Rotate the streak 90° and position the axis of the correcting plus cylinder parallel to the streak. A sweep across this meridian reveals additional *with* motion. Add plus cylinder power until neutrality is achieved.
7. Refine the correcting cylinder axis by sweeping 45° to either side of it. Rotate the axis of the correcting plus cylinder a few degrees toward the "guide" line, the brighter and narrower reflex. Repeat until both reflexes are equal.

8. Refine the cylinder power by moving in closer to the patient to pick up *with* motion in all directions. Back away slowly, observing how the reflexes neutralize. Change sphere or cylinder power as appropriate to make all meridians neutralize simultaneously.

9. Subtract the working distance (measured in diopters). For example, if the working distance is 67 cm, subtract 1.5 D (1.00/0.67).

10. Record the streak retinoscopy findings and, when possible, check the patient's visual acuity with the new prescription.

Corboy JM. *The Retinoscopy Book: An Introductory Manual for Eye Care Professionals.* 4th ed. Thorofare, NJ: Slack; 1995.

Safir A. Retinoscopy. In: Tasman W, Jaeger EA, eds. *Duane's Clinical Ophthalmology.* Philadelphia: Lippincott-Raven; 1995.

Subjective Refraction Techniques

Subjective refraction techniques rely on the patient's responses to determine the refractive correction. If all refractive errors were spherical, subjective refraction would be easy. However, determining the astigmatic portion of the correction is more complex, and a variety of subjective refraction techniques may be used. The Jackson cross cylinder is the most common instrument used in determining the astigmatic correction. However, we will begin with the astigmatic dial technique because it is easier to understand.

Astigmatic Dial Technique

An astigmatic dial is a test chart with lines arranged radially that may be used to determine the axes of astigmatism. A pencil of light from a point source is imaged by an astigmatic eye as a conoid of Sturm. The spokes of the astigmatic dial that are parallel to the principal meridians of the eye's astigmatism will be imaged as sharp lines corresponding to the focal lines of the conoid of Sturm.

Figure 4-15A shows an eye with compound hyperopic astigmatism and how it sees an astigmatic dial. The vertical line of the astigmatic dial is the blackest and sharpest, because the vertical focal line of each conoid of Sturm is closer to the retina than the horizontal focal line. By accommodating, however, the patient might pull both focal lines forward, far enough to make even the horizontal line of the astigmatic dial clear. To avoid accommodation, fogging is used. Enough plus sphere is placed before the eye to pull both the focal lines into the vitreous, creating compound myopic astigmatism, as in Figure 4-15B.

Because accommodating with the eye fogged results in increased blurring of the lines, the patient relaxes accommodation. The focal line closest to the retina can now be identified with certainty as the horizontal line, because it is now the blackest and sharpest line of the astigmatic dial. Note that the terms *blackest* and *sharpest* are more easily understood by patients and should be used instead of the word *clearest*.

After the examiner locates one of the principal meridians of the astigmatism, the interval of Sturm can be collapsed by moving the anterior focal line back toward the posterior focal line. Accomplish this by adding a minus cylinder with axis parallel to the

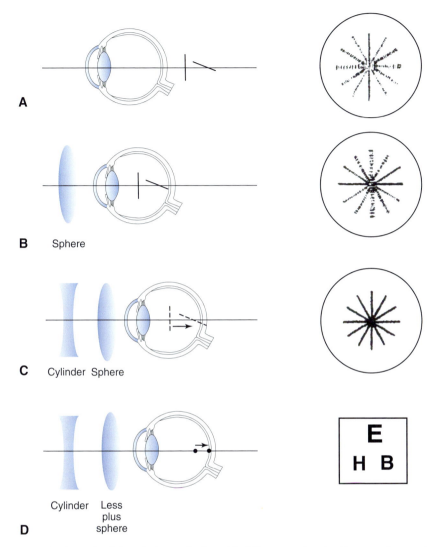

Figure 4-15 Astigmatic dial technique. **A,** Conoid of Sturm and retinal image of an astigmatic dial as viewed by an eye with compound hyperopic astigmatism. **B,** Fogging to produce compound myopic astigmatism. **C,** The conoid of Sturm is collapsed to a single point. **D,** Minus sphere is added (or plus sphere subtracted) to produce a sharp image.

anterior focal line. In Figure 4-15C, the vertical focal line has been moved back to the position of the horizontal focal line and collapsed to a point by the addition of a minus cylinder with axis at 90°. Notice that the minus cylinder is placed with its axis *perpendicular* to the blackest meridian on the astigmatic dial. Also note that as the interval of Sturm is collapsed, the focal lines disappear into a point focus.

All of the lines of the astigmatic dial now appear equally black but still are not in perfect focus, because the eye is still slightly fogged to control accommodation. At this point, a visual acuity chart is used; plus sphere is removed until best visual acuity is obtained (Fig 4-15D).

In summary, the following steps are used in astigmatic dial refraction:

1. Obtain best visual acuity using spheres only.
2. Fog the eye to about 20/50 by adding plus sphere.
3. Note the blackest and sharpest line of the astigmatic dial.
4. Add minus cylinder with axis perpendicular to the blackest and sharpest line until all lines appear equal.
5. Reduce plus sphere (or add minus) until best acuity is obtained with the visual acuity chart.

Astigmatic dial refraction can also be performed with plus cylinder equipment, but it must be used in a way that simulates minus cylinder effect. All of the above steps remain the same except for step 4, which becomes: Add *plus* cylinder with axis *parallel* to the blackest and sharpest line. As each 0.25 D of plus cylinder power is added, change the sphere simultaneously 0.25 D in the minus direction. This simulates minus cylinder effect exactly, moving the anterior focal line posteriorly without changing the position of the posterior focal line.

Michaels DD. *Visual Optics and Refraction: A Clinical Approach.* 3rd ed. St Louis: Mosby; 1985: 319–322.

Cross-Cylinder Technique

The Jackson cross cylinder, in Edward Jackson's words, is probably "far more useful, and far more used" than any other lens in clinical refraction. Every ophthalmologist should be familiar with the principles involved in its use. Although the cross cylinder is usually used to *refine* the cylinder axis and power of a refraction already obtained, it can also be used for the entire astigmatic refraction.

The first step in cross-cylinder refraction is adjusting the sphere to yield best visual acuity with accommodation relaxed. Begin by placing the prescription the patient is wearing into a trial frame or phoropter. Fog the eye to be examined with plus sphere while the patient views a visual acuity chart; then decrease the fog until best visual acuity is obtained. If astigmatism is present, decreasing the fog places the circle of least confusion on the retina, creating a mixed astigmatism. Now, use test figures 1–2 lines larger than the patient's best visual acuity. At this point, introduce the cross cylinder, first for refinement of cylinder axis and then for refinement of cylinder power.

If no cylindrical correction is present initially, the cross cylinder may still be used, placed at 90° and 180°, to check for the presence of astigmatism. If a preferred flip position is found, cylinder is added with axis parallel to the respective plus or minus axis of the cross cylinder until the 2 flip choices are equal. If no preference is found with the cross-cylinder axes at 90° and 180°, then 45° and 135° should always be checked before the assumption is made that no astigmatism is present. Once any cylinder power is found, axis and power are refined in the usual manner.

Always refine cylinder axis before refining cylinder power. This sequence is necessary because the correct axis can be found in the presence of an incorrect power, but the full cylinder power is found only in the presence of the correct axis.

Refinement of cylinder axis involves the combination of cylinders at oblique axes. When the axis of the correcting cylinder is not aligned with that of the astigmatic eye's cylinder, the combined cylinders produce residual astigmatism with a meridian roughly 45° away from the principal meridians of the 2 cylinders. To refine the axis, position the principal meridians of the cross cylinder *45° away from* those of the correcting cylinder. Present the patient with alternative flip choices, and select the choice that is "blackest and sharpest" to the patient. Then, rotate the axis of the correcting cylinder toward the corresponding plus or minus axis of the cross cylinder (plus cylinder axis is rotated toward the plus cylinder axis of the cross cylinder, and minus cylinder axis is rotated toward the minus cylinder axis of the cross cylinder). Low-power cylinders are rotated in increments of 15°; high-power cylinders are rotated by smaller amounts, usually 5°. Repeat this procedure until the flip choices appear equal.

To refine cylinder power, align the cross-cylinder axes with the principal meridians of the correcting lens, as illustrated in Figure 4-16. The examiner changes cylinder power according to the patient's responses; the spherical equivalent of the refractive correction should remain constant to keep the circle of least confusion on the retina. One achieves this by changing the sphere half as much and in the opposite direction as the cylinder power is changed. That is, for every 0.50 D of cylinder power change, the sphere is changed 0.25 D in the opposite direction. Periodically, the sphere power should be adjusted for best visual acuity.

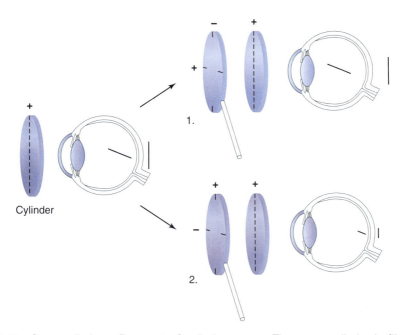

Figure 4-16 Cross-cylinder refinement of cylinder power. The cross cylinder is flipped between positions 1 and 2 as the patient is asked, "Which is better, one or two?" In position 1, the astigmatism is increased; in position 2, it is decreased. Position 2 is chosen because it yields a clearer image. In position 2, the plus axis of the cross cylinder is parallel to the plus cylinder axis, indicating that the plus cylinder should be increased in power.

Continue to refine cylinder power until both flip choices appear equal to the patient. At this point, the 2 flip choices produce equal and opposite mixed astigmatism, blurring the visual acuity chart equally (Fig 4-17).

Remember to use the proper-power cross cylinder for the patient's visual acuity level. For example, a ±0.25 D cross cylinder is commonly used with visual acuity levels of 20/30 and better. A high-power cross cylinder (±0.50 D or ±1.00 D) allows the patient with poorer vision to recognize differences in the flip choices.

The patient may be confused with prior choices during cross-cylinder refinement; giving different numbers to subsequent choices avoids this problem: "Which is better, one or two, three or four?" and so forth. If the patient persists in always choosing either the first or the second number, reverse the order of presentation to check for consistency.

In cross-cylinder refraction, the main points are as follows:

- Adjust sphere to the most plus or least minus that gives best visual acuity.
- Use test figures 1 or 2 lines larger than the patient's best visual acuity.
- If cylindrical correction is not already present, look for astigmatism by testing with the cross cylinder at axes 90° and 180°. If none is found there, test at 45° and 135°.
- Refine axis first. Position the cross-cylinder axes 45° from the principal meridians of the correcting cylinder. Determine the preferred flip choice, and rotate the cylinder axis toward the corresponding axis of the cross cylinder. Repeat until the 2 flip choices appear equal.
- Refine cylinder power. Align the cross-cylinder axes with the principal meridians of the correcting cylinder. Determine the preferred flip choice, and add or subtract cylinder power according to the preferred position of the cross cylinder. Compensate

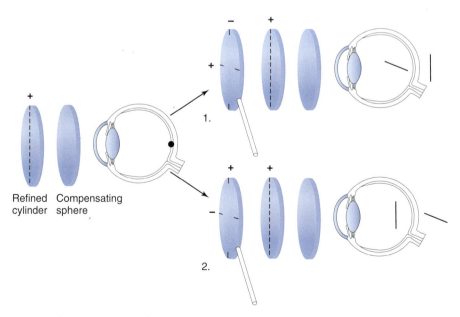

Figure 4-17 Correct endpoint for cross-cylinder refinement of cylinder power. Equal and opposite mixed astigmatism is provided by the 2 flip choices.

for the change in position of the circle of least confusion by adding half as much sphere in the opposite direction each time the cylinder power is changed.

• Refine sphere, cylinder axis, and cylinder power until no further change is necessary.

Guyton DL. *Subjective Refraction: Cross-Cylinder Technique.* Clinical Skills DVD Series [DVD]. San Francisco: American Academy of Ophthalmology; 1987.

Michaels DD. *Visual Optics and Refraction: A Clinical Approach.* 3rd ed. St Louis: Mosby; 1985:322–325.

Wunsh SE. The cross cylinder. In: Tasman W, Jaeger EA, eds. *Duane's Clinical Ophthalmology.* Philadelphia: Lippincott-Raven; 1995.

Refining the Sphere

After cylinder power and axis have been determined using either the astigmatic dial or the cross-cylinder method, the final step of monocular refraction is to refine the sphere. The endpoint in the refraction is the strongest plus, or weakest minus, sphere that yields the best visual acuity. We will briefly consider some of the methods used.

When the cross-cylinder technique has been used to determine the cylinder power and axis, the refractive error is presumed to a single point. Add plus sphere in +0.25 steps until the patient reports decreased vision. If no additional plus sphere is accepted, add minus sphere in –0.25 D steps until the patient achieves maximum acuity.

Using accommodation, the patient can compensate for excess minus sphere. Therefore, it is important to use the *least* minus necessary to reach maximum acuity. Accommodation creates, in effect, a reverse Galilean telescope, whereby the eye generates more plus power as minus power is added to the trial lenses before the eye. As this minus power increases, the patient observes that the letters appear smaller and more distant.

The patient should be told what to look for. Before subtracting each 0.25 D increment, tell the patient that the letters may appear sharper and clearer or smaller and darker, and ask the patient to report any such change. Reduce the amount of plus sphere only when the letters appear more clear.

If the astigmatic dial has been used and the astigmatism is neutralized (all the lines on the astigmatic dial are equally clear or equally blurred), the eye should still be fogged; additional plus will only increase the blur. Therefore, use minus spheres to reduce the sphere power until maximum acuity is achieved. Again, be careful not to overminus the patient.

To verify the spherical endpoint, the *duochrome* (*red-green* or *bichrome*) test is used. A split red-green filter makes the background of the acuity chart appear vertically divided into a red half and a green half. Because of the chromatic aberration of the eye, the shorter wavelengths (green) are focused in front of the longer red wavelengths. The eye typically focuses near the midpoint of the spectrum, between the red and green wavelengths. With optimal spherical correction, the letters on the red and green halves of the chart appear equally clear. The commercial filters used in the duochrome test produce a chromatic interval of about 0.50 D between the red and the green. When the image is clearly focused in white light, the eye is 0.25 D myopic for the green symbols and 0.25 D hyperopic for the red symbols.

Each eye is tested separately for the duochrome test, which is started with the eye slightly fogged (by 0.5 D to relax accommodation). The letters on the red side should appear more clear, and the clinician adds minus sphere until the 2 sides are equal. If the patient responds that the letters on the green side are sharper, the patient is overminused and more plus power should be added. Some clinicians use the RAM-GAP mnemonic— red *add* minus—green *add* plus—to help them with the duochrome test.

Because this test is based on chromatic aberration and not on color discrimination, it is used even with color-blind patients. The eye with overactive accommodation may still require too much minus sphere in order to balance the red and green. Cycloplegia may be necessary. The duochrome test is not used with patients whose visual acuity is worse than 20/30 (6/9), because the 0.50 D difference between the 2 sides is too small to distinguish.

Binocular Balance

The final, important step of subjective refraction is to make certain that accommodation has been relaxed equally in the 2 eyes. Several methods of binocular balance are commonly used. Most require that the corrected visual acuity be nearly equal in the 2 eyes.

Fogging

When the endpoint refraction is fogged using a +2.00 sphere before each eye, the visual acuity should be reduced to 20/200–20/100 (6/60–6/30). Place a –0.25 D sphere first before one eye and then the other, and rapidly alternate cover; the patient should then be able to identify the eye with the –0.25 D sphere before it as having the clearer image at the 20/100 (6/30) or 20/70 (6/20) level. If the eyes are not in balance, sphere should be added or subtracted in 0.25 steps until balance is achieved.

In addition to testing for binocular balance, the fogging method also provides information regarding appropriate sphere power. If either eye is overminused or underplussed, the patient reads farther down the chart, as far as 20/70 (6/20), 20/50 (6/15), or even 20/40 (6/12) with the +2.00 fogging spheres in place. In this case, the refraction endpoints should be reconsidered.

Prism dissociation

The most sensitive test of binocular balance is prism dissociation. For this test, the refractive endpoints are fogged with +1.00 spheres, and vertical prisms of 4 or 5 prism diopters (Δ) are placed before 1 eye. This causes the patient to see 2 charts, one above the other. A single line, usually 20/40 (6/12), is isolated on the chart, with the patient seeing 2 separate lines simultaneously, one for each eye. Differences between the fogged image in the 2 eyes of as little as 0.25 D sphere are readily identified. In practice, +0.25 D sphere is placed before 1 eye and then before the other. In each instance, if the eyes are balanced, the patient will report that the image corresponding to the eye with the additional +0.25 D sphere is more blurred. After a balance is established between the 2 eyes, remove the prism and reduce the fog binocularly until maximum visual acuity is obtained.

Cycloplegic and Noncycloplegic (Manifest) Refraction

Ideally, refractive error is measured with accommodation relaxed. The amount of habitual accommodative tone varies from person to person, and even within an individual it varies at times and with age. Because determining this variable may not always be possible, cycloplegic agents are sometimes used. The indication and appropriate dosage for a specific cycloplegic agent depend on the patient's age, accommodative amplitude, and refractive error.

A practical approach to satisfactory refraction is to perform a careful manifest refraction, ensuring relaxed accommodation with fogging or other nonpharmacologic techniques. If results are inconsistent or variable, a cycloplegic refraction should be performed. If the findings of these 2 refractions are similar, the prescription can be based on the manifest refraction. If there is a disparity, a postcycloplegic evaluation may be necessary. Most children require cycloplegic refraction because of their high amplitude of accommodation.

All cycloplegic agents produce mydriasis as well as cycloplegia. However, not all mydriatic agents produce cycloplegia. For example, sympathomimetic agents such as phenylephrine produce mydriasis without a significant effect on accommodation. Cycloplegic agents are classified on the basis of their intensity and duration of action (Table 4-1). In each instance, cycloplegia lasts somewhat longer than mydriasis.

Adverse effects occasionally occur with the use of all of these agents. The rapid absorption through the nasolacrimal mucosa promotes and augments the occurrence of systemic adverse effects. Atropine can produce dryness, flushing, high fever, and delirium. The most frequent complications of scopolamine are hallucinations and ataxia.

Table 4-1 Commonly Used Cycloplegic Agents

Drug	Concentration (%)	Dosage	Onset of Maximum Cycloplegia	Total Duration of Cycloplegia
Atropine sulfate[1]	0.5, 1.0	2–3 times/day for 3 days	1–2 hr	7–14 days
Scopolamine HBr[2]	0.25	2 drops separated by 5 min	30–60 min	3–4 days
Homatropine HBr[3]	2.0, 5.0		30–60 min	1–2 days
Cyclopentolate[3]	0.5, 1.0, 2.0		20–60 min	1–2 days
Tropicamide	0.5, 1.0, 2.0		20–40 min	4–6 hr

[1]Usually reserved for young children. May be prescribed in ointment or drop form. Adverse effects, such as flushing and fever, may be avoided by applying pressure over the puncta and canaliculi for 1–2 minutes after instilling atropine drops. The same precautions should be used for all cycloplegic-mydriatic drops.
[2]Rarely used for refraction but clinically useful in case of atropine allergy.
[3]The concentration needed will vary with the clinical problem. Higher concentrations of the agents are associated with an increased incidence of undesired side effects.

Overrefraction

Phoropters may be used to refract highly ametropic patients. Variability in the vertex distance of the refraction (the distance from the back surface of the spectacle lens to the cornea) and other induced errors make prescribing directly from the phoropter findings unreliable.

Some of these problems can be avoided if highly ametropic patients are refracted over their current glasses (overrefraction). If the new lenses are prescribed with the same base curve as the current lenses and are fitted in the same frames, many potential difficulties are circumvented, including vertex distance error and pantoscopic tilt error, as well as problems caused by marginal astigmatism and chromatic aberration. Overrefraction may be performed with loose lenses (using trial lens clips such as Halberg trial clips), with a standard phoropter in front of the patient's glasses, or with some automated refracting instruments.

If the patient is wearing spherical lenses, the new prescription is easy to calculate by combining the current spherical correction with the spherocylindrical overrefraction. If the current lenses are spherocylindrical and the cylinder axis of the overrefraction is not at 0° or 90° to the present correction, other methods are used to determine the resultant refraction. Such lens combinations were often determined with a lensmeter used to read the resultant lens power through the combinations of the old glasses and the overrefraction correction. This procedure is awkward and prone to error because the lenses may rotate with respect to each other on transfer to the lensmeter. Manual calculation is possible but complicated. Programmable calculators can be used to perform the trigonometric combination of cylinders at oblique axes, but they may not be readily available in the clinic.

Overrefraction has other uses. For example, a patient wearing a soft toric contact lens may undergo overrefraction for the purpose of ordering new lenses. Overrefraction can also be used in the retinoscopic examination of children.

Spectacle Correction of Ametropias

Ametropia is a refractive error; it is the absence of emmetropia. The most common method of correcting refractive error is by prescribing spectacle lenses.

Spherical Correcting Lenses and the Far Point Concept

The far point plane of the nonaccommodated eye is conjugate with the retina. For a simple lens, distant objects (those at optical infinity) come into sharp focus at the secondary focal point (f_2) of the lens. To correct the refractive error of an eye, a correcting lens must place the image it forms (or its f_2) at the eye's far point. The image at the far point plane becomes the object that is focused onto the retina. For example, in a myopic eye, the far point lies somewhere in front of the eye, between the eye and optical infinity. In this case, the correct *diverging* lens forms a virtual image of distant objects at its secondary focal point, coincident with the far point of the eye (Fig 4-18).

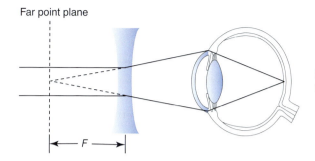

Far point plane

Figure 4-18 A diverging lens is used to correct myopia.

The same principle holds for the correction of hyperopia. However, because the far point plane of a hyperopic eye is behind the retina, a *converging* lens must be chosen in the appropriate power to focus parallel rays of light to the far point plane.

Vertex Distance

For any spherical correcting lens, the distance from the lens to its focal point is constant. Changing the position of the correcting lens relative to the eye will also change the relationship between the secondary focal point of the correcting lens and the far point plane of the eye. With high-power lenses, as used in the spectacle correction of aphakia or high myopia, a small change in the placement of the lens produces considerable blurring of vision unless the lens power is altered to compensate for the new lens position.

With refractive errors greater than ±5 D, the vertex distance must be accounted for in prescribing the power of the spectacle lens. Moving a correcting lens closer to the eye—whether the lens has plus or minus power—reduces its effective plus power (increases the minus power), whereas moving it farther from the eye increases its effective plus power (decreases the minus power).

For example, in Figure 4-19, the +10 D lens placed 10 mm from the cornea (assumed to be at the cornea) provides sharp retinal imagery. Because the secondary focal plane of the correcting lens is identical to the far point plane of the eye and because this lens is placed 1 cm in front of the eye, the far point plane of the eye must be 9 cm behind the cornea. If the correcting lens is moved to a new position 20 mm in front of the eye and the far point plane of the eye is 9 cm, the secondary focal plane of the new lens must be 11 cm, requiring a +9.1 D lens for correction. This example demonstrates the significance of vertex distance in spectacle correction of large refractive errors. Thus, the prescription must indicate not only the lens power but also the vertex distance at which the refraction was performed. The optician must recalculate the lens power as necessary for the actual vertex distance of the chosen spectacle–frame combination.

Cylindrical Correcting Lenses and the Far Point Concept

The far point principles used in the correction of hyperopia and myopia are also employed in the correction of astigmatism with spectacle lenses. However, in astigmatism, the required lens power must be determined separately for each of the 2 principal meridians.

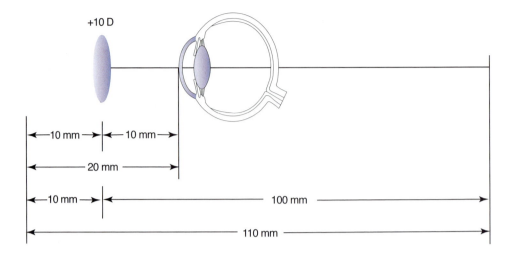

+10 D

10 mm

10 mm

20 mm

10 mm

100 mm

110 mm

Figure 4-19 The importance of vertex distance in the correction of high refractive errors.

Cylinders in spectacle lenses produce both monocular and binocular distortion. The primary cause is *meridional aniseikonia*—that is, unequal magnification of retinal images in the various meridians. Although aniseikonia may be corrected by iseikonic spectacles, such corrections may be complicated and expensive, and most practitioners prefer to prescribe cylinders according to their "clinical judgment." Clinical experience also suggests that adult patients vary in their ability to tolerate distortion, while younger children always adapt to their cylindrical corrections. The following guidelines may prove helpful in prescribing astigmatic spectacle corrections.

- For *children,* prescribe the full astigmatic correction at the correct axis.
- For *adults,* try the full correction initially. Give the patient a "walking-around" trial with trial frames before prescribing, if appropriate. Inform the patient about the need for adaptation.
- To reduce distortion, use minus cylinder lenses (most lenses dispensed today are minus cylinder) and minimize vertex distance.
- Spatial distortion from astigmatic spectacles is a binocular phenomenon. Occlude one eye to verify that this is the cause of the patient's difficulty.
- If necessary, reduce distortion by rotating the axis of the cylinder toward 180° or 90° (or toward the old axis) and/or reduce the cylinder power. Adjust the sphere to maintain spherical equivalent but rely on a final subjective check to obtain the most satisfactory visual result.
- If distortion cannot be reduced sufficiently, consider contact lenses or iseikonic corrections.

For a more detailed discussion of the problem of, and solutions for, spectacle correction of astigmatism, see Appendix: Common Guidelines for Prescribing Cylinders.

Prescribing for Children

The correction of ametropia in children presents several special and challenging problems. In adults, the correction of refractive errors has one measurable endpoint: the best-corrected visual acuity. Prescribing visual correction for children often has 2 goals: providing a focused retinal image and achieving the optimal balance between accommodation and convergence.

In some patients, *subjective refraction* may be impossible or inappropriate, often because of the child's inability to cooperate with subjective refraction techniques. In addition, the optimal refraction in an infant or a small child (particularly with esotropia) requires the *paralysis of accommodation* with complete cycloplegia. (In such cases, objective techniques such as retinoscopy are the best way to determine the refractive correction.) Moreover, the presence of *strabismus* may modify normal prescribing guidelines.

Myopia

Childhood myopia falls into 2 groups: *congenital* (usually high) myopia and *developmental* myopia, usually manifesting itself between ages 7 and 10 years. The latter type of myopia is less severe and easier to manage, as the patients are older and refraction is less difficult. However, both forms of myopia are progressive; frequent refractions (every 6–12 months) and periodic prescription changes are necessary. The following are general guidelines for correction of significant childhood myopia:

- Cycloplegic refractions are mandatory. In infants, esotropic children, and children with very high myopia (>10 D), atropine refraction may be necessary if tropicamide (Mydriacyl) or cyclopentolate fails to paralyze accommodation in the office.
- In general, the full refractive error, including cylinder, should be corrected. Young children tolerate cylinder well.
- Some ophthalmologists undercorrect myopia, and others use bifocals with or without atropine, on the theory that accommodation hastens or increases the development of myopia. However, the results of studies on this theory are inconclusive.
- Intentional undercorrection of a child with myopic esotropia to decrease the angle of deviation is rarely tolerated.
- Intentional overcorrection of a myopic error (or undercorrection of a hyperopic error) can be of some value in controlling intermittent exodeviations.
- Parents should be educated about the natural progression of myopia and the need for frequent refractions and possible prescription changes.
- Contact lenses may be desirable in older children to avoid the problem of image minification found with high-minus lenses.

Hyperopia

The appropriate correction of childhood hyperopia is more complex than that of myopia. First, children who are significantly hyperopic (>5 D) are more visually impaired than their myopic counterparts, who can at least see clearly at near. Second, childhood hyperopia is more frequently associated with strabismus and abnormalities of the accommodative convergence/accommodation (AC/A) ratio. The following are general guidelines for correcting childhood hyperopia:

- Unless there is esodeviation or evidence of reduced vision, it is not necessary to correct low hyperopia. As with myopia, significant astigmatic errors should be fully corrected.
- When hyperopia and esotropia coexist, initial management includes full correction of the cycloplegic refractive error. Reductions in the amount of correction may be appropriate later, depending on the amount of esotropia and level of stereopsis with the full cycloplegic correction in place.
- In a school-aged child, the full refractive correction may cause blurring of distance vision because of the inability to relax accommodation fully. Reducing the amount of correction is sometimes necessary for the child to accept the glasses. A short course of cycloplegia may help a child to accept the hyperopic correction.

Anisometropia

An anisometropic child or infant is typically prescribed the full refractive difference between the 2 eyes, regardless of age, presence or amount of strabismus, or degree of anisometropia.

Anisometropic amblyopia is frequently present and may require occlusion therapy. Amblyopia is more common in conjunction with anisohyperopia than with either anisomyopia or antimetropia. Bilateral amblyopia occasionally occurs when high amounts of hyperopia, myopia, and/or astigmatism occur in both eyes.

Clinical Accommodative Problems

See also Chapter 3, Optics of the Human Eye, for a discussion of the terminology and mechanisms of accommodation.

Presbyopia

Presbyopia is the gradual loss of accommodative response resulting from reduced elasticity of the crystalline lens. Accommodative amplitude diminishes with age. It becomes a clinical problem when the remaining accommodative amplitude is insufficient for the patient to read and carry out near-vision tasks. Fortunately, appropriate convex lenses can compensate for the waning of accommodative power.

Symptoms of presbyopia usually begin after age 40 years. The age of onset depends on preexisting refractive error, depth of focus (pupil size), the patient's visual tasks, and other variables. Table 4-2 presents a simplified overview of age norms.

Accommodative Insufficiency

Accommodative insufficiency is the *premature* loss of accommodative amplitude. This problem may manifest itself by blurring of near visual objects (as in presbyopia) or by the inability to sustain accommodative effort. The onset may be heralded by the development

Table 4-2 Average Accommodative Amplitudes for Different Ages

Age	Average Accommodative Amplitude*
8	14.0 (±2 D)
12	13.0 (±2 D)
16	12.0 (±2 D)
20	11.0 (±2 D)
24	10.0 (±2 D)
28	9.0 (±2 D)
32	8.0 (±2 D)
36	7.0 (±2 D)
40	6.0 (±2 D)
44	4.5 (±1.5 D)
48	3.0 (±1.5 D)
52	2.5 (±1.5 D)
56	2.0 (±1.0 D)
60	1.5 (±1.0 D)
64	1.0 (±0.5 D)
68	0.5 (±0.5 D)

*Under age 40, accommodation decreases by 1 D for each 4 years. Over age 40, accommodation decreases more rapidly. From age 48 on, 0.5 D is lost every 4 years. Thus, one can recall the entire table by remembering the amplitudes at age 40 and age 48.

of asthenopic symptoms, with the ultimate development of blurred near vision. Such "premature presbyopia" may signify concurrent or past debilitating illness, or it may be induced by medications such as tranquilizing drugs or the parasympatholytics used in treating some gastrointestinal disorders. In both cases, the condition may be reversible; however, permanent accommodative insufficiency may be associated with neurogenic disorders such as encephalitis or closed head trauma. In some cases, the etiology may never be determined. These patients require reading add for near vision.

Accommodative Excess

Ciliary muscle spasm, often incorrectly termed *spasm of accommodation,* causes accommodative excess. A ciliary spasm has characteristic symptoms: headache, brow ache, variable blurring of distance vision, and an abnormally close near point. Ciliary spasm may occur as a manifestation of local disease such as iridocyclitis; it may be caused by medications such as the anticholinesterases used in the treatment of glaucoma; or it may be associated with uncorrected refractive errors, usually hyperopia but also astigmatism. In some patients, ciliary spasm exacerbates preexisting myopia. It also occurs after prolonged and intense periods of near work. *Spasm of the near reflex* is a characteristic clinical syndrome often seen in tense or anxious persons presenting with (1) excess accommodation, (2) excess convergence, and (3) miosis.

Accommodative Convergence/Accommodation Ratio

Normally, accommodative effort is accompanied by a corresponding convergence effort (expressed in terms of meter angles). Thus, 1 D of accommodation would be accompanied by a 1-m angle of convergence. For practical purposes, the AC/A ratio is ordinarily expressed in terms of prism diopters of deviation per diopter of accommodation. Using this type of expression, the normal AC/A ratio is 3:1–5:1.

The AC/A ratio is relatively constant for each person, but fortunately there can be some variability among individuals. For example, a patient with an uncorrected 1 D of hyperopia may accommodate 1 D for clear distance vision without exercising a convergence effort. Conversely, a patient with uncorrected myopia must converge without accommodative effort in order to see clearly at the far point of the eye.

The AC/A ratio can be measured by varying the stimulus to accommodation in several ways.

Heterophoria method (moving the fixation target)

The heterophoria is measured at 6 m and again at 0.33 m.

$$\text{AC/A} = \text{PD} + \frac{\Delta n - \Delta d}{\text{D}}$$

where

PD = interpupillary distance in centimeters
Δn = near deviation in prism diopters
Δd = distance deviation in prism diopters
D = diopters of accommodation

Sign convention:
Esodeviations +
Exodeviations –

Gradient method

The AC/A ratio can be measured in 1 of 2 ways using the gradient method. The first way is by *stimulating accommodation*. Measure the heterophoria with the target distance fixed at 6 m. Then remeasure the induced phoria after interposing a –1 D sphere in front of both eyes. The AC/A ratio is the difference between the 2 measurements.

The second way is by *relaxing accommodation*. With the target distance fixed at 0.33 m, measure the phoria before and after interposing +3 D spheres. The phoria difference divided by 3 is the AC/A ratio.

An abnormal AC/A ratio can place stress on the patient's fusional mechanisms at one distance or another, leading to asthenopia or manifest strabismus. Abnormal AC/A ratios should be accounted for when prescribing corrective lenses.

Parks MM. Vergences. In: Tasman W, Jaeger EA, eds. *Duane's Clinical Ophthalmology*. Philadelphia: Lippincott-Raven; 1995.

Effect of Spectacle and Contact Lens Correction on Accommodation and Convergence

Both accommodation and convergence requirements differ between contact lenses and spectacle lenses. The effects become more noticeable as the power of the correction increases.

Let us consider accommodative requirements first. Remember that because of vertex distance considerations, particularly with high-power corrections, the dioptric power of the distance correction in the spectacle plane is different from that at the contact lens plane: For a near object held at a constant distance, the amount that an eye needs to accommodate depends on the location of the refractive correction relative to the cornea. Patients with myopia must accommodate more for a given near object when wearing contact lenses than when wearing glasses. For example, those with myopia in their early 40s who switch from single-vision glasses to contact lenses may suddenly experience presbyopic symptoms. The reverse is true with patients with hyperopia; the spectacle correction requires more accommodation for a given near object than the contact lens correction. Patients with spectacle-corrected high myopia, when presbyopic, need only weak bifocal adds or none at all. For example, a highly myopic patient wearing –20 D glasses needs to accommodate only about 1 D to see an object at 33 cm.

Now let us consider convergence requirements and refractive correction. Because contact lenses move with the eyes and glasses do not, different amounts of convergence are required for viewing near objects. Spectacle correction gives a myopic patient a base-in prism effect when converging and thus reduces the patient's requirement for convergence. (Fortunately, this reduction parallels the lessened requirement for accommodation.) In contrast, the patient with spectacle-corrected hyperopia encounters a base-out prism effect that increases the requirement for convergence. This effect is beneficial in the correction of residual esotropia at near in patients with hyperopia and accommodative esotropia. These effects may be the source of a patient's symptoms on switching between glasses and contact lenses. (See also Chapter 5, Contact Lenses.)

Prescribing Multifocal Lenses

A multifocal lens has 2 or more refractive elements. The power of each segment is prescribed separately.

Determining the Power of a Bifocal Add

The information necessary to prescribe bifocals includes (1) an accurate baseline refraction, (2) the accommodative amplitude, and (3) the patient's social or occupational activities that require near-vision correction (eg, reading, sewing, or computer use).

Measuring accommodative amplitude

Any of the following tests can provide useful information for determining the accommodative amplitude: (1) the near point of accommodation with accurate distance refractive correction in place, (2) the accommodative rule (eg, with a Prince rule), (3) the use of plus and minus spheres at near distance until the fixation target blurs. *Binocular amplitude of accommodation* is normally greater than the measurement for either eye alone by 0.5–1.0 D.

Near point of accommodation A practical method of measuring the near point of accommodation is to have the patient fixate on a near target (most commonly, small print such as 5-point or Jaeger 2 type print) and move the test card toward the eye until the print blurs. If the eye is emmetropic (or rendered emmetropic by proper refractive correction), the far point of the eye will be at infinity, and the near point can be converted into diopters of amplitude.

This method is subject to certain errors, one of which is the apparent increased amplitude resulting from angular magnification of the letters as they approach the eye. In addition, if the eye is ametropic and not corrected for distance, the near point of accommodation cannot be converted into diopters of amplitude. In the following examples, each eye has 3 D of accommodative amplitude:

- A person with emmetropia will have a near point of 33 cm and a far point at optical infinity.
- A patient with an uncorrected 3 D of myopia will have a near point at 16.7 cm, because at the far point of 33 cm no accommodation is needed.
- A patient with an uncorrected 3 D of hyperopia will have a near point at infinity, because all of the available accommodation is needed to overcome the hyperopia.

Accommodative rule   Amplitude of accommodation can be measured with a device such as a Prince rule, which combines a reading card with a ruler calibrated in centimeters and diopters. Placing a +3 D lens before the emmetropic (or accurately corrected ametropic) eye places the far point of accommodation at 33 cm, and the near point will also be brought a corresponding 3 D closer. The amplitude is then determined by subtraction of the far point (in diopters) from the near point (in diopters).

Method of spheres   Amplitude of accommodation may also be measured by having the patient fixate on a reading target at 40 cm. Accommodation is stimulated by the placement of successively stronger minus spheres before the eye until the print blurs; accommodation is then relaxed by the use of successively stronger plus lenses until blurring begins. The difference between the 2 lenses is a measure of accommodative amplitude. For example, if the patient accepted –3 D to blur (stimulus to accommodation) and +2.5 D to blur (relaxation of accommodation), the amplitude would be 5.5 D.

Range of accommodation

Determining the range of accommodation, like measuring the amplitude of accommodation, is valuable in ensuring that a prescribed bifocal add meets the patient's visual needs. The range of accommodation measures the useful range of clear vision when a given lens is employed. For this purpose, a measuring tape, meter stick, or accommodation rule may be used.

Selecting an add

Determine the amount of accommodation required for the patient's near-vision tasks. For example, reading at 40 cm would require 2.5 D of accommodation. From the patient's measured accommodative amplitude, allow one-half to be held in reserve. For instance, if the patient has 2.0 D of accommodation, 1.0 may be comfortably contributed by the patient. (Some patients may use more than one-half of their available accommodation with comfort.) Subtract the patient's available accommodation (1.0 D) from the total amount of accommodation required (2.5 D); the difference (1.5 D) is the approximate additional plus-lens power (add) needed.

Place this add in front of the distance refractive correction, and measure the accommodative *range* (near point to far point of accommodation in centimeters). Does this range adequately meet the requirements of the patient's near-vision activities? If the accommodative range is too close, reduce the add in steps of 0.25 D until the range is appropriate for the patient's requirement.

Because binocular accommodative amplitude is usually 0.5–1.0 D greater than the monocular measurement, using the binocular measurement generally guards against prescribing too high an add.

Types of Bifocal Lenses

Most bifocals dispensed today are 1-piece bifocals, made by generating the different refracting surfaces on a single lens blank (Fig 4-20). *Round segment* 1-piece bifocals have their segment on the concave surface. One-piece molded *plastic bifocals* are available in various shapes, including (1) round top with button on convex surface, (2) flat top with button on convex surface, and (3) Franklin style with split bifocal.

With *fused bifocals,* the increased refracting power of the bifocal segment is produced by fusing a button of glass that has a higher refractive index than the basic crown glass lens into a countersink in the crown glass lens blank. With all such bifocals, the add segment is fused into the convex surface of the lens; astigmatic corrections, when necessary, are ground on the concave surface.

Trifocal Lenses

A bifocal lens may not fully satisfy all the visual needs of an older patient with limited accommodation. Even when near and distant ranges are corrected appropriately, vision will not be clear in the intermediate range, approximately at arm's length. This problem can be solved with trifocal spectacles, which incorporate a third segment of intermediate strength (typically one-half the power of the reading add) between the distance correction and reading segment. The intermediate segment allows the patient to focus on objects beyond the reading distance but closer than 1 m. (See Clinical Example 4-1.)

Progressive Addition Lenses

Both bifocals and trifocals have an abrupt change in power as the line of sight passes across the boundary between one portion of the lens and the next; image jump and diplopia can occur at the segment lines. Progressive addition lenses (PALs) avoid these difficulties by supplying power gradually as the line of sight is depressed toward the reading level. Unlike bifocals and trifocals, PALs offer clear vision at all focal distances. Other advantages of PALs include lack of intermediate blur and absence of any visible segment lines.

The progressive addition lens form has 4 optical zones on the convex surface: a spherical distance zone, a reading zone, a transition zone (or "corridor"), and zones of peripheral distortion. The progressive change in lens power is generated on the convex surface

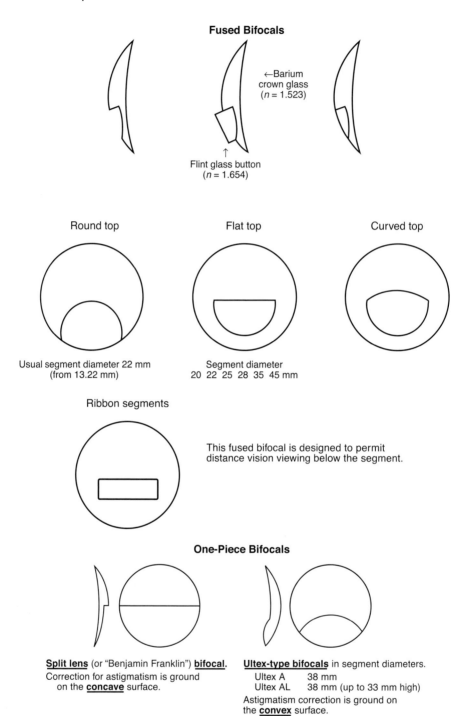

Fused Bifocals

←Barium
crown glass
(*n* = 1.523)

↑
Flint glass button
(*n* = 1.654)

Round top

Usual segment diameter 22 mm
(from 13.22 mm)

Flat top

Segment diameter
20 22 25 28 35 45 mm

Curved top

Ribbon segments

This fused bifocal is designed to permit
distance vision viewing below the segment.

One-Piece Bifocals

Split lens (or "Benjamin Franklin") **bifocal.**
Correction for astigmatism is ground
on the **concave** surface.

Ultex-type bifocals in segment diameters.
  Ultex A   38 mm
  Ultex AL   38 mm (up to 33 mm high)
Astigmatism correction is ground on
the **convex** surface.

Figure 4-20 Bifocal lens styles.

CLINICAL EXAMPLE 4-1

Consider a patient with 1 D of available accommodation. He wears a bifocal with a +2.00 add. His accommodative range for each part of the spectacle lens is:

> *Distance segment:* Infinity to 100 cm
> *Bifocal segment:* 50–33 cm

He now has a blurred zone between 50 and 100 cm. An intermediate segment, in this case +1.00 D (half the power of the reading segment), would provide sharp vision from 50 cm (using all of his available accommodation plus the +1.00 D add) to 100 cm (using the add only). This trifocal combination therefore provides the following ranges:

> *Distance segment:* Infinity to 100 cm
> *Intermediate segment:* 100–50 cm
> *Near segment:* 50–33 cm

of the lens by progressive aspheric changes in curvature from the top to the bottom of the lens. The concave surface is reserved for the sphere and cylinder of the patient's distance lens prescription.

However, there are certain drawbacks to PALs. Most notably, some degree of peripheral distortion is inherent in the design of all PALs. This peripheral aberration is caused by astigmatism resulting from the changing aspheric curves, most pronounced in the lower inner and outer quadrants of the lens. These distortions produce a "swimming" sensation with head movement.

The vertical meridian joining the distance and reading optical centers is free of surface astigmatism and affords maximum visual acuity. To either side of this distortion-free vertical meridian, induced astigmatism and a concomitant degradation of acuity occur. If the lens is designed so that the peripheral distortions are spread out over a relatively wide portion of the lens, there is a concomitant decrease in the distortion-free principal zones. This is the basis of soft-design PALs (Fig 4-21). Conversely, a wider distortion-free zone for distance and reading means a more intense deformity laterally. This is the basis of hard-design PALs. If the transition corridor is lengthened, the distortions are less pronounced, but problems arise because of the greater vertical separation between the distance optical center and the reading zone. Therefore, each PAL design represents a series of compromises. Some manufacturers prefer less distortion at the expense of less useful aberration-free distance and near acuity; others opt for maximum acuity over a wider usable area, with smaller but more pronounced lateral distortion zones.

PALs are readily available from –8.00 to +7.50 D spheres and up to 4.00 D cylinders, with adds from +1.50 to +3.50 D. Some vendors also make custom lenses with parameters outside these limits. Prism can be incorporated into PALs.

The best candidates for PALs are patients with early presbyopia who have not previously worn bifocals, patients who do not require wide near-vision fields, and highly

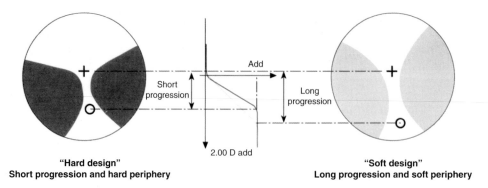

Figure 4-21 Comparison of hard-design and soft-design PALs. These illustrations compare the power progression and peripheral aberration of these 2 PAL designs. *(From Wisnicki HJ. Bifocals, trifocals, and progressive-addition lenses. Focal Points: Clinical Modules for Ophthalmologists. San Francisco: American Academy of Ophthalmology; 1999, module 6.)*

motivated patients. The patient who changes from conventional multifocals to PALs should be advised that distortion will be present and that adaptation will be necessary. The key to successful prescribing is careful patient selection.

The Prentice Rule and Bifocal Design

There are special considerations when prescribing lenses for patients with significant anisometropias.

Prismatic effects of lenses

All lenses act as prisms when one looks through the lens at any point other than the optical center. The amount of the induced prismatic effect depends on the power of the lens and the distance from the optical center. Specifically, the amount of prismatic effect (measured in prism diopters) is equal to the distance (in centimeters) from the optical center multiplied by the lens power (in diopters). This is known as the *Prentice rule*.

$$\Delta = hD$$

where

Δ = prism diopters
h = distance from optical center (in cm)
D = diopters

Image displacement

When reading at near through a point below the optical center, a patient wearing spectacle lenses of unequal power may notice vertical double vision. With a bifocal segment, the gaze is usually directed 8–10 mm below and 1.5–3.0 mm nasal to the distance optical center of the distance lens (in the following examples, we assume the usual 8 mm down and 2 mm nasal). As long as the bifocal segments are of the same power and type, the prismatic displacement is determined by the power of the distance lens alone.

If the lens powers are the same for the 2 eyes, the displacement will be the same (Figs 4-22 and 4-23). However, if the patient is anisometropic, a phoria will be induced by the unequal prismatic displacement of the 2 lenses (Figs 4-24 and 4-25). The amount of *vertical* phoria is determined by subtracting the smaller prismatic displacement from the larger if the lenses are both myopic or both hyperopic (see Fig 4-24) or by adding the two if the patient is hyperopic in one eye and myopic in the other (see Fig 4-25).

For determination of the induced *horizontal* phoria, the induced prisms are added if both eyes are hyperopic or both eyes are myopic; if one eye is hyperopic and the other myopic, the smaller amount of prismatic displacement is subtracted from the larger (see Fig 4-25).

Image displacement is minimized when round-top segment bifocals are used with plus lenses and flat-top segment bifocals are used with minus lenses (Fig 4-26).

Image jump

The usual position of the top of a bifocal segment is 5 mm below the optical center of the distance lens. As the eyes are directed downward through a lens, the prismatic

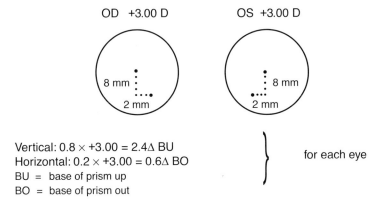

Vertical: 0.8 × +3.00 = 2.4Δ BU
Horizontal: 0.2 × +3.00 = 0.6Δ BO
BU = base of prism up
BO = base of prism out

for each eye

Figure 4-22 Prismatic effect of bifocals in isometropic hyperopia.

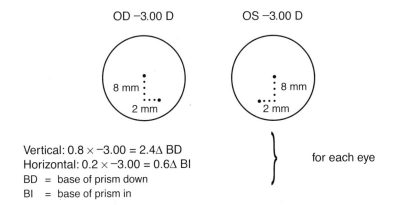

Vertical: 0.8 × −3.00 = 2.4Δ BD
Horizontal: 0.2 × −3.00 = 0.6Δ BI
BD = base of prism down
BI = base of prism in

for each eye

Figure 4-23 Prismatic effect of bifocals in isometropic myopia.

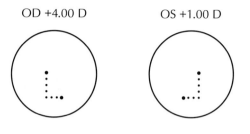

OD +4.00 D   OS +1.00 D

Vertical: OD 0.8 × 4 = 3.2Δ BU   OS 0.8 × 1 = 0.8Δ BU
Horizontal: OD 0.2 × 4 = 0.8Δ BO   OS 0.2 × 1 = 0.2Δ BO
Induced phoria: OD 3.2Δ − 0.8Δ = 2.4Δ BU
                OD 0.8Δ BO + 0.2Δ BO = 1.0Δ BO

Figure 4-24   Prismatic effect of bifocals in anisometropic hyperopia.

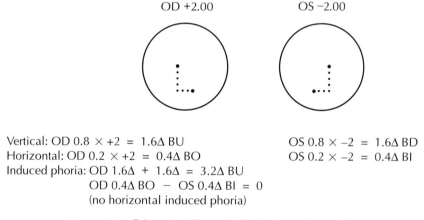

OD +2.00   OS −2.00

Vertical: OD 0.8 × +2 = 1.6Δ BU   OS 0.8 × −2 = 1.6Δ BD
Horizontal: OD 0.2 × +2 = 0.4Δ BO   OS 0.2 × −2 = 0.4Δ BI
Induced phoria: OD 1.6Δ + 1.6Δ = 3.2Δ BU
                OD 0.4Δ BO − OS 0.4Δ BI = 0
                (no horizontal induced phoria)

Figure 4-25   Prismatic effect of bifocals in antimetropia.

displacement of the image increases (downward in plus lenses, upward in minus lenses). When the eyes encounter the top of a bifocal segment, they meet a new plus lens with a different optical center, and the object appears to jump upward unless the optical center of the add is at the very top of the segment (Fig 4-27). Executive-style segments have their optical centers at the top of the segment. The optical center of a typical flat-top segment is located 3 mm below the top of the segment. It is apparent that the closer the optical center of the segment approaches the top edge of the segment, the less the image jump. Thus, flat-top segments produce less image jump than round-top segments because the latter have much lower optical centers.

Patients with myopia who wear round-top bifocals would be more bothered by image jump than patients with hyperopia because it occurs in the direction of image displacement. Thus, it is good practice to avoid prescribing round-top bifocal segments to those with myopia.

Compensating for induced anisophoria

When anisometropia is corrected with spectacle lenses, unequal prism is introduced in all secondary positions of gaze. This prism may be the source of symptoms, even diplopia.

With plus lenses:

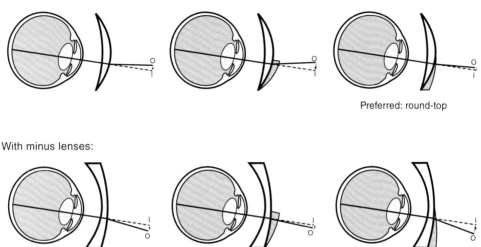

Preferred: round-top

With minus lenses:

Preferred: flat-top

Figure 4-26 Image displacement through bifocal segments. *(From Wisnicki HJ. Bifocals, trifocals, and progressive-addition lenses.* Focal Points: Clinical Modules for Ophthalmologists. *San Francisco: American Academy of Ophthalmology; 1999, module 6. Reprinted with permission from Guyton DL.* Ophthalmic Optics and Clinical Refraction. *Baltimore: Prism Press; 1998. Redrawn by C. H. Wooley.)*

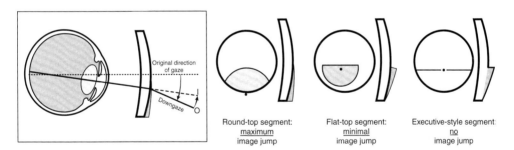

Round-top segment:
maximum
image jump

Flat-top segment:
minimal
image jump

Executive-style segment:
no
image jump

Figure 4-27 Image jump through bifocal segments. If the optical center of a segment is at its top, no image jump occurs. *(From Wisnicki HJ. Bifocals, trifocals, and progressive-addition lenses.* Focal Points: Clinical Modules for Ophthalmologists. *San Francisco: American Academy of Ophthalmology; 1999, module 6. Reprinted with permission from Guyton DL.* Ophthalmic Optics and Clinical Refraction. *Baltimore: Prism Press; 1998. Redrawn by C. H. Wooley.)*

Symptomatic anisophoria occurs especially when a patient with early presbyopia uses his or her first pair of bifocals or when the anisometropia is of recent and/or sudden origin, as occurs following retinal detachment surgery, with gradual asymmetrical progression of cataracts, or after unilateral intraocular lens implantation. The patient usually adapts to horizontal imbalance by increasing head rotation but may have symptoms when looking down, in the reading position. Remember that horizontal vergence amplitudes are large compared to vertical fusional amplitudes, which are typically less than 2Δ. We can calculate the amount of induced phoria by using the Prentice rule (Fig 4-28).

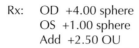

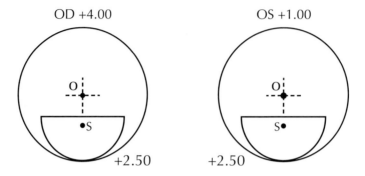

O = optical center, distance
S = optical center of segment
R (= S): Reading position 8 mm below distance optical center

Figure 4-28 Calculating induced anisophoria.

At the reading point, 8 mm below distance optical center:

OD	4.0×0.8	=	3.2Δ BU
OS	1.0×0.8	=	0.8Δ BU
Net difference			2.4Δ BU

In this example, there is an induced right hyperdeviation of 2.4Δ. Conforming to the usual practice in the management of heterophorias, approximately two-thirds to three-fourths of the vertical phoria should be corrected—in this case, 1.75Δ. This correction may be accomplished in several ways.

Press-On prisms With Press-On prisms (3M, St Paul, MN), 2Δ BD may be added to the right segment (in the preceding example) or 2Δ BU to the left segment.

Bicentric grinding ("slab-off") The most satisfactory method of compensating for the induced vertical phoria in anisometropia is the technique of bicentric grinding *(slab-off)* (Fig 4-29). In this method, 2 optical centers are created in the lens having the greater minus (or less plus) power, counteracting the base-down effect of the greater minus lens in the reading position. It is convenient to think of the slab-off process as creating *base-up* prism over the reading area of the lens.

Bicentric grinding is used for single-vision lenses as well as multifocals. By increasing the distance between the 2 optical centers, this method achieves as much as 4Δ of prism compensation at the reading position.

Reverse slab-off Prism correction in the reading position is achieved not only by removing base-down prism from the lower part of the more minus lens (slabbing off) but also by

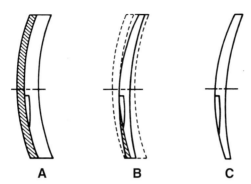

Figure 4-29 Bicentric grinding. **A,** Lens form with a dummy lens cemented to the front surface. **B,** Both surfaces of the lens are reground with the same curvatures but removing base-up prism from the top segment of the front surface and removing base-down prism from the entire rear surface. **C,** The effect is a lens that has had base-down prism removed from the lower segment only.

adding base-down prism to the lower half of the more plus lens. This technique is known as *reverse slab-off*.

Historically, it was easy to *remove* material from a standard lens. Today, with plastic lenses fabricated by molding, it is more convenient to *add* material so as to create a base-down prism in the lower half of what will be the more plus lens. Because plastic lenses account for a majority of the lenses dispensed, reverse slab-off is the most common method of correcting anisometropically induced anisophoria.

When the clinician is ordering a lens that requires prism correction for an anisophoria in downgaze, it is often appropriate to leave the choice of slab-off versus reverse slab-off to the optician by including a statement in the prescription such as, "Slab-off right lens 3Δ (or reverse slab-off left lens)." In either case, the prescribed prism should be measured in the reading position, not calculated, because the patient may have partially adapted to the anisophoria.

Dissimilar segments　In anisometropic bifocal lens prescriptions, vertical prism compensation can also be achieved by the use of dissimilar bifocal segments with their optical centers at 2 different heights. The segment with the lower optical center should be placed in front of the more hyperopic (or less myopic) eye to provide base-down prism. (This method contrasts with the bicentric grinding method, which produces base-up prism and is therefore employed on the lesser plus or greater minus lens.)

In the example shown (Fig 4-30), a 22-mm round segment has been chosen for the right eye, and the top of its segment is at the usual 5 mm below the distance optical center. For the left eye, a 22-mm flat-top segment is used, again with the top of the segment 5 mm below the optical center.

Because the optical center of the flat-top segment is 3 mm below the top of the segment, it is at the patient's reading position and that segment will introduce no prismatic effect. However, for the right eye, the optical center of the round segment is 8 mm below the patient's reading position, and, by the Prentice rule, this 2.5 D segment will produce $2.5 \times 0.8 = 2.0\Delta$ base-down prism.

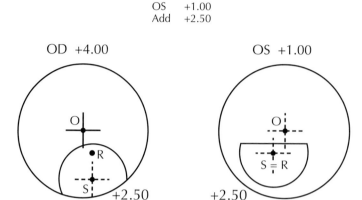

O = optical center, distance
S = optical center of segment
R (= S): Reading position 8 mm below distance optical center

Figure 4-30 Dissimilar segments used to compensate for anisophoria in anisometropic bifocal prescriptions.

Single-vision reading glasses with lowered optical centers Partial compensation for the induced vertical phoria at the reading position can be obtained with single-vision reading glasses, with the optical centers placed 3–4 mm below the pupillary centers in primary gaze. The patient's gaze will be directed much closer to the optical centers of the lenses when reading.

Contact lenses Contact lenses can be prescribed for patients with significant anisometropia that causes a symptomatic anisophoria in downgaze. Reading glasses can be worn over the contacts if the patient is presbyopic.

Refractive surgery Refractive surgery may be an option for some patients with symptomatic anisometropia or anisophoria.

Occupation and Bifocal Segment

The *dioptric power* of a segment depends on the patient's accommodative reserve and the working distance required for each specific job. It must be emphasized that such focal length determinations are a characteristic not of the job but of the individual patient's adaptation to that job. If the patient is allowed to use half of his or her available accommodation (which must be *measured*), the remainder of the dioptric requirement will be met by the bifocal add. For example, if the job is proofreading at 40 cm, the dioptric requirement for that focal length is 2.5 D. If the patient's accommodative amplitude is 2.0 D, and half of that (1.0 D) is used for the job, the balance of 1.5 D becomes the necessary bifocal add.

It is essential that the *accommodative range* (near point to far point) be *measured* and be adequate for the job.

Lens design

The most important characteristic of the bifocal segment is the segment *height* in relation to the patient's pupillary center. The lenses will be unsuitable if the segment is placed too high or too low for the specific occupational need.

Segment *width* is substantially less important. The popular impression that very large bifocals mean better reading capability is not supported by projection measurements. At a 40-cm reading distance, a 25-mm flat-top segment provides a horizontal reading field of 50–55 cm.

At a 40-cm distance, an individual habitually uses face rotation to increase his or her fixation field when it exceeds 45 cm (30° of arc); therefore, a 25-mm-wide segment is more than adequate for all but a few special occupations, such as a graphic artist or an architectural drafter using a drawing board. Furthermore, with a 35-mm segment producing a horizontal field 75 cm wide, the focal length at the extremes of the fixation field would be 55 cm, not 40 cm! Therefore, the split bifocal is useful not because it is a wider bifocal but because of its monocentric construction.

The *shape* of the segment must be considered. For example, round-top segments (Kryptok, Ultex type) require the user to look well down in the segment in order to employ their maximum horizontal dimension. In addition, they exaggerate image jump, especially in myopic corrections.

Segment decentration   To avoid inducing a base-out prism effect when the bifocal-wearing patient converges for near-vision tasks, the reading segment is generally decentered inward. This is especially important in aphakic spectacles. The following are some considerations for proper decentration:

- *Working distance.* Because the convergence requirement increases as the focal length decreases, additional inward decentration of the bifocal segment is required.
- *Interpupillary distance.* The wider the interpupillary distance, the greater the convergence requirement and, correspondingly, the need for inward decentration of the segments.
- *Lens power.* If the distance lens is a high-plus lens, it will create a greater base-out prism effect (ie, induced exophoria) as the viewer converges. Additional inward decentration of the segments may be helpful. The reverse would be true for high-minus lenses.
- *Existing heterophoria.* As with lens-induced phorias, the presence of an existing exophoria suggests increasing the inward decentration; an esophoria would call for the opposite approach.

Prescribing Special Lenses

Some patients require special prescription lenses.

Aphakic Lenses

The problems of correcting aphakia with high-plus spectacle lenses are well known and have been described eloquently by Alan C. Woods (1952). They include

- magnification of approximately 20%–35%
- altered depth perception resulting from the magnification
- pincushion distortion; for example, doors appear to bow inward
- difficulty with hand–eye coordination
- ring scotoma generated by prismatic effects at the edge of the lens (causing the "jack-in-the-box" phenomenon)
- extreme sensitivity of the lenses to minor misadjustment in vertex distance, pantoscopic tilt, and height
- in monocular aphakia, loss of useful binocular vision because of differential magnification

In addition, aphakic spectacles create cosmetic problems. The patient's eyes appear magnified and, if viewed obliquely, may seem displaced because of prismatic effects. The high-power lenticular lens is itself unattractive with its "fried-egg" appearance.

For all these reasons, intraocular lenses and aphakic contact lenses now account for the great majority of aphakic corrections. Nevertheless, spectacle correction of aphakia is sometimes appropriate, as in pediatric aphakia.

Refracting technique

Because of the sensitivity of aphakic glasses to vertex distance and pantoscopic tilt, it is nearly impossible to refract an aphakic eye reliably using a phoropter. The vertex distance and the pantoscopic tilt are not well controlled, nor are they necessarily close to the values for the final spectacles. Rather than a phoropter, trial frames or lens clips are used.

The trial frame allows the refractionist to control vertex distance and pantoscopic tilt. It should be adjusted for minimal vertex distance and for the same pantoscopic tilt planned for the actual spectacles (about 5°–7°, not the larger values appropriate for conventional glasses).

Another good technique is to refract with clip-on trial lens holders placed over the patient's existing aphakic glasses (overrefraction). Care should be taken that the center of the clip coincides with the optical center of the existing lens. Even if the present lens contains a cylinder at an axis different from what is needed, it is possible to calculate the resultant spherocylindrical correction with an electronic calculator, by hand, or with measurement of the combination in a lensmeter.

Guyton DL. *Retinoscopy. Minus Cylinder Technique.* Clinical Skills DVD Series [DVD]. San Francisco: American Academy of Ophthalmology; 1986.

Guyton DL. *Retinoscopy. Plus Cylinder Technique.* Clinical Skills DVD Series [DVD]. San Francisco: American Academy of Ophthalmology; 1986.

Woods AC. Adjustment to aphakia. *Am J Ophthalmol.* 1952;35:118–122. [Editorial originally published anonymously. The author was later acknowledged to be Woods.]

Absorptive Lenses

In certain high-illumination situations, sunglasses allow better visual function in a number of ways.

Improvement of contrast sensitivity

On a bright, sunny day, irradiance from the sun will range from 10,000 to 30,000 foot-lamberts. These high light levels tend to saturate the retina and therefore decrease finer levels of contrast sensitivity. The major function of dark sunglasses (gray, green, or brown) is to allow the retina to remain at its normal level of contrast sensitivity. Most dark sunglasses absorb 70%–80% of the incident light of all wavelengths.

Improvement of dark adaptation

A full day at the beach or on the ski slopes on a sunny day (without dark sunglasses) can impair dark adaptation for more than 2 days. Thus, dark sunglasses are recommended for prolonged periods in bright sun.

Reduction of glare sensitivity

Various types of sunglasses can reduce glare sensitivity. Because light reflected off a horizontal surface is polarized in the horizontal plane, properly oriented *polarized* (Polaroid) lenses reduce the intensity of glare from road surfaces, glass windows, metal surfaces, and lake and river surfaces. *Graded-density sunglasses* are deeply tinted at the top and gradually become lighter toward the lens center. They are effective in removing glare sources above the line of sight, such as the sun. Wide-temple sunglasses work by reducing temporal glare sources.

Improvement of contrast

The range of filters in yellow-orange sunglasses efficiently absorbs wavelengths in the purple through blue-green range, making these colors appear as different shades of dark gray. On the other hand, the wearer clearly sees the spectrum from green through yellow to orange to red. Accordingly, although colors appear slightly unreal, the color contrast is increased (Fig 4-31). Therefore, patients with conditions that decrease color sensitivity, such as cataracts or corneal edema, report improvements in color contrast with such sunglasses.

Use of photochromic lenses

When short-wavelength light (300–400+ nm) interacts with photochromic lenses, the lenses darken by means of a chemical reaction that converts silver ions to elemental silver. This process is similar to the reaction that occurs when photographic film is exposed to light. Unlike photographic film, however, the chemical reaction in photochromic lenses is reversible. Photochromic lenses can darken enough to absorb about 80% of the incident light; when the amount of illumination falls, they can lighten until they absorb only 20% of the incident light. It should be noted that these lenses take longer to lighten than to darken. Because automobile glass absorbs light in the ultraviolet (UV) spectrum,

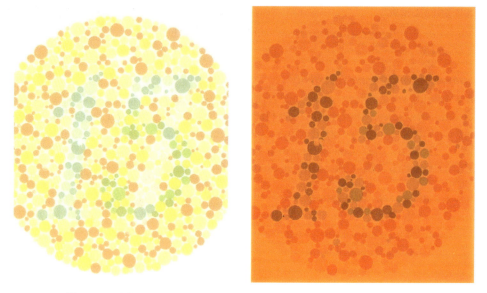

Figure 4-31 Photograph illustrates the color-contrast-enhancing properties of an orange-yellow filter. Although this filter distorts the color, it increases the contrast of the Ishihara plate.

photochromic lenses do not darken inside an automobile. When darkened, these lenses are also excellent UV absorbers.

Ultraviolet-absorbing lenses

The spectrum of UV light is divided into 3 classifications: UV-A contains wavelengths from 400 to 320 nm, UV-B contains wavelengths from 320 to 290 nm, and UV-C contains wavelengths below 290 nm.

The ozone layer of the atmosphere absorbs almost all UV-C coming from the sun. Most exposure to UV-C is from manufactured sources, including welding arcs, germicidal lamps, and excimer lasers. Of the total solar radiation falling on the earth, approximately 5% is UV light, of which 90% is UV-A and 10% UV-B.

The amount of UV light striking the earth varies with season (greatest in the summer), latitude (greatest near the equator), time of day (greatest at noon), and elevation (increases with higher elevation). UV light can also strike the eye by reflection. Fresh snow reflects between 60% and 80% of incident light; sand (beach, desert) reflects about 15% of incident light; and water reflects about 5% of incident light.

Laboratory experiments have shown that UV light damages living tissue in 2 ways. First, chemicals such as proteins, enzymes, nucleic acids, and cell membrane components absorb UV light. In so doing, their molecular bonds (primarily the double bonds) may become disrupted. Second, these essential biochemicals may become disrupted by the action of free radicals (such as the superoxide radical). Free radicals can often be produced by UV light in the presence of oxygen and a photosensitizing pigment. For a fuller discussion of free radicals, see the biochemistry chapters in BCSC Section 2, *Fundamentals and Principles of Ophthalmology*.

Because it may take many years for UV light to damage eye tissue, a tight linkage between cause and effect is difficult to prove. Therefore, proof that UV light damages the eye comes primarily from acute animal experiments and epidemiologic studies covering large numbers of patients.

The available data on the effects of exposure to UV light have suggested a benefit to protecting patients from UV light after cataract surgery. Some surgeons routinely prescribe UV-absorbing glasses after surgery. Today, intraocular lenses incorporating UV-absorbing chromophores are available.

For further information regarding the effects of UV radiation on various ocular structures, see BCSC Section 8, *External Disease and Cornea;* and Section 12, *Retina and Vitreous.*

Almost all dark sunglasses absorb most of the incident UV light. This is also true for certain coated clear glass lenses and the clear plastic lenses made of CR-39 or polycarbonate.

It has been suggested that certain sunglasses (primarily light blue) produce light damage to the eye. The argument contends that the pupil dilates behind dark glasses and that if the sunglasses then do not absorb significant amounts of UV light, they will actually allow more UV light to enter the eye than if no sunglasses were worn. In fact, dark sunglasses reduce light levels striking the eye on a bright, sunny day to the range of 2000–6000 foot-lamberts. Such levels are about 10 times higher than those of an average lighted room. At such light levels, the pupil is significantly constricted. Thus, contrary to the preceding argument, a dark pair of sunglasses used on a bright day will allow pupillary dilation of only a fraction of a millimeter and will not lead to light injury of the eye.

Miller D. *Clinical Light Toxicity to the Eye.* New York: Springer-Verlag; 1987.

Miranda MN. The environmental factor in the onset of presbyopia. In: Stark L, Obrecht G, eds. *Presbyopia: Recent Research and Reviews from the Third International Symposium.* New York: Professional; 1987.

Special Lens Materials

It is important for the ophthalmologist to be aware of the variety of spectacle lens materials available. Four major properties are commonly discussed in relation to lens materials:

1. Index of refraction: As the refractive index increases, the thickness of the lens can be decreased to obtain the same optical power.
2. Specific gravity: As the specific gravity of a material decreases, the lens weight can be reduced.
3. Abbe number (value): This indicates the degree of chromatic aberration or distortion that occurs because of the dispersion of light, primarily at the fringes of the lens. Materials with a higher Abbe number exhibit less chromatic aberration and thus allow higher optical quality.
4. Impact resistance: All lenses dispensed in the United States must meet impact-resistance requirements defined by the Food and Drug Administration (FDA) (in 21CFR801.410), except in special cases where the physician or optometrist communicates in writing that such lenses will not fulfill the visual requirements of

the particular patient. Lenses used for occupational and educational personal eye protection must also meet the impact-resistance requirements defined in the ANSI (American National Standards Institute) high-velocity impact standard (Z87.1). Lenses prescribed for children and active adults should meet the ANSI Z87.1 standard as well, unless the patient is duly warned that he or she is not getting the most impact-resistant lenses available.

Standard glass

Glass lenses provide superior optics and are scratch resistant but also have a number of limitations, including lower impact resistance, increased thickness, and heavy weight. Once the standard in the industry, glass lenses are less frequently used today, with many patients selecting plastic lenses. (Index of refraction: 1.52; Abbe number: 59; Specific gravity: 2.54; Impact resistance: pass FDA 21CFR801.410 if thick enough and chemically or heat treated)

Standard plastic

Because of its high optical quality and light weight, standard plastic (also known as hard resin or CR-39) is the most commonly used lens material. Standard plastic lenses are almost 50% lighter than glass lenses, owing to the lower specific gravity of their material. They offer UV protection and can be tinted easily. A scratch-resistant coating is usually advisable because of the ease with which plastic lenses can be scratched. (Index of refraction: 1.49; Abbe number: 58; Specific gravity: 1.32; Impact resistance: pass FDA 21CFR801.410)

High-impact plastics

Discovered in the 1950s, polycarbonate was the first of the engineering plastics. This material has a low specific gravity and a higher refractive index, making possible a light, thin lens. Polycarbonate is also durable and meets the high-velocity impact standard (ANSI Z87.1). One disadvantage of this material is the high degree of chromatic aberration, as indicated by the low Abbe number (30). Thus, color fringing can be an annoyance, particularly in strong prescriptions. Another disadvantage is that polycarbonate is the most easily scratched of the plastics, so a scratch-resistant coating is required. (Index of refraction: 1.58; Abbe number: 30; Specific gravity: 1.20; Impact resistance: pass FDA 21CFR801.410 and ANSI Z87.1)

Trivex, a newer plastic lens material, delivers strong optical performance and provides clear vision because of its high Abbe number. It is the lightest lens material currently available and meets the high-velocity impact standard (ANSI Z87.1). Trivex material allows a comparably thin lens for the ±3 D prescription range. A scratch-resistant coating is required. (Index of refraction: 1.53; Abbe number: 45; Specific gravity: 1.11; Impact resistance: pass FDA 21CFR801.410 and ANSI Z87.1)

Hi-Index

A lens with a refractive index of 1.60 or higher is referred to as a *hi-index* lens. High-index materials can be either glass or plastic and are most often used for higher-power prescriptions to create thin, cosmetically attractive lenses. The weight, optical clarity, and impact resistance of high-index lenses vary depending on the specific material used and the refractive index, but in general, as the index of refraction increases, the weight of the material increases and the optical clarity (Abbe number) decreases. None of the high-index materials pass the ANSI Z87.1 standard for impact resistance. Plastic high-index materials require a scratch-resistant coating.

Therapeutic Use of Prisms

Small horizontal and vertical deviations can be corrected conveniently in spectacle lenses by the addition of prisms.

Horizontal heterophorias

Patients (usually adults) may develop asthenopic symptoms if fusion is disrupted by inadequate vergence amplitudes; if fusion cannot be maintained, diplopia results. Thus, patients with an exophoria at near develop symptoms when their convergence reserve is inadequate for the task. In some patients, this fusional inadequacy can be compensated for by the improvement of fusional amplitudes. Younger patients may be able to accomplish this through orthoptic exercises, sometimes used in conjunction with prisms that further stimulate their fusional capability (base-out prisms to enhance convergence reserve).

Some patients may have symptoms because of abnormally high accommodative convergence. Thus, an esophoria at near may be improved by full hyperopic correction for distance and/or by the use of bifocals to decrease accommodative demand. In adult patients, orthoptic training and maximum refractive correction may be inadequate, and prisms or surgery may be necessary to restore binocularity.

Prisms are especially useful if a patient experiences an *abrupt* onset of symptoms secondary to a basic heterophoria or heterotropia. The prisms may be needed only temporarily, and the minimum amount of prism necessary to reestablish and maintain binocularity should be used.

Vertical heterophorias

Vertical fusional amplitudes are small ($<2\Delta$). Thus, if a vertical muscle imbalance is sufficient to cause asthenopic symptoms or diplopia, it should be compensated for by the incorporation of prisms into the refractive correction. Once again, the minimum amount of prism needed to eliminate symptoms should be prescribed. In a noncomitant vertical heterophoria, the prism should be sufficient to correct the imbalance in primary gaze. With combined vertical and horizontal muscle imbalance, correcting only the vertical deviation may help improve control of the horizontal deviation as well. If the horizontal deviation is not adequately corrected, an oblique Fresnel prism may be helpful. A brief period of clinical heterophoria testing may be insufficient to unmask a latent muscle imbalance. Often, after prisms have been worn for a time, the phoria appears to increase, and the prism correction must be correspondingly increased.

Methods of prism correction

The potential effect of prisms should be evaluated by having the patient test the indicated prism in trial frames or trial lens clips over the current refractive correction.

Temporary prisms in the form of clip-on lenses or Fresnel Press-On prisms can be used to evaluate and alter the final prism requirement. The Fresnel prisms have several advantages: They are lighter in weight (1 mm thick) and more acceptable cosmetically because they are affixed to the concave surface of the spectacle lens. In addition, they allow much larger prism corrections (up to 40Δ). With higher prism powers, however, it is not unusual to note a decrease in the visual acuity of the corrected eye. Patients may also note chromatic fringes.

Prisms can be incorporated into spectacle lenses within the limits of cost, appearance, weight, and technical skill of the optician. Prisms should be incorporated into the spectacle lens prescription only after an adequate trial of temporary prisms has established that the correction is appropriate and the deviation is stable.

Prism correction may also be achieved by decentering the optical center of the lens relative to the visual axis, although substantial prism effect by means of this method is possible only with higher-power lenses. Aspheric lens designs are not suitable for decentration. (See earlier discussion of lens decentration and the Prentice rule.) Bifocal segments may be decentered *in* more than the customary amount to give a modest additional base-in effect to help patients with convergence insufficiency.

Monocular Diplopia

Monocular diplopia refers to the perception of 2 (or more) images of a single object when only 1 eye is used for viewing. This is a frequently encountered complaint in general ophthalmic practice and, under certain conditions, up to 40% of normal eyes can experience this phenomenon. White letters or lines on a dark background, such as chalk marks on a blackboard, or neon signs at night are most likely to elicit monocular diplopia, often manifested as a ghost image overlapping the true image.

The usual cause of monocular diplopia is optical irregularity in either the cornea or the lens. In some cases, the corneal irregularity may be transient, such as after contact lens wear. Chalazia may induce irregular astigmatism that lasts weeks to months. Such irregularities of the optical system may be lumped together under the term *irregular astigmatism*, which indicates any irregular refractive property of the eye (eg, scissors movement noted on retinoscopy). If the cross section of each bundle of light rays approaching the retina contains 2 areas of concentration of light rays, the result will be monocular diplopia.

Other causes of monocular diplopia, usually obvious, include a decentered contact lens and double reflection in spectacle lenses. Retinal lesions may produce metamorphopsia that the patient occasionally interprets as diplopia.

Optical irregularity as the cause of monocular diplopia may be confirmed by evaluation of the retinoscopic reflex, elimination of the diplopia with a pinhole, or elimination of the diplopia with a trial rigid contact lens. (About 40% of monocular diplopia is caused by corneal pathology.) Irregular astigmatism causes confusion with retinoscopy and with astigmatic dial methods of refraction. Therefore, use of the Jackson cross cylinder is likely the best refractive technique in cases of monocular diplopia.

Treatment of monocular diplopia includes optimizing the refractive correction, use of contact lenses, employment of miotics (such as pilocarpine), and/or increasing light (to constrict the pupil). Sometimes the best approach to monocular diplopia is to provide an explanation and reassure the patient that it does not indicate a more serious health problem. Once reassured, most patients tolerate monocular diplopia, and many can ignore it entirely.

Guyton DL. Diagnosis and treatment of monocular diplopia. *Focal Points: Clinical Modules for Ophthalmologists.* San Francisco: American Academy of Ophthalmology; 1984, module 2.

The authors would like to thank Nathan Troxell for his contributions to this chapter.

CHAPTER 5

Contact Lenses

Introduction

Contact lenses are another device used for correcting refractive errors. One description of contact lens–type devices goes back to the Renaissance, but their first documented use occurred in the 1880s. These lenses were large and made of glass, and they extended to the sclera. Corneal lenses were introduced in the 1940s; they were made of a plastic, polymethylmethacrylate (PMMA), and became a popular alternative to spectacles for refractive correction. Soft hydrogel lenses were introduced in the United States in the 1950s and led to the widespread use of contact lenses. Today, it is estimated that 51% of US adults use some kind of vision correction; a quarter of these use contact lenses. This means that more than 30 million Americans use contact lenses. As a result, all ophthalmologists will, at some time, interact with contact lens users—for fitting, follow-up care, and/or treating complications. Some knowledge of contact lenses, therefore, is essential for all practitioners.

Contact Lens Glossary

It is important that ophthalmologists know the vocabulary related to contact lenses. The 3 most important terms in this vocabulary are base curve, diameter, and power (Fig 5-1):

Base curve The curvature of the central posterior surface of the lens, which is adjacent to the cornea; it is measured by its radius of curvature (mm) or is sometimes converted to diopters (D) by taking the reciprocal of the radius.

Diameter (chord diameter) The width of the contact lens, which typically varies with the lens material; the diameter of soft contact lenses, for example, ranges from 13 to 15 mm, whereas that of rigid gas-permeable (RGP) lenses ranges from 9 to 10 mm.

Power Determined by lens shape and calculated indirectly by Snell's law:

$$D = [n_2 - n_1]/r$$

For measurement of the posterior vertex power (as with spectacles), the lens (convex surface facing the observer) can be placed on a lensmeter.

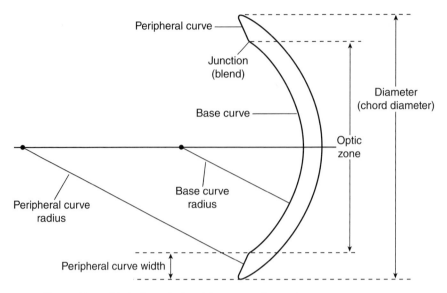

Figure 5-1 Contact lens. Note the relationship among the parts. *(Used with permission from Stein HA, Freeman MI, Stein RM. CLAO Residents Contact Lens Curriculum Manual. New Orleans: Contact Lens Association of Ophthalmologists; 1996. Redrawn by Christine Gralapp.)*

The following terms are also important to know:

Apical zone   The steep part of the cornea, generally including its geometric center; usually 3–4 mm in diameter.

Corneal apex   The steepest part of the cornea.

Dk   A term describing the oxygen permeability of a lens material, where D is the diffusion coefficient for oxygen movement in the material and k is the solubility constant of oxygen in the material.

Dk/L   A term describing the oxygen transmissibility of the lens; dependent on the lens material and the central thickness (L).

Edge lift   Description of the peripheral lens and its position in relation to the underlying cornea. Adequate edge lift (as documented, during fluorescein evaluation, by a ring of fluorescein appearing under the lens periphery) prevents edges from digging into the flatter corneal periphery.

Fluorescein pattern   The color intensity of fluorescein dye in the tear lens beneath a rigid contact lens. Areas of contact appear black; green reflects clearance between the lens and the cornea. (Use of a No. 12 yellow Wratten filter in front of the slit lamp enhances the intensity of the pattern.)

K reading   Keratometry reading; determined by a manual or an automated keratometer.

Lenticular contact lens   A lens with a central optical zone and a nonoptical peripheral zone known as the carrier; designed to improve lens comfort.

Optic zone   The area of the front surface of the contact lens that has the refractive power of the lens.

Peripheral curves   Secondary curves just outside the base curve at the edge of a contact lens. They are typically flatter than the base curve to approximate the normal flattening of the peripheral cornea. Typically, junctions between posterior curves (base curve and peripheral curve, for example) are smooth or "blended" to enhance lens comfort.

Polymethylmethacrylate (PMMA)   The first plastic used in the manufacture of contact lenses.

Radiuscope   A device that measures radius of curvature, such as the base curve of an RGP lens. Flatter surfaces have larger radii of curvature, and steeper surfaces have smaller radii of curvature.

Sagittal depth, or vault   A term describing the depth, or vault, of a lens (Fig 5-2); measuring the distance between the center of the posterior surface (or center of the base curve) to the plane connecting the edges of the lens determines sagittal depth. In general, if the diameter is held constant, the sagittal depth decreases as the base curve increases. Although sagittal depth is critical for determining good fit, designation of the base curve for a particular lens type typically ensures the appropriate sagittal depth.

Tear lens   The optical lens formed by the tear-film layer between the posterior surface of a contact lens and the anterior surface of the cornea. In general, with soft lenses, the tear lens has plano power; with rigid lenses, the power varies, depending on the shape of the lens and the cornea.

Wetting angle   The wettability of a lens surface: a low wetting angle means water will spread over the surface, increasing surface wettability, whereas a high wetting angle means that water will bead up, decreasing surface wettability (Fig 5-3). A lower wetting angle (greater wettability) generally translates into greater lens comfort and better lens optics.

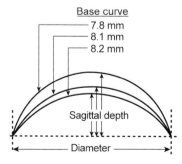

Figure 5-2   Changing the base curve of a contact lens changes the sagittal depth. *(Used with permission from Stein HA, Freeman MI, Stein RM. CLAO Residents Contact Lens Curriculum Manual. New Orleans: Contact Lens Association of Ophthalmologists; 1996. Redrawn by Christine Gralapp.)*

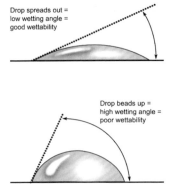

Figure 5-3 The wettability of a lens surface determines whether a wetting angle will be low (greater wettability, greater comfort) or high (less wettability, less comfort). *(Used with permission from Stein HA, Freeman MI, Stein RM. CLAO Residents Contact Lens Curriculum Manual. New Orleans: Contact Lens Association of Ophthalmologists; 1996. Redrawn by Christine Gralapp.)*

Clinically Important Features of Contact Lens Optics

Contact lenses have 4 parameters in common with all conventional lenses: posterior surface curvature *(base curve)*, anterior surface curvature *(power curve)*, diameter, and *power* (see Fig 5-1). However, unlike with spectacle lenses, the shape of their posterior surface is designed to have certain fitting relationships with the anterior surface of the eye.

The refractive performance of contact lenses differs from that of spectacle lenses for 2 primary reasons: (1) contact lenses have a shorter vertex distance and (2) tears, rather than air, form the interface between the contact lens and the cornea.

Key optical considerations related to contact lens use are as follows:

- field of vision
- image size
- accommodation
- convergence demands
- tear lens
- correcting astigmatism
- correcting presbyopia

Field of Vision

Because they are closer to the entrance pupils and lack frames (spectacle frames reduce the field of corrected vision by about 20°), contact lenses provide a larger field of corrected vision and avoid much of the peripheral distortion, such as spherical aberration, created by high-power spectacle lenses.

Image Size

Retinal image size is influenced by the vertex distance of a corrective lens. Contact lenses have shorter vertex distances than do spectacles, so image size is changed less with contact lenses than with spectacles. For example, minus spectacles and contact lenses both reduce the image size, but the latter reduces image size to a lesser extent. Conversely, plus spectacles and contact lenses both increase the image size, but contact lenses do so to a lesser extent.

Anisometropia and image size

The ametropias of eyes with greater (non–surgically induced) refractive errors are predominantly axial. Theoretically, the anisometropic aniseikonia of these eyes is minimized when the corrective lens is placed in the eye's anterior focal plane (see discussion of Knapp's law in Chapter 2), on average, approximately 15.7 mm anterior to the corneal vertex. In axial myopia, moving the corrective lens posterior to the eye's focal plane (closer to the cornea) increases the size of the retinal image compared with that of an emmetropic eye. The reverse is true in axial hyperopia. In practice, however, using contact lenses to correct the refractive error of the eyes is usually best for managing anisometropic aniseikonia, regardless of the dominant type of refractive error present, because this avoids the anisophoria that would be induced by off-axis gaze through a unilateral high-power spectacle lens. In addition, the greater separation of the percipient elements in the stretched retinas of larger myopic eyes may explain the less-than-perceived magnification observed with contact lenses.

Monocular aphakia and aniseikonia

Minimizing aniseikonia in monocular aphakia improves the functional level of binocular vision. An optical model of surgical aphakia can be represented by inserting a neutralizing lens in the location of the crystalline lens and correcting the resulting ametropia with a forward-placed plus-power lens. This in effect creates a Galilean telescope within the optical system of the eye. Accordingly, magnification is reduced as the effective plus-power corrective lens (corrected for vertex distance) is moved closer to the neutralizing minus lens (the former site of the crystalline lens). This model illustrates why contact lens correction of aphakia creates significantly less magnification than a spectacle lens correction, whereas a posterior chamber intraocular lens creates the least magnification of all.

Although the ametropia of an aphakic eye is predominantly refractive, it can also have a significant preexisting axial component. For example, the coexistence of axial myopia would further increase the magnification of a contact lens–corrected aphakic eye (compared with the image size of the spectacle-corrected fellow phakic myopic eye). Even if the image size of the fellow myopic eye were to be increased by fitting this eye with a contact lens, the residual aniseikonia might still exceed the limits of fusion and lead to diplopia (Clinical Example 5-1). Divergent strabismus can develop in the aphakic eye of adults (and esotropia in children) if fusion is interrupted for a significant period of time. If diplopia does not resolve within several weeks, excessive aniseikonia should be suspected and confirmed by demonstration of the patient's inability to fuse images superimposed with the aid of prisms. These patients are usually aware that the retinal image in their aphakic eye is larger than that of the fellow phakic eye.

When the fellow phakic eye is significantly myopic, correcting it with a contact lens will increase its image size and often reduce the aniseikonia sufficiently to resolve the diplopia. If excessive aniseikonia persists, the clinician should direct efforts at further reducing the image size of the contact lens–corrected aphakic eye. Overcorrecting the aphakic contact lens and neutralizing the resulting induced myopia with a forward-placed spectacle lens of appropriate minus power can achieve the additional reduction in image size. In effect, this introduces a *reverse* Galilean telescope into the optical system of that

CLINICAL EXAMPLE 5-1

Fitting a unilateral aphakic eye results in diplopia that persists in the presence of prisms that superimpose the 2 images. The refractive error of the fellow eye is –5.00 D, and the image of the aphakic eye is described as being larger than that of the fellow myopic eye. How can the diplopia be resolved?

The goal is to reduce the aniseikonia of the 2 eyes by magnifying the image size of the phakic eye and/or reducing the image size of the contact lens–corrected aphakic eye. To achieve the former, correct the myopic phakic eye with a contact lens to increase its image size. If this is inadequate, overcorrect the contact lens by 5.00 D and prescribe a spectacle lens of –5.00 D for that eye, thereby introducing a reverse Galilean telescope into the optical system of the eye. (If, however, the phakic eye is hyperopic, its image size would be increased by correcting its refractive error with a *spectacle* rather than a contact lens.)

eye. Empirically, increasing the power of the distance aphakic contact lens by +3 D and prescribing a –3 D spectacle lens for that eye usually suffices. Alternatively, if it is impractical to fit the fellow myopic eye with a contact lens, the clinician can elect to add plus power to the aphakic contact lens by an amount equal to the spherical equivalent of the refractive error of the fellow eye, in effect equalizing the myopia of the 2 eyes.

The resulting decrease in the residual aniseikonia usually improves fusional potential and facilitates the recovery of fusion of even large amounts of aniseikonic exotropia over several weeks. However, the resolution of aphakic esotropia or cyclotropia is less certain.

In contrast with axial myopia, coexisting axial hyperopia *reduces* the magnification of a contact lens–corrected aphakic eye; residual aniseikonia can be further mitigated by correction of the fellow hyperopic eye with a *spectacle lens* (rather than a contact lens) to *maximize* its image size.

Accommodation

Accommodation is defined as the difference in the vergence at the first principal point of the eye (1.35 mm behind the cornea) between rays originating at infinity and those originating at a near point. This creates different accommodative demands for spectacle and contact lenses. Compared with spectacles, contact lenses *increase* the accommodative requirements of myopic eyes and *decrease* those of hyperopic eyes in proportion to the size of the refractive error. The difference in the accommodative efficiency of spectacle and contact lenses results from the effect of these 2 modalities on the vergence of light rays as they pass through the respective lenses. Contact lens correction requires an accommodative effort equal to that of emmetropic eyes. In other words, contact lenses eliminate the accommodative *advantage* enjoyed by those with spectacle-corrected myopia and the *disadvantage* experienced by those with spectacle-corrected hyperopia. This explains the clinical observation that patients with spectacle-corrected high myopia can read through their distance correction at older ages than those with emmetropia, whereas the opposite is true of patients with spectacle-corrected hyperopia.

> *Example:* The myopic refractive error of an eye is –7.00 D at a vertex distance of 15.00 mm, and the object distance is 33.33 cm.
> The vergence of rays exiting the spectacle lens and originating at infinity is –7.00 D.
> The vergence of these rays at the front surface of the cornea (which is approximately the location of the first principal point) is $-1000/[15 + (1000/7)] = -6.33$ D.
> The vergence of rays exiting the spectacle lens originating at a distance of 33.33 cm is –10.00 D (–3.00 – 7.00).
> Therefore, the vergence of these rays at the first principal point is approximately $-1000/[15 + (1000/10)] = -8.70$ D.

Accommodation is the difference in the vergence at the first principal point between rays originating at infinity and those originating at a distance of 33.33 cm, which in this case is 2.37 D (8.70 – 6.33 = 2.37). In contrast, the accommodation required with a contact lens correction is approximately 3.00 D. Therefore, this myopic eye would need 0.63 D more accommodation to focus an object at 33.33 cm when wearing a contact lens compared with correction with spectacles.

Similarly, the accommodative demands of an eye corrected with a +7.00 D spectacle lens would be 4.21 D compared with approximately 3.00 D for a contact lens.

Convergence Demands

Depending on their power, spectacle lenses (optically centered for distance) and contact lenses require different convergences. Myopic spectacle lenses induce base-in prisms for near objects. This benefit is eliminated with contact lenses. Conversely, hyperopic spectacles increase the convergence demands by inducing base-out prisms. In this case, contact lenses provide a benefit by eliminating this incremental convergence requirement.

In summary, correction of myopia with contact lenses, compared with that with spectacle lenses, increases the accommodative *and* convergence demands of focusing near objects proportional to the size of the refractive error. The reverse is true in hyperopia.

Tear Lens

The presence of fluid, rather than air, between a contact lens and the corneal surface is responsible for another major difference in the optical performance of contact and spectacle lenses. The tear layer between a contact lens and the corneal surface is an optical lens in its own right. As with all lenses, the power of this *tear,* or *fluid,* lens is determined by the curvatures of the its anterior surface (formed by the back surface of the contact lens) and its posterior surface (formed by the front surface of the cornea). Because flexible (soft) contact lenses conform to the shape of the cornea and the curvatures of the anterior and posterior surfaces of the intervening tear layer are identical, the power of their fluid lenses is always plano. This is not generally true of rigid contact lenses: the shape of the posterior surface (which defines the anterior surface of the tear lens) can differ from the shape of the underlying cornea (which forms the posterior surface of the tear lenses). Under these circumstances, the tear layer introduces power that is added to the eyes' optical system.

As a rule of thumb, the power of the fluid lens is 0.25 D for every 0.05-mm radius of curvature difference between the base curve of the contact lens and the central curvature of the cornea (K), becoming somewhat greater for corneas steeper than 7.00 mm. Obviously, tear lenses created by rigid contact lenses having base curves steeper (smaller radius of curvature) than K (central keratometry) have plus power, whereas tear lenses formed by base curves flatter than K (larger radius of curvature) have minus power (Fig 5-4). Therefore, the power of a rigid contact lens must account for both the eye's refractive error and the power introduced by the fluid lens. An easy way of remembering this is to use the rules of *steeper add minus (SAM)* and *flatter add plus (FAP)* (Clinical Example 5-2).

Because the refractive index of the fluid lens (1.336) is almost identical to that of a cornea (1.3765), the anterior surface of the fluid lens virtually masks the optical effect of the corneal surface. If the back surface of a contact lens is spherical, the anterior surface of the fluid lens will also be spherical, regardless of the corneal topography. In other words, the tear layer created by a spherical rigid contact lens neutralizes more than 90% of regular and irregular corneal astigmatism. This principle simplifies the calculation of the tear lens power on astigmatic corneas: Because the powers of the steeper corneal meridians are effectively neutralized, they can be ignored and only the flattest meridians need to be considered. The refractive error along the flattest meridian is represented by the spherical component of refractive errors expressed in *minus cylinder form.* For this reason, *clinicians should use only the minus cylinder format when dealing with contact lenses* (Clinical Example 5-3).

Correcting Astigmatism

Because rigid (and toric soft) contact lenses neutralize astigmatism at the corneal surface, the meridional aniseikonia created by the 2 different powers incorporated within each spectacle lens is avoided. This explains why contact lens–wearing patients with significant corneal astigmatism often experience an annoying change in spatial orientation

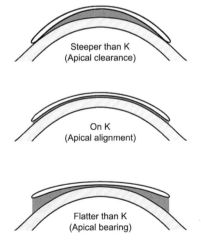

Figure 5-4 A rigid contact lens creates a tear, or fluid, lens, whose power is determined by the difference in curvature between the cornea and the base curve of the contact lens (K). *(Courtesy of Perry Rosenthal, MD. Redrawn by Christine Gralapp.)*

CLINICAL EXAMPLE 5-2

The refractive error of an eye is –3.00 D, the K measurement is 7.80 mm, and the base curve chosen for the rigid contact lens is 7.95 mm. What is the anticipated power of the contact lens?

The power of the resulting tear lens is –0.75 D. This corrects –0.75 D of the refractive error. Therefore, the remaining refractive error that the contact lens is required to correct is –2.25 D (FAP). (Conversely, with a hyperopic eye, the plus power of the rigid contact lens would have to be increased in order to correct for both the hyperopic refractive error and the minus power introduced by the tear lens.) A rigid contact lens that does not provide the expected correction despite verification of its power suggests that its base curve differs from that which was ordered, thereby introducing an unanticipated tear lens power.

CLINICAL EXAMPLE 5-3

The refractive correction is –3.50 +0.75 × 90, and the K measurements along the 2 principal meridians are 7.80 mm horizontal (43.25 D @ 180°) by 7.65 mm vertical (43.12 D @ 90°). The contact lens base curve is chosen to be 7.65 mm. What is the anticipated power of the contact lens?

The refractive correction along the flattest corneal meridian (7.80) is –2.75 D (don't forget to convert the refractive error to minus cylinder form), and the lens has been fitted steeper than flat K (7.80 – 7.65 = 0.15 mm), creating a tear lens of +0.75 D. Thus, a corresponding amount of minus power must be added (SAM). Accordingly, the power of the contact lens should be –3.50 D [(–2.75) + (–0.75)].

when they switch to spectacles. However, refractive astigmatism is the sum of corneal and lenticular astigmatism. Lenticular astigmatism, if present, is not corrected by spherical contact lenses. Because lenticular astigmatism usually has an against-the-rule orientation (vertical axis minus cylinder), it persists as residual astigmatism when the corneal astigmatism component is neutralized by rigid contact lenses. This finding is more common among older patients and often explains why their hard contact lenses fail to provide the anticipated vision correction. These cases can be identified via spherocylinder refraction over the contact lens. However, the presence of against-the-rule lenticular astigmatism can be inferred when the against-the-rule *refractive* astigmatism (adjusted to reflect the power at the corneal surface) exceeds the keratometric corneal astigmatism. Such eyes may have less residual astigmatism when the refractive error is corrected with soft rather than rigid spherical contact lenses.

For example, a patient's refraction is –3.50 –0.50 × 180 and the K measurements of the eye are 42.5 D (7.94 mm) horizontal and 44.0 D (7.67 mm) vertical. Would a soft or rigid contact lens provide better vision (less residual astigmatism)? The disparity between the corneal astigmatism of 1.50 D and the refractive astigmatism of 0.50 D reveals the presence of 1.00 D of against-the-rule lenticular astigmatism that neutralizes a similar amount of with-the-rule corneal astigmatism. Neutralizing the corneal component of the refractive astigmatism with a rigid contact lens exposes the lenticular residual astigmatism. Therefore, a spherical soft contact lens would provide better vision, because the residual astigmatism is 0.50 D compared with 1.00 D for a rigid contact lens.

Correcting Presbyopia

Correcting presbyopia with contact lenses can be done in several different ways:

- reading glasses over contact lenses
- alternating vision contact lenses (segmented or annular)
- simultaneous vision contact lenses (aspheric [multifocal] or diffractive)
- monovision
- modified monovision

From an optical point of view, using reading glasses or alternating vision contact lenses is most like standard spectacle correction for presbyopia. Simultaneous vision contact lenses direct light from 2 points in space—one near, one far—to the retina, resulting in a loss of contrast. Distant targets are "washed out" by light coming in through the near segment(s). Near objects are "washed out" by light coming in through the distance segment(s). Monovision allows one eye to have better distance vision and the other to have better near vision, but this arrangement interferes with binocular function, and the patient will have reduced stereopsis.

Contact Lens Materials and Manufacturing

A variety of materials has been used to fashion contact lenses. The choice of material can affect contact lens parameters, such as wettability, oxygen permeability, and lens deposits. In addition, material choice will affect flexibility, contact lens comfort, and stability and quality of vision. Manufacturing techniques primarily address the ability to make reproducible lenses in a cost-effective manner.

Materials

Contact lens materials can be described by flexibility (hard, rigid gas-permeable, soft, or hybrid) (Tables 5-1, 5-2). The first popular corneal contact lenses were made of PMMA, a plastic that is durable but is not very oxygen permeable. Gas-permeable materials are rigid but usually more flexible than PMMA. RGP lenses allow some oxygen permeability; this can vary from Dk 15 to over Dk 100, which has allowed some RGP lenses to be approved for overnight or extended wear. Some of the original RGP lenses were made of cellulose acetate butyrate (CAB); CAB, however, has poor wettability, so it is now rarely used for RGP lenses. Most RGP lenses today are made of silicone acrylate. Silicone acrylate provides the hardness needed for sharp vision, which was associated with PMMA lenses, and the oxygen permeability associated with silicone material; however, wettability is still an issue.

Table 5-1 Monomers and USAN for Common Hydrogel Contact Lens Materials

Commercial Name	Manufacturer	USAN	Water Content	Monomers	FDA Group
Frequency 38	CooperVision	polymacon	38.0	HEMA	I
Optima FW	Bausch & Lomb	polymacon	38.0	HEMA	I
Preference	CooperVision	tetrafilcon	42.5	HEMA, MMA, NVP	I
Biomedics 55	Ocular Sciences	ocufilcon D	55.0	HEMA, MA	IV
Focus (1–2 wks)	CIBA Vision	vifilcon	55.0	HEMA, PVP, MA	IV
1-Day Acuvue	Vistakon	etafilcon	58.0	HEMA, MA	IV
Acuvue 2	Vistakon	etafilcon	58.0	HEMA, MA	IV
Focus Dailies	CIBA Vision	nelfilcon	69.0	Modified PVA	II
Soflens One Day	Bausch & Lomb	hilafilcon	70.0	HEMA, NVP	II
Precision UV	CIBA Vision	vasurfilcon	74.0	MMA, NVP	II

Key: HEMA (2-hydroxyethyl methacrylate), MA (methacrylic acid), MMA (methyl methacrylate), NVP (*N*-vinyl pyrrolidone), PVA (polyvinyl alcohol), PVP (polyvinyl pyrrolidone), USAN (United States Adopted Names).

Jones L, Tighe B. Silicone hydrogel contact lens materials update—part 1. *Silicone Hydrogels* (editorial online). July 2004.

Table 5-2 Silicone-Hydrogel Lens Materials

Proprietary name (United States)	PureVision	Focus Night&Day	Acuvue Advance	Acuvue Oasys
Adopted name	Balafilcon A	Lotrafilcon A	Galyfilcon A	Senofilcon A
Manufacturer	Bausch & Lomb	CIBA Vision	Vistakon	Vistakon
Center thickness (@ –3.00 D) mm	0.09	0.08	0.07	0.07
Water content	36%	24%	47%	38%
Oxygen permeability ($\times 10^{-11}$)	99	140	60	98
Oxygen transmissibility ($\times 10^{-9}$)	110	175	86	96
Modulus (psi)*	148	238	65	104 ±8
Surface treatment	Plasma oxidation, producing glassy islands	25-nm plasma coating with high refractive index	No surface treatment; internal wetting agent (PVP)	No surface treatment; internal wetting agent (PVP)
FDA group	3	1	1	1
Principal monomers	NVP + TPVC + NCVE + PBVC	DMA + TRIS + siloxane macromer	Unpublished	Benzotriazole UV

Key: DMA (*N,N*-dimethylacrylamide), NVP (*N*-vinyl pyrrolidone), TPVC (tris-[trimethylsiloxysilyl] propylvinyl carbamate), NCVE (*N*-carboxyvinyl ester), PBVC (poly[dimethysiloxy] di [silylbutanol] bis[vinyl carbamate]), PVP (polyvinyl pyrrolidone).
*Modulus data provided by Johnson & Johnson.

Updated with permission from Jones L, Tighe B. Silicone hydrogel contact lens materials update—part 1. *Silicone Hydrogels* (editorial online). July 2004.

The newest lenses are made of fluoropolymer, which provides greater oxygen permeability. The disadvantage to the fluoropolymer lens is the discomfort that many patients experience because of the rigidity of this lens. The gas permeability of a material is related to (1) the size of the intermolecular voids that allow the transmission of gas molecules and (2) the gas solubility of the material. Silicon monomers are used most commonly because their characteristic bulky molecular structure creates a more open polymer architecture. Adding fluorine increases the gas solubility of polymers and somewhat counteracts the tendency of silicon to bind hydrophobic debris (such as lipid-containing mucus) to the contact lens surfaces. In general, polymers that incorporate more silicon offer greater gas permeability at the expense of surface biocompatibility.

Soft contact lenses are typically made of a soft hydrogel polymer, hydroxyethyl-methacrylate. The surface characteristics of hydrogels can change instantaneously, depending on their external environment. When hydrogel lenses are exposed to water, the hydrophilic elements are attracted to (and the hydrophobic components are repelled away from) the surface, which becomes more wettable. On the other hand, drying of the surface repels the hydrophilic elements inward, making the lens surfaces less wettable. The hydrophobic surface elements have a strong affinity for nonpolar lipid tear components through forces known as *hydrophobic interaction*. This process further reduces surface wettability, accelerates evaporative drying, and compromises the clinical properties of soft lenses.

The oxygen and carbon dioxide permeability of traditional hydrogel polymers is directly related to their water content. Because tear exchange under soft lenses is minimal, corneal respiration is almost totally dependent on the transmission of oxygen and carbon dioxide through the polymer matrix. Although the oxygen permeability of hydrogel polymers increases with their water content, so does their tendency to dehydrate. To maintain the integrity of the tear compartment and avoid corneal epithelial desiccation in dry environments, these lenses are made thicker, thus limiting their oxygen transmissibility.

High-Dk, low-water-content silicone hydrogels are used for extended wear. The oxygen transmission of these lenses is a function of their silicon (rather than water) content and is sufficient to meet the oxygen needs of most corneas during sleep. The surfaces of these lenses require special coatings to mask their hydrophobic properties.

Other clinically important properties of contact lens hydrogels include light transmission, modulus (resistance to flexure), rate of recovery from deformation, elasticity, tear resistance, dimensional sensitivity to pH and the osmolality in the soaking solution and tears, chemical stability, deposit resistance, and surface water-binding properties.

Manufacturing

Several methods are used to manufacture contact lenses. Some contact lenses are spin-cast, a technique popularized with the first soft contact lenses. With this technique, the liquid plastic polymer is placed in a mold that is spun on a centrifuge; the shape of the mold and the rate of spin determine the final shape of the contact lens. Soft contact lenses can also be made on a lathe, starting with a hard, dry plastic button; this is similar to the way that RGP lenses are made. Once the soft lens lathe process is complete, the lens is hydrated in saline solution to create the "softness" associated with these lenses. Lathes are manually operated or automated. In either case, very complex, variable shapes can be made that provide correction for many different types of refractive error; lenses can even be customized to meet individual needs.

With the introduction of disposable contact lenses—and thus the need to manufacture large quantities of lenses—cast molding was developed. With this technique, different metal dies, or molds, are used for specific refractive corrections. Liquid polymer is injected into the mold and then polymerized to create a soft contact lens of the desired dimensions. This process is completely automated from start to finish, enabling cost-effective production of large quantities of lenses.

Scleral contact lenses have very large diameters and touch the sclera 2–4 mm beyond the limbus. They have been available for years but, because they were originally made of PMMA—and thus oxygen impermeable—the lenses were not comfortable. With newer RGP materials, interest in these lenses resurfaced, especially for fitting abnormal corneas. These lenses are made from a mold taken of the anterior surface of the eye; an alginate mix is used, which hardens in the shape of the ocular surface. This alginate mold is then used to make a plaster mold, which, in turn, is used to make the actual scleral lens.

Patient Examination and Contact Lens Selection

As in all patient care, a complete history and eye examination are needed to rule out serious ocular problems such as glaucoma and macular degeneration.

Patient Examination

Specific information is needed to select a contact lens for a particular patient. This includes the patient's daily activities (desk work, driving, and so on) and reason for using contact lenses (eg, full-time vision, sports only, social events only, changing eye color, avoiding use of reading glasses). If a patient is already a lens user, the fitter must also find out the following: the number of years the patient has worn contact lenses, the current type of lens worn, the wear schedule, and the care system used. In addition, the fitter must determine whether the patient currently has or previously had any problems with lens use.

Patient history that could suggest an increased risk for complications with contact lens use includes diabetes mellitus, especially if uncontrolled; immunosuppression—for example, from AIDS; use of systemic medications, such as oral contraceptives, antihistamines, antidepressants, immunosuppressants (eg, prednisone); long-term use of topical medications such as corticosteroids; or environmental exposure to dust, vapors, or chemicals. Other relative contraindications to contact lens use include an inability to handle and/or care for contact lenses; monocularity; abnormal eyelid function, such as with Bell's palsy; severe dry eye; and corneal neovascularization.

Key areas to note during the slit-lamp examination include the eyelids (to rule out blepharitis), the tear film, and the ocular surface (to rule out dry eye). Eyelid movement and blink, corneal neovascularization, allergy, and so on, should also be noted. Through refraction and keratometry, the ophthalmologist can determine whether there is significant corneal and/or lenticular astigmatism or irregular astigmatism, which could suggest other pathologies, such as keratoconus, that would require further evaluation.

Contact Lens Selection

Soft contact lenses are currently the most frequently prescribed and worn lenses in the United States. They can be classified according to a variety of characteristics (Tables 5-3, 5-4). With this variety, selecting the appropriate lens for each patient may be difficult. Typically, an experienced fitter knows the characteristics of several lenses that cover the needs of most patients.

The main advantages of soft contact lenses are their shorter period of adaptation and high level of comfort (Table 5-5). They are available with many parameters so that all regular refractive errors are covered. Also, the ease of fitting soft lenses makes them the first choice of many practitioners.

The decision about a replacement schedule may be made on a cost basis. Conventional lenses (changed every 6 to 12 months) are often the least expensive, but disposable lenses and conventional lenses that are replaced more frequently are typically associated with less irritation, such as red eyes, and more consistent quality of vision. One-day daily disposable lenses require the least amount of care, and thus less expense is involved for lens care solutions.

Daily wear (DW) is the most favored wear pattern in the United States. Extended wear (EW)—that is, leaving the lens in while sleeping—is less popular, primarily because of reports from the 1980s of the increased incidence of keratitis with EW lenses. However, newer materials have been approved for EW that have far greater oxygen permeability (Dk = 60 to 140), which may decrease the risk of infection compared to that with earlier materials (although it is difficult to document the incidence because serious infections are rare with all lenses used today). Patients who want EW lenses should understand the risks and benefits of this modality. Patients are at increased risk of bacterial keratitis and other ocular infections. Risk factors for EW complications include previous history of eye infections, lens use while swimming, and any exposure to smoke. To avoid complications associated with EW lenses, the clinician should make sure that the lens fits properly, that it feels comfortable to the patient, and, most importantly, that the patient's vision is good. Patients should understand the need for careful contact lens care and replacement, as well as the signs and symptoms of eye problems that require the attention of their physician.

Rigid contact lenses continue to be used today, but by a small percentage of lens wearers in the United States (<20%). The original hard contact lenses, made of PMMA, are rarely used now due to their oxygen impermeability. Today, commonly used RGP materials include fluorinated silicone acrylate with Dks from the 20s to over 250 and manufactured with a great variety of parameters. Modern RGP lenses are approved for DW—and some even for extended, overnight wear. Because of the manufacturing costs and the many parameters available, RGP lenses are not usually offered in disposable packs, but yearly replacement is recommended. The main advantages of RGP lenses are the quality of vision they offer and the ease with which they correct astigmatism (see Table 5-5). The main disadvantages are initial discomfort, a longer period of adaptation, and greater difficulty in fitting. Today, RGP lenses are more likely to be provided by individual practitioners with experience and an interest in fitting more-challenging patients and not by chain optical stores.

Table 5-3 Soft Lens Characteristics

Wear schedule	Daily wear (DW), extended wear (EW), flexible
Replacement schedule	Conventional, daily disposable, disposable (1 to 2 weeks), frequent replacement (1 to 3 months)
Manufacturing method	Cast-molded, lathe-cut, spin-cast
Water content	Low (under 45%), medium (46%–58%), high (59%–79%)
Oxygen transmissibility	Dk/L: greater with higher water and/or silicone content
FDA classification (see Table 5-4)	4 groups based on ionic characteristics and water content
Lens parameters	Base curve, diameter, thickness
Refractive correction	Spherical, toric, bifocal
Color	Handling tint, or enhancing or changing eye color
UV blocking	With or without UV blocker

Table 5-4 FDA Contact Lens Classification

Group 1	Low water content (<50%), nonionic polymers
Group 2	High water content (>50%), nonionic polymers
Group 3	Low water content (<50%), ionic polymers
Group 4	High water content (>50%), ionic polymers

Table 5-5 Comparative Advantages of Soft and RGP Contact Lenses

Soft Contact Lenses	RGP Contact Lenses
Immediate comfort	Clear and sharp quality of vision
Shorter adaptation period	Correction of small and large amounts of astigmatism, as well as irregular astigmatism
Flexible wear schedule	Ease of handling
Less sensitivity to environmental foreign bodies, dust	Acceptable for dry-eye patients, ocular surface disease abnormalities, and so on
Variety of lens types (disposable lens; available for frequent lens replacement use)	Stability and durability
Ability to change eye color	Ease of contact lens care

Contact Lens Fitting

The goals of lens fitting include patient satisfaction—good vision that does not fluctuate with blinking or eye movement—and good fit—the lens is centered and moves slightly with each blink. The specifics of what constitutes a good fit vary between soft and RGP lenses and involve the "art" of contact lens fitting. For example, a patient who wants contact lenses only for skiing or tennis is probably best fitted with soft contact lenses because of the rapid adaptation possible with these lenses. On the other hand, a patient with 3 D of astigmatism will likely get the best vision with RGP contact lenses.

Soft Contact Lenses

Soft contact lenses are comfortable primarily because the material is soft and the diameter is large, extending beyond the cornea to the sclera. Most manufacturers make a specific style lens that varies in only 1 parameter, such as a lens that comes in 3 base curves, with all other parameters being the same. The first lens is fit empirically; often the lens chosen is one that the manufacturer reports "will fit 80% of patients." Then, based on the patient's comfort and vision and the slit-lamp evaluation of the fit, the lens may be changed for another base curve and then reevaluated.

A good soft contact lens fit is often described as having "3-point touch," meaning the lens touches the surface of the eye at the corneal apex and at the limbus on either side of the cornea. (In cross section, the lens would touch the limbus at 2 places.) To find a light 3-point touch and reach this goal, one may need to choose a lens with a different sagittal depth. Changing the lens diameter and/or changing the base curve can alter the sagittal depth of a lens. If the base curve is kept unchanged, as the diameter is increased, the sagittal depth increases and the lens will fit more tightly—that is, there will be less lens movement. If the diameter is kept constant and the base curve is decreased, the sagittal depth increases and, again, the fit is tightened (Table 5-6).

In evaluating the soft lens fit, note the lens movement and centration. In a good fit, the lens will move about 0.5–1.0 mm with upward gaze or blink or with gentle pressure on the lower eyelid to move the lens. A tight lens will not move at all and a loose lens will move too much. By evaluating a patient's vision and comfort, slit-lamp findings (lens movement, lens edge, limbal injection), and keratometry mires, clinicians can determine whether the fit is adequate, too loose, or too tight (Table 5-7).

Once a fit is deemed adequate, an overrefraction is performed to check the contact lens power. The power is changed if necessary while other parameters are kept the same.

When the initial fitting process is complete, the patient needs to be taught how to insert and remove the contact lenses, instructed in their use and care, and taught the signs and symptoms of eye emergencies. Follow-up care includes assessing symptoms and vision and performing a slit-lamp examination. The follow-up appointment is usually scheduled for 1 week after the initial fitting (for EW, an additional visit is usually scheduled for 24 to 48 hours after the first use of the lens); a second office visit is often scheduled for 1 to 6 months later, depending on the type of lens, the patient's experience with contact lenses, and the patient's ocular status.

At the end of the soft contact lens fitting process, the final lens parameters should be clearly identified (Table 5-8). Also, the chart should note any signs and symptoms of eye infection, any recommendation for lens wear (eg, DW, EW) and lens care, and any follow-up plans.

RGP Contact Lenses

RGP lenses, with their small overall diameter, should center over the cornea but move freely with each blink in order to allow tear exchange. Unlike with soft contact lenses, the lens parameters are often not determined by the manufacturer but are individualized for

Table 5-6 Adjusting Soft Contact Lens Fit

To create a looser fit	To create a tighter fit
• Decrease the sagittal depth	• Increase the sagittal depth
• Choose a flatter base curve	• Choose a steeper base curve
• Choose a smaller diameter	• Choose a larger diameter

Table 5-7 Evaluating Soft Contact Lens Fit

Loose Fit	Tight Fit
Excessive movement	No lens movement
Poor centration; lens easily dislocates off the cornea	Centered lens
Lens edge standoff	"Digging in" of lens edge
Blurred mires after a blink	Clear mires with blink
Fluctuating vision	Good vision initially
Continuing lens awareness	Initial comfort, but increasing lens awareness with continued use
Air bubbles under the lens	Limbal–scleral injection at lens edge

Table 5-8 Soft Lens Parameters

Parameter	Common Abbreviation	Typical Range of Values
Overall diameter	OAD	12.5 to 16.0 mm
Base curve	BC	8.0 to 9.5 mm
Center thickness	CT	0.04 to 0.20 mm (varies with the power of the lens and is set by the manufacturer)
Prescription	RX	Sphere and astigmatism, if any, in D
Manufacturer		Company name and lens style

each patient—this makes RGP fitting more challenging. However, for a normal eye, standard parameters are typically used and, as with soft lenses, a patient is fit from trial lenses. The fit is optimized first; then the vision is optimized by overrefraction (Table 5-9).

Some of the key issues in RGP fitting are briefly reviewed in the following sections, but a complete coverage of the topic is beyond the scope of this chapter.

Base curve

Because RGP lenses maintain their shape when placed on a cornea (unlike soft contact lenses), a tear layer is formed between the cornea and the RGP lens that varies in shape, depending on the base curve and whether or not there is corneal astigmatism. The tear layer, usually called the *tear lens,* is one of the parameters used to determine best contact lens fit as well as needed contact lens power.

Table 5-9 RGP Lens Parameters

Parameter	Common Abbreviation	Range of Normal Values
Overall diameter	OAD	8.0–11.5 mm
Optic zone diameter	OZD	7.0–8.5 mm
Peripheral curve width	PCW	0.1–1.0 mm
Base curve	BC	7.0–8.5 mm
Center thickness	CT	0.08–0.30 mm
Prescription	RX	Any power required

The type of fit is determined by the relationship of the base curve to the cornea's curvature (K; see Fig 5-4). For selection of the initial base curve, the following options are available:

- Apical alignment (on K): The base curve matches that of the cornea (see Fig 5-4).
- Apical clearance (steeper than K): The base curve has a steeper fit (smaller radius of curvature, smaller number in millimeters, and thus more curved) than the cornea (see Fig 5-4).
- Apical bearing (flatter than K): The base curve has a flatter fit (larger radius of curvature, larger number in millimeters, and thus less curved) than the cornea (see Fig 5-4).

Position

The most common type of RGP fit is the apical alignment fit (see Fig 5-4), where the upper edge of the lens fits under the upper eyelid (Fig 5-5), thus allowing the lens to move with each blink, enhancing tear exchange, and decreasing lens sensation because the eyelid does not "hit" the lens edge with each blink.

A central or interpalpebral fit is achieved when the lens rests between the upper and lower eyelids. To achieve this fit, the lens is given a steeper fit than K (apical clearance; see Fig 5-4) to try to minimize lens movement and keep the lens centered over the cornea. Typically with this type of fit, the diameter of the lens is smaller than in an apical alignment fit, the base curve is steeper than K, and the lens has a thin edge. There is also greater

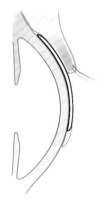

Figure 5-5 The most common and most comfortable type of RGP fit is apical alignment, where the upper edge of the lens fits under the upper eyelid. *(Reprinted from Albert DM, Jakobiec FA, eds.* Principles and Practice of Ophthalmology. *Philadelphia: Saunders; 1994;5:3630. Redrawn by Christine Gralapp.)*

lens sensation because the eyelid "hits" the lens with each blink. The resulting sensation discourages normal blinking and often leads to an unconscious incomplete blinking pattern and reduced blink rate. Peripheral corneal staining at the 3 o'clock and 9 o'clock positions may be a consequence of poor wetting. This type of fit is best if a patient has a very large interpalpebral opening and/or astigmatism greater than about 1.75 D, and/or against-the-rule astigmatism.

A flatter than K fit (apical bearing) is not typically used with normal eyes.

Other lens parameters

With an RGP lens, the diameter needs to be chosen so that when the lens moves, it does not ride off the cornea; typically the diameter is approximately 2 mm less than the corneal diameter. Central thickness and peripheral curves can also be selected, but often the lens laboratory will assume standard parameters. The lens edge is important in enhancing tear exchange and maintaining lens position, as well as providing comfort. A thicker edge helps maintain the lens position under the upper eyelid in apical alignment fitting; a thin edge maintains centration and comfort for an interpalpebral fit.

Power

The tear lens, as previously noted, is the lens formed by the posterior surface of the RGP lens and the anterior surface of the cornea. Its "power" is determined by the base curve:

- on K: The tear lens has plano power.
- steeper than K: The tear lens has + power.
- flatter than K: The tear lens has – power.

This leads to the rule of thumb for calculating the needed contact lens power from the spectacle sphere power and the base curve of the RGP lens:

- SAM = steeper add minus
- FAP = flatter add plus

For example, if the spectacle prescription is –3.25 –0.75 × 180, and the Ks are 42.25/43.00 @ 90, and the base curve is slightly flatter than K at 41.75 D (ie, 0.50 D flatter), then, per the FAP rule, the contact lens power should be: –3.75 + 0.50 = –3.25 D.

The lens power can also be determined empirically: a trial lens of known power is placed on the eye, the overrefraction determined, and then the lens power and the overrefraction power are added.

Fit

Three criteria are used to determine a good fit: (1) quality of vision, (2) lens movement, and (3) fluorescein evaluation. Overrefraction determines whether a power change is needed. Vision should be stable before and immediately after a blink. Stable vision ensures that the lens is covering the optical axis, even when it moves with normal blinking.

Because the peripheral zone of the cornea flattens toward the limbus, the central vault of a contact lens is determined by its base curve and diameter. Steepening the base curve (ie, decreasing its radius of curvature) obviously increases the vault of a contact lens. However, increasing the diameter of a lens also increases its central vault (see Fig 5-2).

Lens position in the alignment fitting should be such that the lens rides high, with the upper one-third or so of the contact lens under the upper eyelid (see Fig 5-5). With each blink, the lens should move as the eyelid moves. Insufficient movement means the lens is too tight, so the base curve should be flattened (larger number [in millimeters]) or the diameter made smaller. Excessive movement means the lens is too loose, so the base curve should be steepened (smaller number [in millimeters]) or the lens diameter made larger.

Evaluating the fluorescein pattern with a cobalt blue light at the slit lamp can help in assessing RGP fit (Fig 5-6). If there is apical clearing of the cornea, pooling or a bright green area will be noted; if the RGP lens is touching the cornea, dark areas will be observed (Fig 5-7).

Once the lens parameters are determined, the information is given to a laboratory, which then makes the lens to these specifications, typically on a lathe. When the lens is received, the major parameters must be checked: base curve (use an optic spherometer, such as Radiuscope), lens diameter, and lens power (use a lensmeter).

Although RGP lens fitting can be more challenging than soft lens fitting, the use of trial lenses and consultation with the laboratory that will make the lens can lead to a good fit on most patients with a normal anterior segment.

Toric Soft Contact Lenses

It is estimated that 20% of the US population has significant astigmatism, but with today's contact lenses, the astigmatism can be corrected.

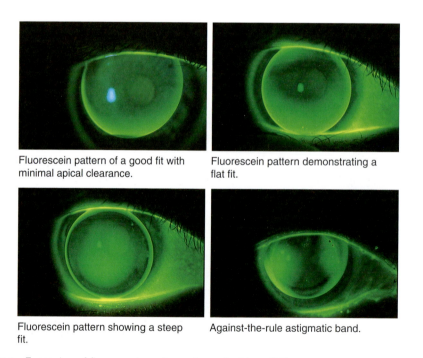

Fluorescein pattern of a good fit with minimal apical clearance.

Fluorescein pattern demonstrating a flat fit.

Fluorescein pattern showing a steep fit.

Against-the-rule astigmatic band.

Figure 5-6 Examples of fluorescein patterns in contact lens fitting. *(Courtesy of Perry Rosenthal, MD.)*

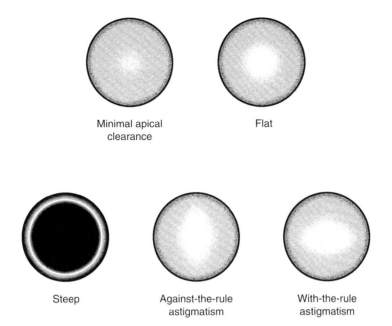

Minimal apical clearance

Flat

Steep

Against-the-rule astigmatism

With-the-rule astigmatism

Figure 5-7 Schematic illustrations of fluorescein patterns. See also Figure 5-6. *(Courtesy of Perry Rosenthal, MD.)*

When the clinician is considering a contact lens for a patient with astigmatism, the first question to ask is whether a toric lens is needed. The type of lens usually depends on the amount of astigmatism, although there is no hard-and-fast rule for when to correct astigmatism. In general, more than 0.75 D of astigmatism is significant enough to correct (Table 5-10).

Soft toric contact lenses are readily available in several fitting designs. The astigmatic correction can be on the front lens surface—*front toric contact lenses*—or on the back surface—*back toric contact lenses.* To prevent lens rotation, several manufacturing techniques are used: adding prism ballast—that is, placing extra lens material on the bottom edge of the lens; truncating or removing the bottom of the lens to form a straight edge that will align with the lower eyelid; or creating thin zones—that is, making lenses with a thin zone on the top and bottom so that eyelid pressure can keep the lens in the appropriate position. Most toric soft lenses use either prism ballast or thin zones to provide stabilization and comfort.

Table 5-10 Astigmatism and Lens Fitting

Amount of Astigmatism	First Choice of Lens
Under 1 D	Spherical soft or RGP
1 D to 2 D	Toric soft contact lens or spherical RGP
2 D to 3 D	Custom soft toric or spherical RGP
Over 3 D	Toric RGP or custom soft toric

Fitting soft toric lenses is similar to fitting other soft lenses, except that lens rotation must also be evaluated. Toric lenses typically have a mark to note the 6 o'clock position. If the lens fits properly, the lens will be in that position. Note that the mark does not indicate the astigmatic axis; it is used only to determine proper fit. If slit-lamp examination shows that the lens mark is rotated away from the 6 o'clock axis, the amount of rotation should be noted, in degrees (1 clock-hour equals 30°) (Fig 5-8). The rule of thumb for adjusting for lens rotation is LARS (left add, right subtract). When ordering a lens, use the adjusted axis (using LARS—that is, adding or subtracting from the spectacle refraction axis), instead of the cylinder axis of the refraction. (See Clinical Example 5-4.)

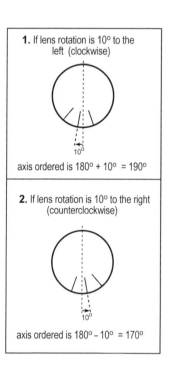

1. If lens rotation is 10° to the left (clockwise)

axis ordered is 180° + 10° = 190°

2. If lens rotation is 10° to the right (counterclockwise)

axis ordered is 180° − 10° = 170°

Figure 5-8 Evaluating lens rotation in fitting soft toric contact lenses using the LARS rule of thumb (left add, right subtract). The spectacle prescription in this example is −2.00 −1.00 × 180°. *(Used with permission from Key JE II, ed.* The CLAO Pocket Guide to Contact Lens Fitting. *2nd ed. Metairie, LA: Contact Lens Association of Ophthalmologists; 1998. Redrawn by Christine Gralapp.)*

CLINICAL EXAMPLE 5-4

A patient with a refraction of –3.00 –1.00 × 180 is fitted with a toric contact lens with astigmatic axis given as 180°. Slit-lamp examination shows the lens is well centered, but lens markings show that the "6 o'clock mark" is located at the 7 o'clock position. What axis should be ordered for this eye?

Because the trial contact lens rotated 1 clock-hour, or 30°, to the left, the contact lens ordered (with LARS used) should be 180° + 30° = 210° or 30°: –3.00 –1.00 × 30°.

Contact Lenses for Presbyopia

Presbyopia affects everyone older than age 40. Thus, as contact lens wearers age, their accommodation needs must be considered as well. Three options are available for these patients: (1) use of reading glasses with contact lenses, (2) monovision, and (3) bifocal contact lenses.

The first option of using reading glasses over the contact lenses has the advantages of being simple and inexpensive. The second option, monovision, involves correcting one eye for distance and the other eye for near. Many patients tolerate this without difficulty, although some note monocular blurring initially. Successful adaptation requires interocular suppression, which is easier to achieve with patients who have only 1.00 or 1.50 D difference between their eyes. Typically, the dominant eye is corrected for distance, although often trial and error is needed to determine which eye is best for distance correction. For most tasks, no overcorrection is needed, but for driving and other critical functions, overcorrection is recommended in order to provide the best-corrected vision in each eye.

The third option for patients with presbyopia is to use bifocal contact lenses. There are 2 types of bifocal lenses: alternating vision lenses (segmented or concentric) and simultaneous vision lenses (aspheric or diffractive).

Alternating vision bifocal contact lenses are similar in function to bifocal spectacles in that there are separate areas for distance and near, and the retina receives light from only 1 image location at a time (Fig 5-9). *Segmented contact lenses* have 2 areas, top and bottom, like bifocal spectacles, whereas *concentric contact lenses* have 2 rings, or tines, one for far and one for near. For segmented contact lenses, the position on the eye is critical and must change as the patient switches from distance to near viewing. The lower eyelid controls the lens position so that as a person looks down, the lens stays up and the visual axis moves into the reading portion of the lens. Maintenance of the proper lens position is critical, and therefore such lens designs do not work for all patients.

Simultaneous vision bifocal contact lenses provide the retina with light from both distance and near points in space at the same time, requiring the patient's brain to ignore

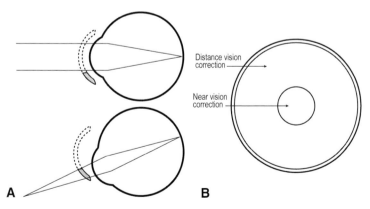

Figure 5-9 Alternating vision bifocal contact lenses. **A,** Segmented. **B,** Concentric (annular). *(Used with permission from Key JE II, ed. The CLAO Pocket Guide to Contact Lens Fitting. 2nd ed. Metairie, LA: Contact Lens Association of Ophthalmologists; 1998. Redrawn by Christine Gralapp.)*

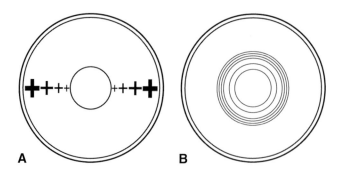

Figure 5-10 Simultaneous vision bifocal contact lenses. **A,** Aspheric, or multifocal. **B,** Diffractive. *(Used with permission from Key JE II, ed.* The CLAO Pocket Guide to Contact Lens Fitting. *2nd ed. Metairie, LA: Contact Lens Association of Ophthalmologists; 1998. Redrawn by Christine Gralapp.)*

the reduction in contrast (Fig 5-10; see also Fig 5-9B). Usually there is some compromise, either of the distance or the near vision; the compromise is greater for higher adds.

The optical design of 1 type of simultaneous vision contact lens is *aspheric,* or *multifocal,* as with IOLs. Aspheric surfaces change power from the center to the periphery—minus lenses decrease in power from the center to the periphery, whereas plus lenses increase (see Fig 5-10A).

Another type of simultaneous vision lens has a *diffractive* design (see Fig 5-10B). This lens has concentric grooves on its back surface, such that the light rays are split into 2 focal packages: near and far. The diffractive surfaces reduce incoming light by 20% or more, which reduces vision in dim lighting. These lenses are less sensitive to pupil size than are aspheric multifocal designs, but they must be well centered for best vision.

No one style works for all patients, and most require highly motivated patients and fitters for success. Most fitters must be experienced with at least 2 styles in order to offer alternatives for the best vision and comfort for their patients. Despite the availability of presbyopia contact lenses, however, monovision is still the most common approach, probably because of the ease of fitting and the high acceptance among patients with presbyopia.

Keratoconus and the Abnormal Cornea

Contact lenses often provide better vision than spectacles by masking irregular astigmatism (higher orders of aberration). For mild or moderate irregularities, soft, soft toric, or custom soft toric contact lenses are used. Large irregularities typically require RGP lenses to "cover" the abnormal surface. As with nonastigmatic eyes, fitters should first find the best alignment fit and then determine the optimal power. Three-point touch can be successfully used for larger cones to ensure lens centration and stability: slight apical and paracentral touch or bearing (dark areas on the fluorescein evaluation; Fig 5-11). To have a lens vault slightly over the cone, the apical clearance fitting technique can also be tried. Fitting the abnormal cornea takes an experienced fitter, an understanding patient, and willingness on the part of both the patient and the fitter to spend the time needed to optimize the fit. When these lenses are ordered, it is best to request a warranty or exchange option, because typically several lenses will be tried before the final lens parameters are found.

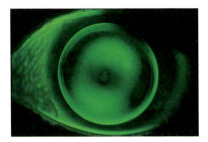

Figure 5-11 Three-point touch in keratoconus. *(Courtesy of Perry Rosenthal, MD.)*

Some specialized RGP lenses have been developed specifically for keratoconus. Most provide a steep central posterior curve to vault over the cone and flatter peripheral curves to approximate the more normal peripheral curvature. Examples of these lenses are the Soper cone lens, McGuire lens, NiCone lens, and Rose-K lens. Larger RGP contact lenses with larger optical zones (diameters >11 mm) are available for keratoconus and post-transplant fitting (intralimbic contact lenses). Some RGPs designed for keratoconus are made of new materials that have high-oxygen permeability, allowing a more comfortable fit (Menicon lens, Boston XO lens).

An alternative approach is to use a hybrid contact lens comprising a rigid center and a soft skirt. The hybrid lens provides the good vision of an RGP lens and the comfort of a soft lens. One example, SoftPerm (CIBA Vision, Duluth, GA), often ends up too tight (little lens movement and tear exchange) for long-term use.

A new generation of hybrid contact lenses, including one designed specifically for patients with keratoconus (SynergEyes-KC, SynergEyes Inc, Carlsbad, CA), became available in the United States in January 2008. In addition to patients with keratoconus or other degenerative conditions, SynergEyes lenses, which are the first FDA-approved hybrid contact lenses, can be used for all types of refractive errors, in patients with corneal trauma, and in patients following refractive surgery (SynergEyes-PS) or penetrating keratoplasty. The lens has an RGP center (Dk 145) and an outer ring whose material is similar to that of a soft lens—a combination providing optimal vision and comfort. In patients with keratoconus, these lenses are extremely beneficial. There is no toric rotation; the lenses do not become dislodged; an optimal level of oxygen is provided to the cornea; and the vision is consistent after each blink.

Another alternative is piggyback lenses, where a soft lens is fitted to the cornea and an RGP lens is placed on top of it; the 2 lenses are used together in each eye. For a very abnormal cornea that is unable to accommodate any of these designs, scleral contact lenses made of gas-permeable materials have come back into use. For some patients, these lenses provide good vision and comfort and preclude the need for transplant or other eye surgery (see the following section).

Gas-Permeable Scleral Contact Lenses

Scleral lenses have unique advantages over other types of contact lenses in rehabilitating the vision of eyes with damaged corneas: Because these lenses are entirely supported by the sclera, their centration and positional stability are independent of distorted corneal topography, and they avoid contact with a damaged corneal surface. Moreover, these lenses create an artificial tear-filled space over the cornea, thereby providing a protective function for corneas suffering from ocular surface disease.

Scleral lenses consist of a central optic that vaults the cornea and a peripheral haptic that rests on the scleral surface (Fig 5-12). The shape of the posterior optic surface is chosen so as to minimize the volume of the fluid compartment while avoiding corneal contact after the lenses have settled. The posterior haptic surface is configured to minimize localized scleral compression; the transitional zone that joins the optic and haptic surfaces is designed to vault the limbus.

Unfortunately, the advantages of PMMA scleral lenses as a vision rehabilitating modality were outweighed by the damage they caused through corneal asphyxiation. The introduction of highly oxygen-permeable rigid polymers provided an opportunity to overcome this limitation. However, a second obstacle to safe use of scleral lenses is their propensity to become sucked onto the eye. This occurs when some of the fluid behind the lens is squeezed out during eye movement and forceful blinking, thereby generating negative pressure that pulls the lens onto the eye. Unless it is immediately relieved, this process becomes self-perpetuating and leads to massive chemosis and corneal edema.

In traditional scleral lenses, holes drilled in the periphery of the optic enabled suction to be avoided. These holes permit the aspiration of air bubbles that replace the volume of fluid lost by lens compression and thereby prevent suction. These lenses are known as *air-ventilated lenses*. However, air bubbles desiccate the underlying corneal epithelium, which is especially damaging to corneas suffering from ocular surface disease. Furthermore, air-ventilated scleral lenses require a more precise lens–cornea relationship to avoid the intrusion of air bubbles in the visual axis.

Fluid-ventilated gas-permeable scleral lenses depend on tear–fluid interchange to prevent suction. Their posterior haptic surfaces are designed to create channels large enough to allow tears to be aspirated into the fluid compartment of the lens between the haptic and scleral surfaces but small enough to exclude air. In every case, the requisite tear–fluid interchange must be confirmed via observation of fluorescein dye placed outside the lens seeping under the haptic into the fluid compartment after the lenses have been worn for at least 2 hours. The fitting method for these lenses uses a series of diagnostic lenses with known vaults, diameters, powers, and haptic design.

Figure 5-12 Scleral contact lens. *(Reprinted from Albert DM, Jakobiec FA, eds.* Principles and Practice of Ophthalmology. *Philadelphia: Saunders; 1994;5:3643. Redrawn by Christine Gralapp.)*

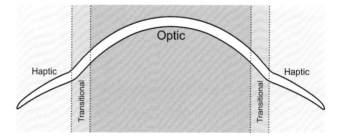

Indications

Gas-permeable scleral lenses have 2 primary indications: (1) correcting abnormal regular and irregular astigmatism in eyes that preclude the use of rigid corneal contact lenses and (2) managing ocular surface diseases that benefit from the constant presence of a protective, lubricating layer of oxygenated artificial tears.

Whenever possible, it is more convenient and less costly to correct irregular astigmatism with rigid corneal contact lenses. However, the abnormal corneal topography of many eyes may preclude adequate corneal centration, stability, or tolerance. Conditions under which this may occur include pellucid degeneration, Terrien marginal degeneration, keratoconus, Ehlers-Danlos syndrome, elevated corneal scars, and astigmatism following penetrating keratoplasty.

Fluid-ventilated gas-permeable scleral contact lenses are especially useful in managing ocular surface diseases, many of which have no other definitive treatment options. These include complications of neurotrophic corneas, ocular complications of Stevens-Johnson syndrome, tear layer disorders, and ocular cicatricial pemphigoid. The improvement in the quality of life that these lenses offer is most dramatic for patients with Stevens-Johnson syndrome. When the fragile epithelium of diseased corneas is protected from the abrasive effects of the keratinized eyelid margins associated with distichiasis and trichiasis and from exposure to air, the disabling photophobia is remarkably attenuated. Moreover, these lenses have proven to be especially valuable in accelerating the healing of persistent epithelial defects that are refractory to all other available treatment strategies. For these patients, the accompanying improvement in vision is a bonus.

Therapeutic Lens Usage

Therapeutic, or bandage, contact lenses are used to enhance epithelial healing, prevent epithelial erosions, or control surface-generated pain; they are not used for their optical properties. Usually, soft contact lenses with plano power are used. To decrease irritation to the ocular surface, they are worn on an extended basis without removal. Because the lenses are used on an EW basis and fit on abnormal corneas, Dk is high to prevent hypoxia. Fitting principles are similar to those of other soft lenses, although for therapeutic use, a tighter fit is usually sought—any lens movement could injure the healing epithelium further. Some fitters prefer high-water-content lenses, but probably high Dk is the critical factor in lens selection. The use of disposable lenses allows for easy lens replacement, such as during follow-up examinations.

Conditions and circumstances in which bandage contact lenses might be useful include

- bullous keratopathy (for pain control)
- recurrent erosions
- Bell's palsy
- keratitis, such as filamentary, post–chemical exposure, and so on
- corneal dystrophy with erosions

- postsurgery (corneal transplant, laser in situ keratomileusis, photorefractive keratectomy, and so on)
- nonhealing epithelial defect, such as geographic herpes keratitis, slow-healing ulcer, or abrasion
- eyelid abnormalities (entropion, eyelid lag, trichiasis, and so on)
- bleb leak posttrabeculectomy

During the fitting, patients should be made aware of the signs and symptoms of infection, because the risk of infection will be increased, given the abnormal surface covered by a foreign body, the lens.

Orthokeratology and Corneal Reshaping

Orthokeratology generally refers to the process of reshaping the cornea and thus reducing myopia by wearing RGP contact lenses designed to flatten the central cornea for a period of time after the lenses are removed. The shape change is similar to that resulting from laser procedures for myopia. Orthokeratology, however, is reversible and noninvasive, and no tissue is removed. Experience in the 1970s with this procedure was disappointing: orthokeratology was unpredictable, the amount of correction that resulted (up to 1.5 D) was small, the procedure induced irregular astigmatism, the lenses were difficult to fit, multiple lenses were needed per patient per eye, and extensive follow-up was required. These problems led to unfavorable publicity about this procedure, and it was only rarely used.

However, advances in the 1990s in lens design and material led to a resurgence of interest in orthokeratology, and the Food and Drug Administration (FDA) approved lenses for myopia correction. The introduction of the so-called *reverse-geometry designs* and the strategy of overnight wear improved results. The shape of the central zone (molding surface) of these lenses is calculated to be somewhat flatter than is needed for the cornea to correct the eye's myopia. The intermediate zones are steeper to provide a peripheral bearing platform, and the peripheral zones are designed to create the necessary clearance and edge lift.

Lens centration is key to the effectiveness of these lenses. It requires them to be supported by circumferential peripheral bearing at the junction of the intermediate and peripheral zones. It also requires that the lenses incorporate a design mechanism that enables the fitter to adjust the molding pressure independently of the central shape of the molding surfaces. Because the lenses are worn overnight, their oxygen transmissibility must be high; consequently, they are generally made of very high Dk materials (100 or greater).

In 2002, the FDA approved the corneal refractive lens (Paragon CRT, Paragon Vision Sciences, Mesa, AZ) for overnight wear to correct myopia up to 6.00 D ± 0.75 D of astigmatism. The fitting is simple and is based on the manifest refraction and keratometry readings and a nomogram. Typically, once a good fit is achieved—that is, centered, with a bull's-eye fluorescing pattern—that lens is the right one for the patient. Refractive change is rapid, usually occurring after less than 2 weeks of wear. The lens is worn only during sleep and provides good vision at night, if needed, and good vision all day without correction. It is not entirely clear how the CRT lens works, but central corneal thinning is noted with epithelial thinning or compression.

Although the CRT lens is approved for all ages, and FDA data show a high safety and effi-cacy record, corneal ulcers have been reported with other overnight orthokeratology lenses.

A new development in the field of orthokeratology is using soft contact lenses as a means of reshaping the corneal curvature. In traditional orthokeratology, the reverse-geometry lens design creates positive pressure in the center of the cornea and negative pressure in the midperiphery. With the soft lens, however, it is the reverse: nega-tive pressure is created in the corneal center; positive pressure, in the midperiphery. This is achieved by the reverse-geometry soft lens design, which flattens the midperiphery and steepens the central curvature, making these lenses suitable for patients interested in hy-peropic orthokeratology.

See also BCSC Section 13, *Refractive Surgery*.

Custom Contact Lenses and Wavefront Technology

A normal cornea is generally steepest near its geometric center; beyond this, the surface flattens. The steep area is known as the *apical zone* (or *optic cap*), and its center is the *corneal apex*. Outside the apical zone, which is approximately 3–4 mm in diameter, the rate of peripheral flattening can vary significantly in the different corneal meridians of the same eye, between the eyes of the same patient, and in the eyes of different patients. This variation is important because peripheral corneal topography significantly affects the position, blink-induced excursion patterns, and, therefore, wearing comfort of corneal contact lenses, especially gas-permeable lenses.

In addition to addressing contact lens fitting in relation to corneal shape, custom contact lenses can address the correction of optical aberrations, especially higher-order aberrations, in much the same way that custom laser surgery attempts to improve the optics of the eye.

The availability of corneal topographers and wavefront aberrometers, together with desktop graphics programs, allows contact lenses to be designed that are unique for each eye. (For greater discussion of wavefront technology, see Chapters 7 and 8 in this volume and BCSC Section 13, *Refractive Surgery*.) Combining these unique designs with comput-erized lathes that can produce custom, nonsymmetrical shapes has opened the possibility of creating contact lenses that are individualized to each specific cornea, thus offering patients better vision and increased comfort.

However, before this can happen, significant obstacles need to be overcome:

- *Vertical lens movement.* Some contact lens movement is considered integral to good lens fit. With each blink, though, this movement may negate or even worsen cus-tom optics. Because movement is typically less with soft as opposed to rigid lenses, soft contact lenses may be better for creating custom contact lenses.
- *Rotational movement.* A wavefront-designed contact lens needs rotational stability to maintain the benefit of aberration correction, but even toric contact lenses rotate about 5° with each blink.

- *Variability of the optical aberration.* Variations in aberrations occur based on pupil size, accommodation, lens changes, age, and probably other factors as well. Deciding which aberrations to correct may be yet another challenge.
- *Maintenance of corneal health.* Tear film exchange is important for good, long-lasting contact lens health; yet it is contrary to the requirements for stability and nonmovement needed for optimal correction of optical aberrations.
- *Manufacturing issues.* Even with custom lathes and the ability to make nonsymmetrical curves, challenges remain in creating lens shapes that will correct aberrations, provide comfortable lenses, and allow identical copies to be made on demand.

Despite these challenges, there has been significant interest in using new technology to evaluate aberrations and in new methods of lens manufacturing and design to deliver custom contact lenses—perhaps first for abnormal eyes, such as those with keratoconus, and then for the patient who has standard refractive errors and desires "supervision."

Contact Lens Care and Solutions

Most contact lenses are removed after use, cleaned, stored, and used again (1-day disposable lenses are the exception). Lens care systems have been developed to remove deposits and microorganisms from lenses, enhance lens comfort, and decrease the risk of eye infection and irritation associated with lens use. Although the specific components of these systems vary with the type of lens to be cleaned (soft or RGP), most include a lens cleaner, rinsing solution, and disinfecting and storing solution (Table 5-11). Multipurpose solutions, which perform several of these functions, are popular because of their ease of use and convenience. Enzymatic cleaners, which remove protein deposits from the lens surface, provide additional cleaning. These cleaners typically include papain, an enzyme derived from papaya; pancreatin, an enzyme derived from pancreatic tissue; or enzymes derived from bacteria. In addition, lubricating drops can be used when the lenses are on the eyes. Recently, serious infectious keratitis (*Fusarium*; *Acanthamoeba*) related to the use of certain contact lens solutions was reported; these products were withdrawn from the market.

Table 5-11 Contact Lens Care Systems

Type	Purpose	Lens Use	Comments
Saline	Rinsing and storing	All types	Use with disinfecting systems.
Daily cleaner	Cleaning	All types	Use with disinfecting and storage systems.
Multipurpose solution	Cleaning, disinfecting, rinsing, and storing	All types	May not be ideal for RGP comfort.
Hydrogen peroxide solution	Cleaning, disinfecting, rinsing, and storing	All types	Lenses should be rinsed with saline before use.

Several methods have been developed for disinfecting lenses, including the use of

- heat
- chemicals
- hydrogen peroxide
- UV exposure

The care system selected depends on the personal preference of the fitter and patient, the simplicity and convenience of use, cost, and possible allergies to solution components. Today, multipurpose solutions are the most popular care systems in the United States.

The fitter should instruct the patient in the care of contact lenses. The following are important guidelines:

- Clean and disinfect a lens whenever it is removed.
- Follow the advice included with the lens care system that is selected—do not "mix and match" solutions.
- Do not use tap water for storing or cleaning lenses because it is not sterile.
- Do not use homemade salt solutions, which also are not sterile.
- Do not use saliva to wet a lens.
- Do not reuse contact lens care solutions.
- Do not allow the dropper tip to touch any surface; close the bottle tightly when not in use.
- Clean the contact lens case daily and replace it every 2–3 months; the case can be a source of contaminants.
- Pay attention to labels on contact lens care solutions, because solution ingredients may change without warning to the consumer.

In addition to teaching appropriate contact lens and case care, the fitter should instruct the patient in proper lens insertion and removal techniques, determine a wear schedule (DW or EW), and decide if and when the lens should be disposed of or replaced. The insertion and handling of lenses vary significantly between soft and RGP lenses, and many manufacturers provide written information and videos to instruct professional staff and patients in appropriate insertion and removal techniques.

Contact Lens–Related Problems and Complications

Cornea

Corneal infections secondary to lens use are rare today, but, when they occur, they are potentially serious and vision threatening. To reduce risk, contact lenses should be fitted properly, contact lens care systems used regularly, and follow-up care provided. In addition, patients should understand the signs and symptoms of serious eye problems and know where to seek medical assistance, if needed. Today, with the increased use of disposable lenses, better patient education, more convenient care systems, and the use of more oxygen-permeable lens materials, serious eye infections from lens use are unusual. However, practitioners should be aware of unusual infections that can occur, such as *Acanthamoeba* keratitis. Diagnosis and treatment of corneal infections are covered in BCSC Section 8, *External Disease and Cornea*.

Following is a list of corneal changes that can occur with contact lens use:

- *Infectious keratitis/corneal ulcers.* This can be related to a poor lens fit, as well as improper contact lens care/hygiene. (See also BCSC Section 8, *External Disease and Cornea.*)
- *Corneal abrasions.* These can result from foreign bodies under a lens, a poor insertion/removal technique, or a damaged contact lens. Because contact lens use can increase the risk of infection, most clinicians treat abrasions with antibiotic eyedrops and no patching.
- *Punctate keratitis.* This finding can be related to a poor lens fit, a toxic reaction to lens solutions, or dry eyes.
- *3 o'clock and 9 o'clock staining.* This specific superficial punctate keratitis (SPK) staining pattern can be seen in RGP contact lens users and is probably related to poor wetting in the horizontal axis (Fig 5-13). The paralimbal staining is characteristic of low-riding lenses and is associated with an abortive reflex blink pattern, insufficient lens movement, inadequate tear meniscus, and a thick peripheral lens profile. Sometimes refitting the lens and/or initiating regular use of wetting drops can decrease the finding.
- *Sterile infiltrates.* Typically these are seen in the peripheral cornea; often there is more than one spot, and the epithelium over the spots is intact. Discontinuing lens use can resolve the problem, but clinicians often prescribe an antibiotic, although cultures tend to show no growth.
- *Contact lens superior limbic keratoconjunctivitis (CLSLK).* This finding is similar to superior limbic keratoconjunctivitis, with injection of the superior bulbar conjunctiva and palpebral changes in the overlying upper eyelid. Discontinuing lens use leads to resolution.
- *Dendritic keratitis.* The slit-lamp appearance is like that of herpes simplex virus (HSV) keratitis, but the fluorescein staining is typically less intense. A follow-up

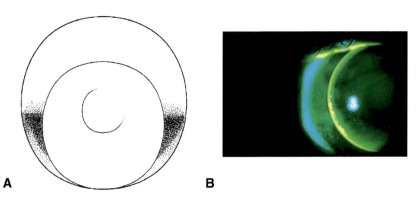

A **B**

Figure 5-13 Three o'clock and 9 o'clock corneal staining. **A,** Schematic illustration showing inferior corneal desiccation of the tear film. **B,** Peripheral corneal desiccation. *(Part B courtesy of Perry Rosenthal, MD.)*

examination, after discontinuation of lens use, usually confirms the rapid resolution of this condition and its noninfectious cause.

- *Corneal neovascularization.* This is usually a sign of hypoxia. Refitting with lenses of higher Dk material and/or a looser fit and/or fewer hours of lens wear per day and/or switching to disposable lenses can prevent further progression. If neovascularization is extensive, it can lead to corneal scarring and lipid deposition or intracorneal hemorrhage.
- *Corneal warpage.* Change in corneal shape from contact lens use has been reported with both soft and RGP lenses, but it is more commonly associated with hard lenses. Most warpage will resolve after the patient discontinues wearing the lens. To evaluate corneal shape on an ongoing basis, part of the contact lens follow-up examination should include a standard evaluation by keratometry or corneal topography and manifest refraction, and the findings should be compared with previous ones.
- *Spectacle blur.* Corneal warpage and more temporary changes in corneal shape can change the normal spectacle-corrected vision immediately after lens removal. If patients complain of spectacle blur, the contact lens fit should be reevaluated and discontinuation of lens use for a period should be considered.
- *Ptosis.* This problem is related not to corneal changes but possibly to dehiscence of the levator aponeurosis secondary to long-term use of RGP lenses.

Most of these problems can be treated in one of the following ways: discontinuing lens use; refitting at a later date after changing lens parameters, material, and Dk; switching to disposable lenses; or decreasing lens wear.

The Red Eye

Red eye in contact lens wearers can have multiple etiologies, including poor contact lens fit and eye infection. Understanding the differential diagnosis is important for determining the correct etiology and appropriate treatment and management. Also, because contact lenses can be associated with vision-threatening infections, patient reports of "red eye" should include recommendations for discontinuing contact lens use and an eye examination if symptoms persist or are associated with loss of vision and if symptoms recur. Red eye can be caused by a number of conditions, including the following:

- *Poor fit.* Both tight and loose fits can cause red eye. With a *tight fit,* inadequate lens movement is noted on slit-lamp examination. Typically, when the patient first inserts the lens, he or she experiences a good degree of comfort, but this declines over hours of use. With continued use of a tight lens, the patient can develop a "tight lens syndrome," in which the soft lens becomes dehydrated and fits even more tightly on the eye; hypoxia sets in because of poor tear exchange; and severe eye redness, pain, and corneal edema are noted.

  With a *loose fit,* too much lens movement is noted on slit-lamp examination, along with possible lens decentration, and—if soft lenses—edge standoff. The patient complains of varying vision with each blink and increased lens awareness.

- *Hypoxia.* The sequelae of inadequate oxygen reaching the anterior cornea are less common today because of the higher Dk (greater oxygen permeability) of both soft and RGP materials. However, patients who do not replace lenses and/or use them beyond the recommended wearing time may present with red eyes, eye irritation, and slit-lamp findings of punctate staining, epithelial microcysts, corneal edema, and/or corneal neovascularization. Treatment can include discontinuing lens use and/or refitting with a lens of higher Dk and reducing hours of lens use.
- *Deposits on contact lenses.* Lens deposits can usually be noted at the slit lamp. With the increased use of disposable lenses, as well as an increase in the rate of lens replacement, deposits are less of an issue; nevertheless, they are seen and can be the cause of red eyes, discomfort with lens use, and allergic reactions such as *giant papillary conjunctivitis (GPC).* In terms of treatment, dry eyes, ocular allergies, and poor lens care should first be ruled out as possible causes of lens deposit formation. Increasing the rate of contact lens replacement, improving lens care, and/or switching to another lens material (lower water content) may all help decrease lens deposit formation.
- *Damaged contact lenses.* Damaged lenses are problematic. For example, a damaged edge (torn if a soft lens, chipped if an RGP lens) can cause pain upon insertion. Inspection at the slit lamp can help in diagnosing such problems.
- *Toxic reaction or allergy to ingredients in the lens care solutions.* This type of toxic reaction or allergy may be hard to diagnose. Typically, reactions to lens care products are a degree of redness and discomfort when lenses are inserted that decreases over the time the lens remains in the eye. Conjunctivitis with possible sterile corneal infiltrates can be seen that resolves when lens use is discontinued. Switching lens care products can confirm the diagnosis if the reactions disappear.
- *Preexisting history of systemic and/or ocular allergies.* Patients with this history may have increased symptoms of the red eye with lens use. The symptoms can be reduced with the use of disposable lenses or an increase in the rate of lens replacement, because deposits on the surface may be a source of allergens that stimulate the reaction. GPC typically occurs in an established lens user with no history of problems who now has red and itchy eyes, increased lens awareness, and mucus discharge. Slit-lamp examination of the upper tarsus will demonstrate papillae, reminiscent of findings in vernal keratoconjunctivitis. With GPC, immediate resolution of symptoms comes with discontinuing lens use. If a patient prefers to continue lens wear, disposable contact lenses, an improved lens care regimen, and the use of mast-cell stabilizers and topical nonsteroidal anti-inflammatory medications may be considered.
- *Dry eye.* Evaluating a patient for dry eyes should be part of the prefitting eye examination. If a patient has severe dry eyes, he or she is probably not a candidate for contact lens use; a properly fitting lens rides on the tear film, which is essential for comfort and allows fluid exchange under the lens to remove debris and bring in oxygen. Patients with moderate to mild dry eyes, however, may do well with contact lenses. Some soft lenses are marketed for dry-eye patients; these lenses often have lower water content and/or better wettability and/or are made of material that is less

prone to lens deposit formation. Some patients may respond to placement of punctal plugs. Sometimes the signs and symptoms of dry eyes result from incomplete or infrequent blinking (fewer than 12 times per minute). The clinician may diagnose this condition by simply observing patients during the examination. Some fitters feel that it is helpful to instruct the patient on how to blink.

- *Infectious keratitis/corneal ulcers.* These conditions can also cause red eyes and therefore should be considered as part of the differential diagnosis.

HIV Transmission in Contact Lens Care

HIV has been isolated from ocular tissues, tears, and soft contact lenses used by patients with AIDS. However, no documented case of HIV transmission through contact with human tears or contaminated contact lenses has been reported. The CDC advisory of 1985 recommended the following disinfection methods for trial contact lenses:

- *Hard lenses.* Use a commercially available hydrogen peroxide contact lens disinfecting kit (the type used for soft lenses); other hydrogen peroxide preparations may cause lens discoloration. Heat disinfection (78°–80°C for 10 minutes), as used for soft lens care, can also be used but may damage a lens.
- *RGP lenses.* Same as above, but heat disinfection is not recommended because it can cause lens warpage.
- *Soft lenses.* Same as above, although heat should be used only if the lens is approved for such a care system.

The most commonly used disinfection systems for contact lenses today are chemical. Published studies suggest that chemical disinfection is effective against HIV-contaminated contact lenses, but these studies have not been reviewed by the FDA. As a result, although the FDA requires demonstration of virucidal activity in treatments for herpes simplex virus, there is no such requirement for HIV.

American Academy of Ophthalmology. Minimizing transmission of bloodborne pathogens and surface infectious agents in ophthalmic offices and operating rooms. Information Statement. San Francisco: AAO; 2002.

Centers for Disease Control Morbidity and Mortality Weekly Report. Recommendations for preventing possible transmission of human T-lymphotropic virus type III/lymphadenopathy-associated virus from tears. Atlanta, GA: Centers for Disease Control; 1985;34:533–534. (www.cdc.gov/mmwr/preview/mmwrhtml/00000602.htm) (Additional information on CDC guidelines can be obtained by viewing the CDC website for the Division of Healthcare Quality Promotion (http://www.cdc.gov/ncidod/dhqp/index.html).

Slonim CB. AIDS and the contact lens practice. *CLAO J.* 1995;21(4):233–235.

Federal Law and Contact Lenses

The Federal Fairness to Contact Lens Consumers Act (PL 108-164) was passed by Congress and became effective on February 4, 2004. The law is intended to make it easier for consumers to obtain contact lenses from providers other than the individual who fitted the lenses. Once the fitting process is complete, the patient must automatically be provided with a free copy of the prescription, regardless of whether the patient requested it. Also, the provider must verify the prescription information—within a reasonable period (typically defined as 8 hours during the normal business day)—to anyone designated to act on behalf of the patient (eg, an Internet contact lens seller). The Federal Trade Commission (FTC) can impose sanctions for noncompliance on both prescribers and sellers of up to $11,000 per offense. For further details of this law, see the FTC website: www.ftc.gov.

Amano S, Tanaka S, Shimizu K. Topographical evaluation of centration of excimer laser myopic photorefractive keratectomy. *J Cataract Refract Surg.* 1994;20(6):616–619.

Amm M, Duncker GI, Schroder E. Excimer laser correction of high astigmatism after keratoplasty. *J Cataract Refract Surg.* 1996;22(3):313–317.

Aquavella JV, Rao GN. *Contact Lenses.* Philadelphia: Lippincott; 1987.

Arrowsmith PN, Marks RG. Visual, refractive, and keratometric results of radial keratotomy. Five-year follow-up. *Arch Ophthalmol.* 1989;107(4):506–511.

Bennett E. Contemporary orthokeratology. *Contact Lens Spectrum.* February 2005. http://www.clspectrum.com. Accessed February 14, 2008.

Chang DC, Grant GB, O'Donnell K, et al. Multistate outbreak of Fusarium keratitis associated with use of a contact lens solution. *JAMA.* 2006;296(8):953–963.

Continuous wear contact lenses for the new millennium: challenges, controversies, and new opportunities. *Eye & Contact Lens: Science and Clinical Practice.* Suppl. 2003;29.

Cornea: The Journal of Cornea and External Disease. Philadelphia: Lippincott Williams & Wilkins. Published 8 times per year.

Eye & Contact Lens: Science and Clinical Practice. Philadelphia: Lippincott Williams & Wilkins. Published quarterly.

Jain S, Arora I, Azar DT. Success of monovision in presbyopes: review of the literature and potential applications to refractive surgery. *Surv Ophthalmol.* 1996;40(6):491–499.

Kastl PR, ed. *Contact Lenses: The CLAO Guide to Basic Science and Clinical Practice.* 4 vols. Dubuque, Iowa: Kendall-Hunt; 1995.

Laibson PR, Cohen EJ, Rajpal RK. Conrad Berens Lecture. Corneal ulcers related to contact lenses. *CLAO J.* 1993;19(1):73–78.

McDermott ML, Chandler JW. Therapeutic uses of contact lenses. *Surv Ophthalmol.* 1989;33(5):381–394.

Mountford J, Ruston D, Dave T. *Orthokeratology: Principles and Practice.* London: Butterworth-Heinemann; 2004.

Pilskalns B, Fink BA, Hill RM. Oxygen demands with hybrid contact lenses. *Optometry & Vision Science.* 2007;84(4):334–342.

Refojo MF. Polymers, Dk, and contact lenses: now and in the future. *CLAO J.* 1996;22(1):38–40.

Rosenthal P, Cotter JM. Contact lenses. In: Albert DM, Jakobiec FA, eds. *Principles and Practice of Ophthalmology.* Philadelphia: Saunders; 1994;5:3621–3648.

Ruben M. *A Color Atlas of Contact Lenses & Prosthetics.* 2nd ed. St Louis: Mosby-Year Book; 1990.

Schein OD, Glynn RJ, Poggio EC, Seddon JM, Kenyon KR. The relative risk of ulcerative keratitis among users of daily-wear and extended-wear soft contact lenses. A case-control study. Microbial Keratitis Study Group. *N Engl J Med.* 1989;321(12):773–778.

Stein HA, Freeman MI, Stein RM. *CLAO Residents Contact Lens Curriculum Manual.* New York: CLAO; 1996.

Williams BT. Ortho-K for presbyopia. *The Corrected View: Journal of the Orthokeratology Academy of America.* 2006;spring/summer. http://d19988442.k91.kchostserver.com/pdf/CV2006SpringSummer.pdf. Accessed February 14, 2008.

CHAPTER 6

Intraocular Lenses

The history of intraocular lenses (IOLs) began in 1949, when English ophthalmologist Harold Ridley implanted the first polymethylmethacrylate (PMMA) IOL in London. He made 2 decisions that were fortuitous for the development of IOL implantation: he used extracapsular cataract extraction (ECCE), and he placed the IOL in the posterior chamber. In addition, he experienced the first IOL complication, a power error of 16 diopters (D). Initially, there was strong opposition to the use of IOLs, and it took years of development and perseverance for the IOL to become the standard it is today. For his pioneering contributions, Ridley was knighted by Queen Elizabeth II in 2000.

This chapter discusses optical considerations relevant to IOLs. For surgical and historical information, see BCSC Section 11, *Lens and Cataract*.

Theoretically, implanting an artificial lens is the optimal form of aphakic correction. Correction with aphakic spectacles can produce a number of difficulties, including image magnification, ring scotomata, peripheral distortion, a "jack-in-the-box" phenomenon (in which images pop in and out of view), and a decreased useful peripheral field. Most of these aberrations and distortions derive from placement of the spectacles, anterior to the pupillary plane.

Intraocular Lens Designs

Classification

Intraocular lenses can be categorized by

- implantation site (anterior chamber, posterior chamber, or prepupillary [no longer used]; Fig 6-1)
- optic profile (biconvex, planoconvex, or meniscus; see Fig 6-1)
- optic material (PMMA, glass, silicone, acrylic, collamer, or hydrogel)
- haptic style (plate or loops)
- sphericity (spheric, aspheric, or toric)
- wavelength feature (UV or blue-light blocking)
- focality (monofocal, bifocal, or multifocal)
- degree of accommodation
- edge finish (ridge, square, or sharp)
- power (plus, minus, or plano)
- the type of correction

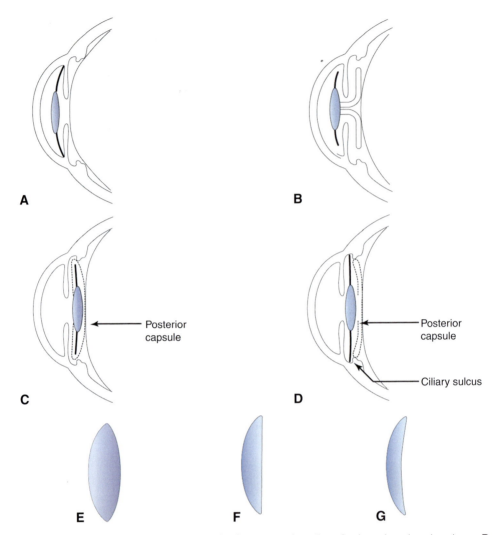

Figure 6-1 The major types of intraocular lenses and optics. **A,** Anterior chamber lens. **B,** Prepupillary lens (no longer used). **C,** Posterior chamber lens in the capsular bag. **D,** Posterior chamber lens in the ciliary sulcus. **E,** Biconvex optic. **F,** Planoconvex optic. **G,** Meniscus optic. *(Redrawn by C. H. Wooley.)*

The number of factors to consider is daunting and requires that the surgeon know how to select the best IOL design for each patient's needs.

Background

In the 1970s, surgeons implanting IOLs were divided primarily into those who used intracapsular cataract extraction (ICCE) and those who used small-incision phacoemulsification (phaco). The IOL optic was made from PMMA, with supporting haptics of metal, polypropylene, or PMMA. The rigidity of these materials required that the small phaco incision be enlarged for IOL insertion. However, with the introduction of a foldable optic (made from silicone) in the late 1980s, enlargement was no longer required and the combination of phacoemulsification and IOL implantation became the standard of care.

The effect of lens material on factors such as posterior capsular opacification (PCO) has been investigated, with earlier studies suggesting that IOLs made from acrylic are associated with lower rates of PCO than are those made from silicone or PMMA. However, more recent studies suggest that lens edge design is a more important factor in PCO than is lens material, as Hoffer proposed in 1979 in the lens edge barrier theory. IOLs with an annular ridge or a square, truncated edge create a barrier effect at the optic edge that reduces cell migration behind the optic and thus reduces PCO (Figs 6-2 through 6-4). The

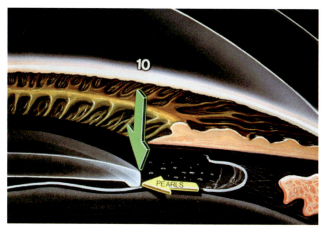

Figure 6-2 Diagram illustrating the concept of increased pressure at the edge of the IOL. *(Courtesy of Kenneth J. Hoffer, MD.)*

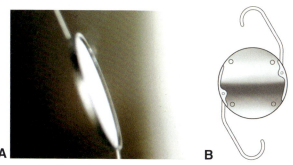

Figure 6-3 **A,** Hoffer annular ridge IOL. **B,** Kratz-Johnson PCIOL. *(Courtesy of Kenneth J. Hoffer, MD. Part B redrawn by C. H. Wooley.)*

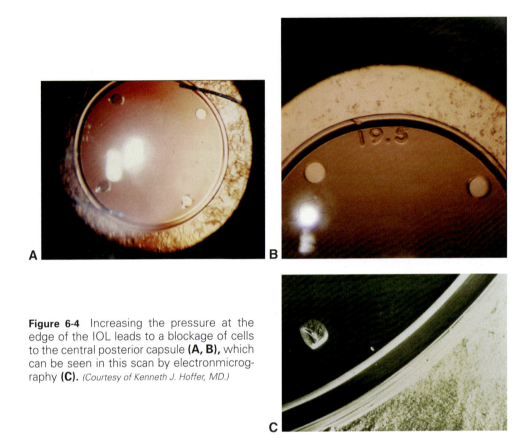

Figure 6-4 Increasing the pressure at the edge of the IOL leads to a blockage of cells to the central posterior capsule **(A, B),** which can be seen in this scan by electronmicrography **(C).** *(Courtesy of Kenneth J. Hoffer, MD.)*

ridge concept led to the development of partial-ridge and meniscus IOLs, which were used for a time, and the sharp-edge designs used today.

Lens material may also play a role in the amount of condensation that develops on the posterior surface of an IOL (especially after a capsulotomy). During vitrectomy, there is less condensation and better visibility with IOLs of acrylic material than with those of silicone. Silicone oil condenses more easily on silicone IOLs than on IOLs made from other materials; thus, silicone IOLs may be contraindicated for cases in which silicone oil will be used. Some have suggested not using silicone IOLs in eyes that may be at risk for later vitrectomy, such as in persons with diabetes or high myopia.

Although the role of UV light in retinal damage is unclear, UV filters have been proven safe and are routinely included in most IOLs. Some IOLs filter out higher-frequency (blue) visible light, with the intention of reducing phototoxicity to the macula.

Plano IOLs are available for those eyes that require zero power in the aphakic state (patients with very high myopia). Studies have shown that the presence of an IOL is beneficial in maintaining the structural integrity of the anterior segment and reducing the long-term incidence of retinal tears and detachment.

"Piggyback" lenses (2 IOLs in 1 eye, biphakia), implanted either simultaneously or sequentially, may be used in 2 situations: (1) when the postoperative IOL power is incorrect;

and (2) when the needed IOL power is higher than what is commercially available. Minus-power IOLs can be used to correct extreme myopia and (as piggybacks) IOL power errors.

Over the years, the designs for and location of IOL fixation have changed considerably. The early success of prepupillary lens designs in the 1970s was sufficient to allow IOL implantation to progress. An early IOL design for ICCE, the prepupillary Binkhorst *iris clip lens,* floated freely but maintained centrality by pupil fixation of its anterior and posterior loops (Fig 6-5A). The Binkhorst prepupillary *iridocapsular 2-loop lens* had posterior loops fixated in the capsular bag after ECCE (Fig 6-5B). Later designs (eg, Epstein, Fig 6-6; Medallion and Platina, Fig 6-7A) were sutured or clipped to the iris for fixation. The Fyodorov Sputnik was an extremely popular lens (Fig 6-7B). Prepupillary lenses are no longer used; however, one early loopless design, the Worst "iris claw" lens (Fig 6-8; renamed the Artisan lens in 1997), which imbricates the iris stroma, has been FDA approved for insertion in phakic eyes to correct high degrees of ametropia.

The 2 basic lens designs in use today are differentiated by the plane in which the lens is placed (posterior chamber or anterior chamber) and the tissue supporting the lens (capsule/ciliary sulcus or chamber angle) (see Fig 6-1).

Apple DJ. Influence of intraocular lens material and design on postoperative intracapsular cellular reactivity. *Trans Am Ophthalmol Soc.* 2000;98:257–283.

Hoffer KJ. Five years' experience with the ridged laser lens implant. In: *Current Concepts in Cataract Surgery: Selected Proceedings of the Eighth Biennial Cataract Surgical Congress.* Emery JM, Jacobson AC, eds. New York, NY: Appleton-Century Crofts; 1983:chap 96, pp 296–299.

Hoffer KJ. Hoffer barrier ridge concept [letter]. *J Cataract Refract Surg.* 2007;33(7):1142–1143; author reply 1143.

Nagamoto T, Fujiwara T. Inhibition of lens epithelial cell migration at the intraocular lens optic edge: role of capsule bending and contact pressure. *J Cataract Refract Surg.* 2003;29(8): 1605–1612.

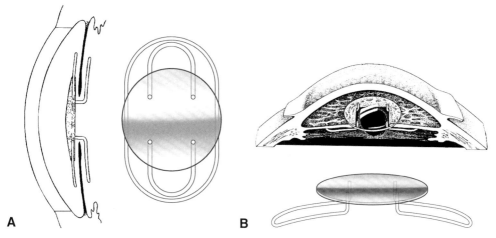

A **B**

Figure 6-5 Prepupillary IOL styles. **A,** Illustrations showing the Binkhorst iris clip lens and its position in the eye. **B,** Iridocapsular 2-loop IOL by Binkhorst. *(Courtesy of Kenneth J. Hoffer, MD. IOLs redrawn by C. H. Wooley.)*

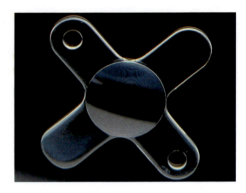

Figure 6-6 The prepupillary Epstein lens by Copeland. *(Courtesy of Robert C. Drews, MD.)*

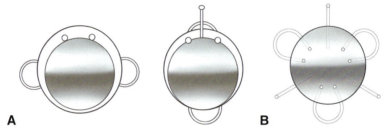

A   **B**

Figure 6-7 **A,** The prepupillary Medallion *(left)* and Platina *(right)* lenses by Worst. **B,** Sputnik lens by Fyodorov. *(Courtesy of Kenneth J. Hoffer, MD. Redrawn by C. H. Wooley.)*

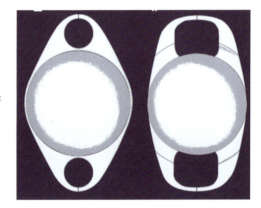

Figure 6-8 "Lobster claw" aphakic and phakic IOLs by Worst. *(Courtesy of Kenneth J. Hoffer, MD.)*

Posterior Chamber Lenses

The Ridley lens (Fig 6-9) and other early IOL styles were associated with serious complications, prompting ophthalmologists in the 1950s to turn their attention to anterior chamber IOLs, as well as prepupillary lenses. In the late 1970s, posterior chamber intraocular lenses (PCIOLs) were reintroduced with a planar 2-loop design and continued to evolve, resulting in a number of successful designs. The first 2 design changes were angulation of the loop haptics to prevent pupillary capture, which remains a feature of current designs, and the addition of a posterior annular ridge peripherally to prevent PCO. Today, PCIOLs

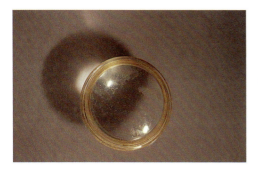

Figure 6-9 The original Ridley lens. *(Courtesy of Robert C. Drews, MD.)*

are by far the most widely used IOLs and are generally employed following ECCE, usually with phacoemulsification (Fig 6-10).

With a PCIOL, the optic and supporting haptics are intended to be placed entirely within the capsular bag; in patients with a torn or an absent posterior capsule, placement is in the ciliary sulcus. The PCIOL has also been sutured in place (with a *nonabsorbable* suture) in cases with poor or no remaining capsular support. Alternatively, some prefer using a well-placed, properly sized, quality modern anterior chamber lens to suturing PC lenses.

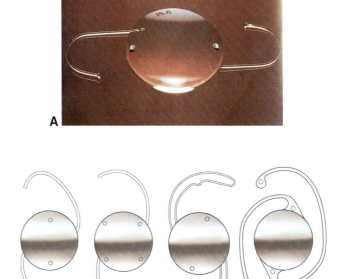

Figure 6-10 Posterior chamber IOLs. **A,** J-loop design. **B,** Kratz-Sinskey modified J-loop lens. **C,** Simcoe modified C-loop lens. **D,** Knolle lens. **E,** Arnott lens. *(Part A courtesy of Robert C. Drews, MD. All other parts courtesy of Kenneth J. Hoffer, MD, and redrawn by C. H. Wooley.)*

Anterior Chamber Lenses

Anterior chamber intraocular lenses (ACIOLs) (eg, Strampelli and Mark VIII lenses; Fig 6-11) sit entirely within the anterior chamber, but the optical portion of the lens is supported by solid "feet" or loops resting in opposite sides of the chamber angle. ACIOLs may be inserted with or without capsular support and are a popular style for secondary lens insertion in ICCE aphakic eyes. A particular problem with the use of rigid ACIOLs is inaccurate estimation of the size of the lens required to span the anterior chamber. The haptics must rest lightly in the chamber angle without tucking the iris (too large) or "propellering" in the anterior chamber from unstable fixation (too small). The "one-size-fits-all" (eg, Azar 91Z and Copeland lenses; Fig 6-12) and closed-loop designs of the 1970s and 1980s led to many complications (persistent uveitis, hyphema, cystoid macular edema, iris atrophy, corneal decompensation, and glaucoma), while poor manufacturing led to the *UGH* (*uveitis-glaucoma-hyphema*) *syndrome*.

These severe problems led to a bias against ACIOLs that persists to this day. One change manufacturers made that helped improve the status of ACIOLs was maintaining a supply of these lenses in several diameter sizes. Charles Kelman, MD, resolved other,

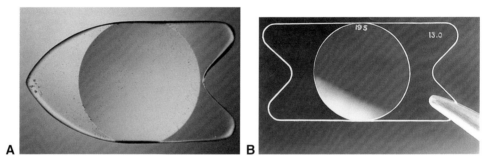

Figure 6-11 Anterior chamber IOLs. **A,** Angle-supported lens by Strampelli. **B,** Mark VIII lens by Choyce. *(Courtesy of Robert C. Drews, MD.)*

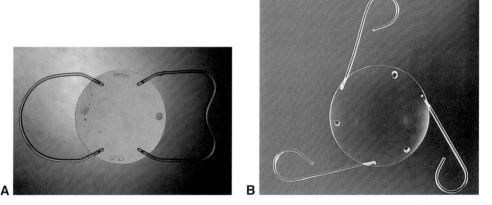

Figure 6-12 One-size-fits all ACIOLs. **A,** Azar 91Z lens. **B,** Copeland lens. *(Courtesy of Robert C. Drews, MD.)*

more critical problems by designing lathe-cut, single-piece PMMA ACIOLs with haptics that absorbed minor compression in the plane of the optic; in previous designs, the optic moved anteriorly, toward the cornea, to absorb compression. The original Kelman Tripod (Fig 6-13A) was replaced by the present-day quadripodal Multiflex II (Fig 6-13B) and other similar designs (Fig 6-14).

In addition, Kelman strongly urged clinicians to measure horizontal corneal diameter carefully and to check the status and position of the haptics with gonioscopy in the operating room immediately after lens placement. When properly followed, these concepts make modern ACIOL implantation an excellent alternative when a PCIOL is not advisable. One drawback is that an eye implanted with an ACIOL will be tender if rubbed vigorously. Thus, rubbing the eye should be discouraged.

Optical Considerations for IOLs

IOL Power Calculation

The aim of accurate power calculation is to provide an IOL that fits the specific needs and desires of the individual patient, not the "routine" of the surgeon. It is the surgeon's responsibility to determine the patient's needs through examining and questioning the patient.

In IOL power calculation, a formula is used that requires accurate biometric measurements of the eye, the visual axial length (AL), and the central corneal power (K). The desired "target" postoperative refraction and the estimated vertical position of the IOL

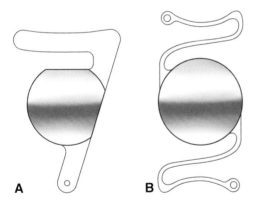

Figure 6-13 Anterior chamber lens designs by Kelman. **A,** Original Tripod, also known as the "Pregnant 7." **B,** Multiflex II. *(Courtesy of Kenneth J. Hoffer, MD. Redrawn by C. H. Wooley.)*

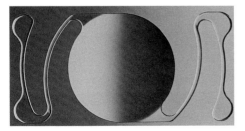

Figure 6-14 Kelman open-looped lens. *(Courtesy of Robert C. Drews, MD.)*

(estimated lens position [ELP]) are added to these for power calculation. It is better to err slightly on the side of a myopic error unless a multifocal IOL is to be implanted, where emmetropia is required. The advantage of selecting a slightly myopic lens power is that it reduces image magnification.

Power prediction formulas

Intraocular lens power prediction formulas are termed *theoretical* because they are based on theoretical optics, the basis of which is the Gullstrand eye (see Chapter 3, Optics of the Human Eye). In the 1980s, regression formulas (eg, SRK I and II) were popular because they were simple to use. However, power error often resulted from the use of these formulas, which subsequently became the major reason IOLs were removed, and in the 1990s, regression formulas were largely replaced by the more accurate theoretical formulas.

Geometric optics was used to create basic theoretical formulas for IOL power calculation, an example of which is shown below. The pseudophakic eye can be modeled as a 2-element optical system (Fig 6-15). Using Gaussian reduction equations, the IOL power that produces emmetropia may be given by

$$P = [n_V/(AL - C)] - [K/(1 - K \times C/n_A)]$$

where

P = power of the target IOL (in diopters [D])
K = average dioptric power of the central cornea (in D)
AL = visual axial length (in millimeters)
C = ELP (in millimeters), the distance from the anterior corneal surface to the principal plane of the IOL
n_V = index of refraction of the vitreous
n_A = index of refraction of the aqueous

Most of the developments in later theoretical formulas (Haigis, Hoffer Q, Holladay, and SRK/T) concerned improved methods of predicting the ELP, as described later in this chapter. These formulas are complex and cannot be easily used for calculation by hand. However, programmable calculators and computer programs (Hoffer Programs, Holladay

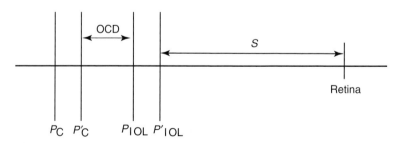

Figure 6-15 Schematic eye. P_C and P'_C are the front and back principal planes of the cornea, respectively. Similarly, P_{IOL} and P'_{IOL} are the front and back principal planes of the IOL. S is the distance between the back principal plane of the IOL and the retina. (The drawing is not to scale.) *(Redrawn by C. H. Wooley.)*

IOL Consultant) are widely available, obviating this disadvantage. These formulas are also programmed into the IOLMaster, Lenstar LS 900 (discussed in the section "Biometric formula requirements"), and most modern ultrasonographic instruments, thus eliminating any need for regression formulas. In all such cases, make sure that the formula author has verified the programming and accuracy of his or her particular formula.

Biometric formula requirements

Axial length The AL is the most important factor in the formula. A 1-mm error in AL measurement results in a refractive error of approximately 2.35 D in a 23.5-mm eye. The refractive error drops to only 1.75 D/mm in a 30-mm eye but rises to 3.75 D/mm in a 20-mm eye. Therefore, accuracy in AL measurement is more important in short eyes than in long eyes.

ULTRASONIC MEASUREMENT OF AL When *A-scan ultrasonography* is used to measure AL, we either assume a constant ultrasound velocity through the entire eye *or* measure each of the various ocular structures at their individual velocities. A-scans do not measure distance but rather the time required for a sound pulse to travel from the cornea to the retina. Sound travels faster through the crystalline lens and the cornea (1641 m/s) than through aqueous and vitreous (1532 m/s). Even within the lens itself, the speed of sound can vary in different layers of nuclear sclerosis. The sound transit time measured is converted to a distance using the formula

$$d = t/V$$

where

d = the distance in meters
t = the time in seconds
V = the velocity in meters per second

The average velocity through a phakic eye of normal length is 1555 m/s; however, it is 1560 m/s for a short (20-mm) eye and 1550 m/s for a long (30-mm) eye. This variation is due to the presence of the crystalline lens; thus, 1554 m/s is accurate for an aphakic eye of any length. One method that can be used to correct for this velocity difference is measuring the eye at 1532 m/s and adding 0.34 to the result to account for the effect of the lens.

The following formula can be used to easily correct any AL measured with an incorrect average velocity:

$$AL_C = AL_M \times V_C/V_M$$

where AL_M is the resultant AL at the incorrect velocity, V_C is the correct velocity, and V_M is the incorrect velocity used.

In eyes with AL greater than 25 mm, *staphyloma* should be suspected, especially when multiple disparate readings are obtained. The errors occur because the macula is located sometimes at the deepest part of the staphyloma and at other times on the "side of the hill." To measure these eyes and obtain the true measurement to the fovea, a B-scan technique must be used. The IOLMaster is very useful in such cases (see the following section).

When ultrasonography is used to measure the AL in *biphakic* eyes (phakic IOL in a phakic eye), it is often difficult to eliminate the effect of the sound velocity through the phakic lens. To correct for this potential error, the following published formula can be used:

$$AL_{corrected} = AL_{1555} + C \times T$$

where

AL_{1555} = the measured AL of the eye at a sound velocity of 1555 m/s
C = the material-specific correction factor, which is +0.42 for PMMA, –0.59 for silicone, +0.11 for collamer, and +0.23 for acrylic
T = the central thickness of the phakic IOL

Published tables list the central thickness of every phakic IOL on the market today (for each dioptric power; see the references in the next section). The least error (in terms of AL error) is seen with a very thin myopic collamer lens (eg, Visian ICL [Implantable Collamer Lens], STAAR Surgical, Monrovia, CA) and the greatest error is seen with a thick hyperopic silicone lens (eg, PRL [Phakic Refractive Lens], Zeiss Meditec, Jena, Germany).

The 2 primary A-scan techniques—*applanation* (contact) and *immersion* (noncontact)—often give unpredictably different results (Figs 6-16, 6-17). The applanation method has been proven to give a shorter AL measurement that is also inconsistent and unpredictable. An artificially shortened AL measurement occurs with inadvertent corneal indentation. In the immersion method, accepted as the more accurate of the 2 techniques, space is maintained between the probe and the cornea, eliminating corneal indentation. See also Chapter 8, Telescopes and Optical Instruments.

OPTICAL MEASUREMENT OF AL   Another method of measuring AL was introduced in 1999. The IOLMaster (Zeiss Meditec, Dublin, CA) uses a partial coherence laser for AL measurement (Fig 6-18). In a manner analogous to ultrasonography, the IOLMaster measures the time required for infrared light to travel to the retina. Because light travels at too high

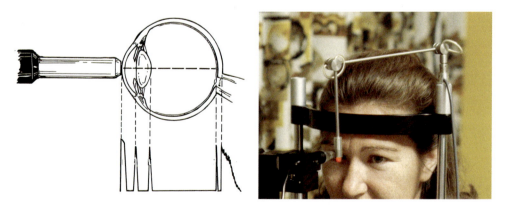

Figure 6-16 In applanation ultrasonography, the probe must contact the cornea, which causes corneal depression and shortening of the axial length reading. *(Courtesy of Kenneth J. Hoffer, MD.)*

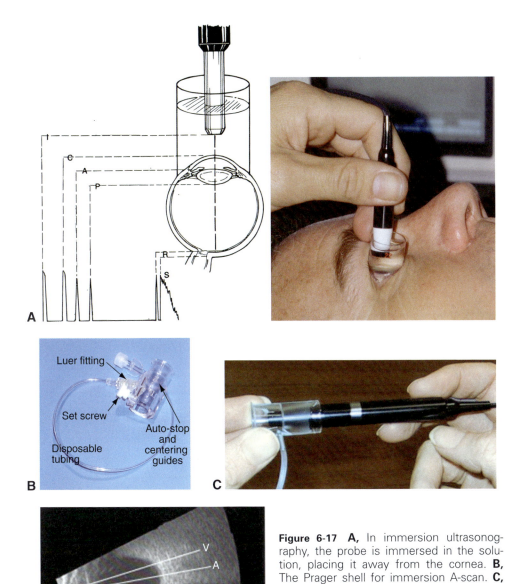

Figure 6-17 A, In immersion ultrasonography, the probe is immersed in the solution, placing it away from the cornea. **B,** The Prager shell for immersion A-scan. **C,** Ultrasound probe and Kohn shell. **D,** B-scan of an eye with staphyloma showing the difference between the anatomical length *(A)* and the visual length *(V). (Courtesy of Kenneth J. Hoffer, MD.)*

a speed to be measured directly, light interference methodology is used to determine the transit time and thus the AL. This technique does not require contact with the globe, so corneal compression artifacts are eliminated. The instrument was set so that its readings would be equivalent to those of the immersion technique. The IOLMaster requires the

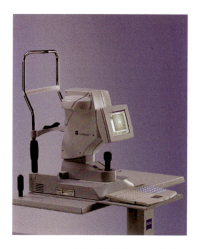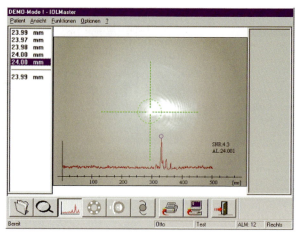

Figure 6-18 The IOLMaster *(left)* and view of its axial length screen *(right)*. *(Courtesy of Kenneth J. Hoffer, MD.)*

patient to fixate on a target; thus, the length measured is the path the light takes to the fovea, the "visual" AL. Because the ocular media must be clear enough to allow voluntary fixation and light transmission, in dense cataracts (especially posterior subcapsular), ultrasound biometry is still necessary (in 10%–15% of cataract patients). Compared with ultrasonography, the IOLMaster provides more accurate, reproducible AL measurement. In addition, measurement with the IOLMaster is ideal in 2 situations that are difficult with ultrasonography: eyes with staphyloma and eyes filled with silicone oil.

In 2008, Haag-Streit (Koeniz, Switzerland) introduced an optical measuring device similar to the IOLMaster, the Lenstar LS 900.

Drexler W, Findl O, Menapace R, et al. Partial coherence interferometry: a novel approach to biometry in cataract surgery. *Am J Ophthalmol.* 1998;126(4):524–534.

Hoffer KJ. Addendum to ultrasound axial length measurement in biphakic eyes: factors for Alcon L12500–L14000 anterior chamber phakic IOLs. *J Cataract Refract Surg.* 2007;33(4): 751–752.

Hoffer KJ. Modern IOL power calculations: Avoiding error and planning for special circumstances. *Focal Points: Clinical Modules for Ophthalmologists.* San Francisco: American Academy of Ophthalmology; 1999, module 12.

Hoffer KJ. Ultrasound axial length measurement in biphakic eyes. *J Cataract Refract Surg.* 2003; 29(5):961–965.

Hoffer KJ. Ultrasound velocities for axial eye length measurement. *J Cataract Refract Surg.* 1994; 20(5):554–562.

Shammas HJ. A comparison of immersion and contact techniques for axial length measurement. *J Am Intraocul Implant Soc.* 1984(4);10:444–447.

Corneal power   The central corneal power is the second important factor in the calculation formula, with a 1.0 D error in corneal power resulting in a 1.0 D postoperative refractive error. Central corneal power can be measured by keratometry or corneal topography, neither of which measures corneal power directly. The standard manual

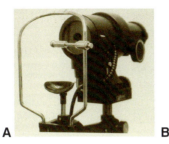
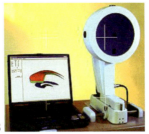

Figure 6-19 **A,** Manual keratometer. **B,** Oculus Pentacam. *(Part A courtesy of Kenneth J. Hoffer, MD. Part B courtesy of Oculus Optikgeräte GmbH.)*

keratometer (Fig 6-19A) measures only a small portion (3.2-mm diameter) of the central cornea, viewing the cornea as a convex mirror. From the size of the reflected image, the corneal radius of curvature is calculated. Both front and back corneal surfaces contribute to corneal power, but the keratometer measures only the front surface, using assumptions regarding the posterior surface.

The Pentacam (Oculus Optikgeräte GmbH, Wetzlar, Germany; Fig 6-19B) is a relatively new imaging system that uses a single Scheimpflug camera to measure the radius of curvature of the anterior and posterior corneal surfaces, as well as the corneal thickness, for the calculation of corneal power. Early studies have been equivocal as to the accuracy of the Pentacam in eyes that have undergone laser corneal refractive procedures. Steps are being taken to improve it. Another device, the Galilei (Ziemer Ophthalmic Systems AG, Port, Switzerland), measures corneal power in a similar fashion and is based on a dual Scheimpflug camera and a Placido disk.

Estimated lens position   All formulas require an estimation of the distance that the principal plane of the IOL will sit behind the cornea—a factor now known as the ELP. Initially, most IOLs were either AC or prepupillary IOLs. Thus, in the original theoretical formulas, this factor was called the anterior chamber depth (ACD), and it was a constant value (usually 2.8 or 3.5 mm). This value became incorporated in the *A* constant of the regression formulas of the 1980s, such as the SRK.

In 1983, using pachymetry studies of PCIOLs as a basis, Hoffer introduced an ACD prediction formula for PC lenses, based on the eye's AL:

$$ACD = 2.93 \times AL - 2.92$$

Other authors followed with formula adjustments based on AL (second-generation formulas). The Holladay 1 formula used the K reading and AL as factors (in a corneal height formula by Fyodorov), as did the later SRK/T formula, whereas the Hoffer Q used the AL and a tangent factor of K (third generation). Olsen added other measurements of the anterior segment, such as the preoperative ACD, "lens thickness," and corneal diameter (CD) (fourth generation); and then Holladay used these, as well as patient age and preoperative refraction, in his unpublished Holladay 2 formula. Haigis eliminated the K as a prediction factor and replaced it with the preoperative ACD measurement. These newer formulas were shown to be more accurate than those of the first and second generation, and all are used today.

The most accurate way to measure the preoperative ACD or the postoperative ELP is to use an optical pachymeter (Haag-Streit, Bern, Switzerland) (Fig 6-20). Ultrasonography is usually less precise and provides a shorter reading. The IOLMaster is fairly accurate. The ACMaster (Carl Zeiss Meditec AG, Jena, Germany), based on the partial coherence interferometry technique, has recently been introduced.

Most formulas use only one constant, such as the ACD, the A constant, or the surgeon factor (one exception is the Haigis, which uses 3 constants). The A constant, developed as a result of regression formulas, was widely used in the 1980s, so much so that every lens design was assigned a specific A constant, as well as an ACD value, by the manufacturer. Even though regression formulas are no longer recommended and are rarely used today, A constants still exist.

Holladay developed 2 formulas that convert a lens's A constant. One of these converts it to a surgeon factor (SF) for the Holladay formula:

$$SF = (0.5663 \times A) - 65.6$$

where A is the IOL-specific A constant and SF is the Holladay surgeon factor.

The other converts a lens's A constant to a personalized ACD (pACD) for the Hoffer Q formula:

$$pACD = [(0.5663 \times A) - 62.005]/0.9704$$

where A is the IOL-specific A constant, and pACD is the Hoffer personalized ACD (ELP). So, for example, A constants of 113.78, 116.35, and 118.92 convert to pACDs of 2.50 mm, 4.00 mm, and 5.50 mm, respectively.

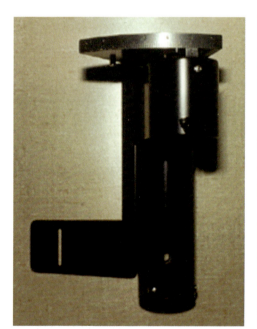
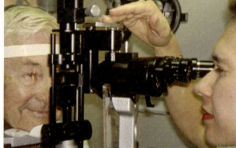
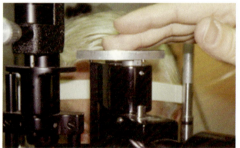

Figure 6-20 Haag-Streit optical pachymeter mounted on the slit lamp. *(Courtesy of Kenneth J. Hoffer, MD.)*

In emergencies, the *A* constant can be used to adjust the power of an alternate IOL (eg, an ACIOL used instead of a PCIOL; placement in the sulcus instead of the capsular bag). However, it is more prudent to calculate the power of an alternate IOL before surgery. If not calculated in advance, the power of an IOL intended for bag placement can be decreased for sulcus placement with subtraction of 0.75–1.25 D, depending on AL.

Formula choice

Several studies have indicated that the Hoffer Q formula is more accurate for eyes less than 24.5 mm; the Holladay 1, for eyes from 24.5 to 26.0 mm; the SRK/T, for eyes greater than 26.0 mm (very long eyes). The Haigis may be superior to these formulas, for all eyes, but only after 3 personalized constants (a_0, a_1, and a_2) have been generated based on 500–1000 eyes implanted with IOLs of a single design (triple optimization)—a difficult undertaking for the average ophthalmic surgeon.

The choice of formula is, of course, up to the surgeon, but whatever the method, every effort should be made to ensure that the biometry is as accurate as possible. Preoperative ALs and K readings should be reviewed by the operating surgeon. If a reading is suspicious because it lies outside normal limits, biometry should be repeated during or immediately after the initial reading. Similarly, it is prudent to measure both eyes and recheck the readings if there is a large discrepancy between the 2 eyes. Great care should be taken in the measurement of eyes that have undergone previous refractive surgery (corneal or phakic IOL), as well as in those that have had an encircling band treatment of a retinal detachment.

Haigis W. The Haigis formula. *Intraocular Lens Power Calculations.* Shammas HJ, ed. Thorofare, NJ: Slack Inc; 2003:chap 5, pp 41–57.

Hoffer KJ. Biometry of the posterior capsule: a new formula for anterior chamber depth of posterior chamber lenses. In: *Current Concepts in Cataract Surgery* (8th Congress). Emery JC, Jacobson AC, eds. New York, NY: Appleton-Century Crofts; 1983:chap 21, pp 56–62.

Hoffer KJ. Clinical results using the Holladay 2 intraocular lens power formula. *J Cataract Refract Surg.* 2000;26(8):1233–1237.

Hoffer KJ. The Hoffer Q formula: a comparison of theoretic and regression formulas. *J Cataract Refract Surg.* 1993;19(6):700–712. [Published corrections appear in *J Cataract Refract Surg.* 1994;20:677 and *J Cataract Refract Surg.* 2007;33(1):2–3.]

Hoffer KJ. Intraocular lens calculation: the problem of the short eye. *Ophthalmic Surg.* 1981; 12(4):269–272.

Holladay JT, Prager TC, Chandler TY, Musgrove KH, Lewis JW, Ruiz RS. A three-part system for refining intraocular lens power calculations. *J Cataract Refract Surg.* 1988;14(1):17–24.

Retzlaff JA, Sanders DR, Kraff MC. Development of the SRK/T intraocular lens implant power calculation formula. *J Cataract Refract Surg.* 1990;16(3):333–340. [Published correction appears in *J Cataract Refract Surg.* 1990;16(4):528.]

Piggyback IOLs

When an IOL is inserted in an eye that already has an IOL, it is called a *piggyback* IOL. The piggyback IOL can be inserted at the time the first IOL is implanted to produce a high power that is commercially unavailable. It can also be inserted secondarily to correct a postoperative refractive error. Computer programs can be used to calculate the power of the second IOL and also to make adjustments, which may be needed if the posterior IOL is displaced posteriorly. However, these adjustments are minor, and using one of the following formulas is the easiest way to calculate them:

Myopic correction: P = 1.0 × Error
Hyperopic correction: P = 1.5 × Error

where

P = the needed power in the piggyback lens
Error = the residual refractive error that needs to be corrected

Findl O, Menapace R. Piggyback intraocular lenses [letter]. *J Cataract Refract Surg.* 2000;26(3): 308–309.

Findl O, Menapace R, Rainer G, Georgopoulos M. Contact zone of piggyback acrylic intraocular lenses. *J Cataract Refract Surg.* 1999;25(6):860–862.

IOL Power Calculation After Corneal Refractive Surgery

Intraocular lens power calculation is a problem in eyes that have undergone radial keratotomy (RK) or laser corneal refractive procedures such as photorefractive keratectomy (PRK), laser in situ keratomileusis (LASIK), and laser subepithelial keratomileusis (LASEK). The difficulty stems from 3 errors: (1) instrument error, (2) index of refraction error, and (3) formula error.

Instrument Error

This was first described by Koch in 1989. The instruments used by ophthalmologists to measure the corneal power (keratometers, corneal topographers) cannot obtain accurate measurements in eyes that have undergone corneal refractive surgery. Most manual keratometers measure at the 3.2-mm zone of the central cornea, which often misses the central flatter zone of effective corneal power. The flatter the cornea, the larger the zone of measurement and the greater the error. Topography units do not correct this problem either; rather, they usually overestimate the corneal power, leading to a hyperopic refractive error postoperatively.

Index of Refraction Error

The assumed index of refraction (IR) of the normal cornea is based on the relationship between the anterior and posterior corneal curvatures. This relationship is changed in PRK, LASIK, and LASEK eyes but not in RK eyes. RK causes a relatively proportional equal flattening of both corneal surfaces, leaving the IR relationship essentially the same. The other procedures flatten the anterior surface but not the posterior surface, thus changing the IR calculation. This leads to an overestimation of the corneal power by approximately 1 D for every 7 D of correction obtained. A manual keratometer measures only the front surface curvature and converts the radius of curvature (r) obtained to diopters, usually using an IR of 1.3375. The following formula can be used to convert diopters to radius:

r = 337.5/D

To convert radius to diopters:

D = 337.5/r

Formula Error

With the exception of the Haigis formula, all of the modern IOL power formulas (Hoffer Q, Holladay 1 and 2, and SRK/T) use the AL and K reading to predict the position of the IOL postoperatively (ELP). The flatter than normal K in RK, PRK, LASIK, and LASEK eyes causes an error in this prediction because the anterior chamber dimensions do not really change in these eyes commensurately with the much flatter K.

Power Calculation Methods for the Postkeratorefractive Eye

In 2002, Aramberri developed the Double-K method, which uses the pre-LASIK corneal power (or 43.50 D if unknown) for the calculation of the ELP, and the post-LASIK (much flatter) corneal power for the calculation of the IOL power. This can be done automatically (for the Hoffer Q, Holladay 1, SRK/T formulas) in the Hoffer Programs and (for the Holladay 2) in the Holladay IOL Consultant program.

Aramberri's method is just one of more than 20 methods proposed over the years to either calculate the true corneal power or adjust the calculated IOL power to account for the errors discussed in the preceding sections. Some require knowledge of prerefractive surgery values such as refractive error or K reading. The earliest of these methods is the "clinical history method":

$K = K_{pre} + R_{pre} - R_{po}$

where

K = calculated corneal power
K_{pre} = preoperative average K
R_{pre} = preoperative refractive error
R_{po} = postoperative refractive error

The earliest method not needing historical values is the "contact lens method":

$K = B + P + R_{CL} - R_{bare}$

where

K = calculated corneal power
B = base curve (in D) of hard PMMA contact lens (CL)
P = power of CL
R_{CL} = refraction with CL on the eye
R_{bare} = bare refraction without the CL

It is not possible here to describe the remaining methods, but all methods are included in the Hoffer/Savini LASIK IOL Power Tool, which can be downloaded free of charge. The tool requests the data needed to calculate each method, and the results appear automatically for every method for which complete data have been entered. The ultimate choice is left to the surgeon. The entire sheet can be printed out on a single page and entered in the patient's chart.

Perhaps in the future, there will be a more satisfactory method of measuring true corneal power using topography and the latest measuring techniques. But at the present time, the ideal method of handling post–refractive surgery patients has yet to be proven.

Hoffer KJ. The EyeLab website. Available at http://www.EyeLab.com or http://www.IOLPower Club.org. Accessed July 4, 2008.

Koch DD, Liu JF, Hyde LL, Rock RL, Emery JM. Refractive complications of cataract surgery after radial keratotomy. *Am J Ophthalmol.* 1989;108(6):676–682.

IOL Power in Corneal Transplant Eyes

It is very difficult to predict the ultimate power of the cornea after the eye has undergone penetrating keratoplasty. Thus, in 1988, Hoffer recommended that the surgeon wait for the cornea to completely heal before implanting an IOL. The safety of intraocular surgery today allows for such a double-procedure approach in all but the rarest cases. Subsequent authors have proven the validity of this approach, with posttransplant eyes having better uncorrected visual acuity (68% with 20/40 or better) and with the range of IOL power error decreasing, from 10 D to 5 D (95% within ±2.00 D).

If simultaneous IOL implantation and corneal transplant are necessary, it has been suggested that surgeons use either the K reading of the fellow eye or the average postoperative K of a previous series of transplants. When there is corneal scarring in an eye but no need for a corneal graft, it might be best to use the corneal power of the other eye or even a power that is commensurate with the eye's AL and refractive error.

Geggel HS. Intraocular lens implantation after penetrating keratoplasty. Improved unaided visual acuity, astigmatism, and safety in patients with combined corneal disease and cataract. *Ophthalmology.* 1990;97(11):1460–1467.

Hoffer KJ. Triple procedure for intraocular lens exchange. *Arch Ophthalmol.* 1987;105(5): 609–610.

Silicone Oil Eyes

The ophthalmologist considering IOL implantation in eyes filled with silicone oil encounters 2 major problems. The first is obtaining an accurate AL measurement with the ultrasonic biometer. Recall that the ultrasonic biometer measures the transit time of the ultrasound pulse and, using estimated ultrasound velocities through the various ocular media, calculates the distance. This concept needs to be taken into consideration when velocities differ from the norm, as the velocity does when silicone oil fills the posterior chamber (980 m/sec for silicone oil versus 1532 m/sec for vitreous). Using the IOLMaster to measure AL solves this problem. It is recommended that retinal surgeons perform an immersion AL measurement before silicone oil placement.

The second problem is that the oil filling the vitreous cavity acts like a negative lens power in the eye when a biconvex IOL is implanted. This must be offset by an increase in IOL power of 3–5 D.

Pediatric Eyes

There are several issues that make IOL power selection for children much more complex than that for adults. The first is obtaining accurate AL and corneal measurements, usually with the patient under general anesthesia. Second, because shorter AL causes greater IOL power errors, the small size of a child's eye compounds power calculation errors, particularly if the child is very young. The third problem is selecting an appropriate target IOL power, one that will not only provide adequate visual acuity to prevent amblyopia but also allow adequate vision in adulthood.

A possible solution to the latter problem is to implant 2 (or more) IOLs simultaneously: one with the predicted adult emmetropic power and the other (or others) with the power that provides childhood emmetropia. When the patient reaches adulthood, the obsolete IOL(s) can be removed. Alternatively, hyperopic corneal refractive surgery could be used to treat the myopia developed in adulthood. Several recent studies have shown that the best modern formulas perform less accurately for children's eyes than for adults' eyes.

Image Magnification

Image magnification of as much as 20%–35% is the major disadvantage of aphakic spectacles. Contact lenses magnify images only 7%–12%, while IOLs magnify by 4% or less. An IOL implanted in the posterior chamber produces less image magnification than an IOL in the anterior chamber. However, the issue of magnification is further complicated by the correction of residual postsurgical refractive errors. A Galilean telescope is in effect created when spectacles are worn over pseudophakic eyes. Clinically, each diopter of spectacle overcorrection at a vertex of 12 mm causes a 2% magnification or minification (for plus or minus lenses, respectively). Thus, a pseudophakic patient with a PCIOL and a residual refractive error of –1 D will have 2% magnification from the IOL and 2% minification from the spectacle lens, resulting in little change in image size.

Aniseikonia is defined as a difference in image size between the 2 eyes and can lead to disturbances in stereopsis. Generally, a person can tolerate spherical aniseikonia of 5%–8%. In clinical practice, aniseikonia is rarely a significant problem; however, it should be considered in patients with unexplained visual complaints.

Lens-Related Visual Disturbances

The presence of IOLs may lead to the occurrence of a number of optical phenomena. Various light-related visual phenomena encountered by pseudophakic (and phakic) patients have been termed *dysphotopsias*. These have been further subdivided into positive and negative dysphotopsias. Positive dysphotopsias are characterized by *brightness, streaks,* and *rays* emanating from a central point source of light, sometimes with a diffuse hazy *glare*. Negative dysphotopsias are characterized by subjective darkness or *shadowing*. Such optical phenomena may be related to light reflection and refraction along the edges of the IOL. High-index acrylic lenses with square or truncated edges produce a more intense edge glare (Fig 6-21A). These phenomena may also be due to internal re-reflection within the IOL itself, which is more likely to occur with materials that have a higher index of refraction, such as acrylic (Fig 6-21B). With a less steeply curved anterior surface, the lens may be more likely to have internal reflections that are directed toward the fovea and that are therefore more distracting (Figs 6-21C, D).

Davison JA. Positive and negative dysphotopsia in patients with acrylic intraocular lenses. *J Cataract Refract Surg.* 2000;26(9):1346–1355.

Erie JC, Bandhauer MH. Intraocular lens surfaces and their relationship to postoperative glare. *J Cataract Refract Surg.* 2003;29(2):336–341.

Farbowitz MA, Zabriskie NA, Crandall AS, Olson RJ, Miller KM. Visual complaints associated with the AcrySof acrylic intraocular lens (1). *J Cataract Refract Surg.* 2000;26(9):1339–1345.

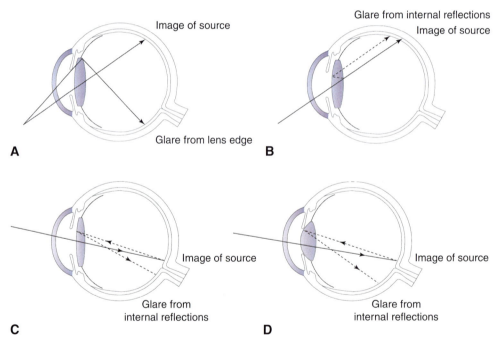

Figure 6-21 **A,** Light may reflect back from the surface of the retina and reach the anterior surface of the IOL. This acts as a concave mirror, reflecting back an undesirable dysphotopsic image. When the anterior surface of the IOL is more curved, the annoying image is displaced relatively far from the fovea. **B,** When the anterior IOL surface is less steeply curved, the annoying image appears closer to the true image and is likely to be more distracting. **C,** Light striking the edge of the IOL may be reflected to another site on the retina, resulting in undesirable dysphotopsias. This occurs less with smoother-edged IOLs. **D,** Light may be internally re-reflected within an IOL, producing an undesirable second image or halo. This may be more likely to occur as the index of refraction of the IOL increases. *(Redrawn by C. H. Wooley.)*

Franchini A, Gallarati BZ, Vaccari E. Computerized analysis of the effects of intraocular lens edge design on the quality of vision in pseudophakic patients. *J Cataract Refract Surg.* 2003;29(2): 342–347.

Tester R, Pace NL, Samore M, Olson RJ. Dysphotopsia in phakic and pseudophakic patients: incidence and relation to intraocular lens type. *J Cataract Refract Surg.* 2000;26(6):810–816.

Nonspherical Optics

IOLs with more complex optical parameters have become available. It may be possible to offset the positive spherical aberration of the cornea in pseudophakic patients by implanting an IOL with the appropriate negative spherical aberration on its anterior surface. To correct astigmatism, IOLs with a *toric* surface are available. Studies have shown that rotational stability may be more of a concern when plate-haptic toric lenses are implanted in the vertical axis than when they are implanted in the horizontal axis. As a toric lens rotates from the optimum desired angular orientation, the benefit of the toric correction diminishes. A toric IOL that is more than 31° off-axis increases the residual astigmatism of an eye; if it is 90° off-axis, the residual astigmatism will be doubled. Fortunately, some benefit remains even with lesser degrees of axis error, though the axis of residual cylinder will change.

Recently, investigators developed an IOL whose optical power can be altered by laser after lens implantation. This would be useful in correcting both IOL power calculation errors and residual astigmatism.

Mester U, Dillinger P, Anterist N. Impact of a modified optic design on visual function: clinical comparative study. *J Cataract Refract Surg.* 2003;29(4):652–660.

Ruhswurm I, Scholz U, Zehetmayer M, Hanselmayer G, Vass C, Skorpik C. Astigmatism correction with a foldable toric intraocular lens in cataract patients. *J Cataract Refract Surg.* 2000; 26(7):1022–1027.

Sun XY, Vicary D, Montgomery P, Griffiths M. Toric intraocular lenses for correcting astigmatism in 130 eyes. *Ophthalmology.* 2000;107(9):1776–1781.

Multifocal IOLs

Conventional IOLs are *monofocal* and correct the refractive ametropia associated with removal of the crystalline lens. Since a standard plastic IOL has no accommodative power, its focus is essentially for a single distance only. Of course, the improved visual acuity resulting from IOL implantation may allow a patient to see with acceptable clarity over a range of distances. This ability may be further augmented if the patient is left with a residual refractive cylinder such as a myopic astigmatism. If one endpoint of the astigmatic conoid of Sturm corresponds to distance focus while the other represents several diopters of myopia and, thus, a near focus, satisfactory visual clarity may be possible if the object in view is focused between these 2 endpoints. In bilateral asymmetric oblique myopic astigmatism, the brain ignores the blurred axis images and chooses the clearest axis images to form one clear image for distance vision, selecting the opposite images for near. It is difficult to replicate this process clinically. Thus, even standard IOLs may provide some degree of depth of focus and "bifocal" capabilities. An alternate approach to this problem is to correct one eye for distance and the other for near vision, which is called *monovision*. Nevertheless, most patients who receive IOLs are corrected for distance vision and wear reading glasses as needed.

Multifocal IOLs are designed to provide patients with both near and distance vision to decrease the patient's dependence on glasses. They differ from spectacles in the way they attempt to correct presbyopic symptoms. Bifocal, trifocal, and "blended bifocal" spectacles provide (in effect) different lenses in the same spectacle frame. The patient chooses which area to look through, depending on the visual task. At any time, the distance or near correction (or an intermediate correction) is used, but not both (or all) simultaneously. The brain processes one clear image at a time.

With a multifocal IOL, the correcting lens is placed in a fixed location within the eye, and the patient cannot voluntarily change the focus. Depending on the type of multifocal IOL and the viewing situation, both near and far images may be presented to the eye at the same time. The brain must process the clearest image, ignoring the other(s). Most patients can adapt to this, but not all.

The performance of certain types of IOLs is greatly impaired by decentration if the visual axis does not pass through the center of the IOL. However, in general, the use of modern surgical techniques results in adequate lens centration. Pupil size, on the other hand, is an active variable, but it can be employed in some situations to improve multifocal function.

Other disadvantages of a multifocal IOL are image degradation, "ghost" images (or *monocular diplopia*), decreased contrast sensitivity, and reduced performance in lower-light (eg, trouble with night vision), making them less desirable in eyes with impending macular disease.

Accuracy of IOL power calculation is very important for multifocal IOLs, because their purpose is to reduce the patient's dependence on glasses. Preoperative and postoperative astigmatism should be low.

Types of Multifocal IOLs

Bifocal IOL

The bifocal IOL is conceptually the simplest of the various designs. The bifocal concept was based on the idea that when there are 2 superimposed images on the retina, the brain always selects the clearer image and suppresses the blurred one. The first bifocal IOL implanted in a human was the Hoffer *split bifocal* in 1984. In this simple design, which was independent of pupil size, half the optic was for distance vision and the other half for near (Fig 6-22A). The additional power needed for near vision is not affected by the AL or the corneal power but is affected by the ELP. A PCIOL requires more near add than does an ACIOL for the same focal distance. About 3.75 D of added power is required in order to provide the 2.75 D of myopia needed.

A later design was the *"bullet" bifocal* (Fig 6-22B), which had a central zone for near power, with the surrounding zone being for distance. When the pupil constricted for near vision, its smaller size reduced or eliminated the contribution from the distance portion of the IOL. For viewing distant objects, when the pupil dilated, more of the distance portion of the IOL was exposed and contributed to the final image. Obviously, lens decentration

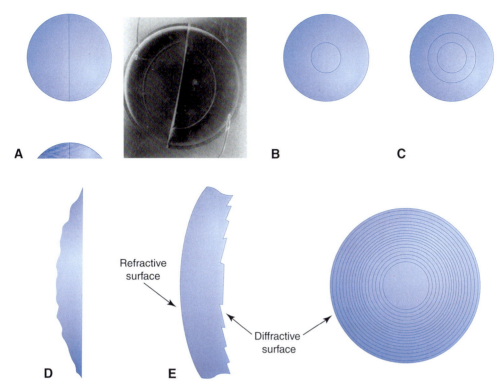

Figure 6-22 Multifocal IOLs. **A,** Split bifocal *(left)* and photo of lens implanted in 1984 *(right).* **B,** Bullet bifocal. **C,** Three-zone multifocal design. **D,** Multifocal IOL designed with several annular zones. **E,** Diffractive multifocal IOL with magnified cross section of central portion (the depth of the grooves is exaggerated). *(Photograph courtesy of Kenneth J. Hoffer, MD. All other parts redrawn by C. H. Wooley.)*

could have a deleterious effect on the IOL's optical performance. One problem with the design itself was that the patient's pupil size did not always correspond to the desired visual task. For this reason, the bullet bifocal IOL fell into disuse.

Multiple-Zone IOL

To overcome the problems associated with pupil size, a *3-zone bifocal* (Fig 6-22C) was introduced. The central and outer zones are for distance vision; the inner annulus is for near. The diameters were selected to provide near correction for moderately small pupils and distance correction for both large and small pupils.

Another design uses several *annular zones* (Fig 6-22D), each of which varies continuously in power over a range of 3.5 D. The advantage is that whatever the size, shape, or location of the pupil, all the focal distances are represented.

Diffractive multifocal IOL

The *diffractive multifocal* IOL designs (Fig 6-22E) use Fresnel diffraction optics to achieve a multifocal effect. The overall spherical shape of the surfaces produces an image for distance vision. The posterior surface has a stepped structure, and the diffraction from these multiple rings produces a second image, with an effective add power. At a particular point along the axis, waves diffracted by the various zones add in phase, giving a focus for that wavelength. About 20% of the light entering the pupil is absorbed in this process, and optical aberrations with diffractive IOLs can be particularly troublesome.

Second-generation diffractive multifocal IOL

Today, 3 newer diffractive multifocal IOLs are available that have increased independence from spectacles and decreased the incidence of optical side effects.

The *AcrySof ReSTOR* IOL (Alcon, Ft Worth, TX) is an apodized diffractive lens (Fig 6-23A). Apodization refers to the gradual tapering of the diffractive steps from the center to the outside edge of a lens to create a smooth transition of light between the distance, intermediate, and near focal points.

The *ReZoom* lens (Advanced Medical Optics [AMO], Santa Ana, CA) (Fig 6-23B) has 5 anterior surface zones for distance and near, and the grading between the zones provides intermediate vision.

The *TECNIS ZM* 900 lens (AMO) adds an aspheric surface, whereas the ReSTOR and ReZoom lenses do not.

Clinical Results of Multifocal IOLs

Some multifocal IOLs perform better for near vision; others, for intermediate. Studies have shown a benefit to using a combination of these lenses in the same patient.

The best-corrected visual acuity may be less with a multifocal IOL than with a monofocal IOL; this difference increases in low-light situations. However, the need for additional spectacle correction for near vision is greatly reduced in patients with multifocal IOLs. Some patients are quite pleased with multifocal IOLs; others have requested their removal and replacement with monofocal IOLs. Interestingly, patients with a multifocal

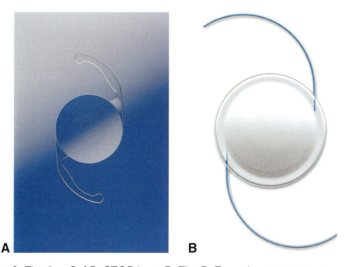

A   **B**

Figure 6-23   **A,** The AcrySof ReSTOR lens. **B,** The ReZoom lens. *(Part A courtesy of Alcon Laboratories; part B courtesy of Advanced Medical Optics.)*

IOL in one eye and a monofocal in the other seem to be less tolerant of the multifocal than are those with bilateral multifocal IOLs.

Patient selection is crucial for successful adaptation to multifocal IOLs. Patients must be willing to accept the trade-off of decreased performance at distance (and at near, compared with that of a monofocal IOL and reading glasses)—particularly in low-light situations—in exchange for the possibility of seeing well enough at all distances to be able to dispense with spectacles altogether. This technology will continue to evolve.

Ford JG, Karp CL. *Cataract Surgery and Intraocular Lenses: A 21st-Century Perspective*. 2nd ed. Ophthalmology Monograph 7. San Francisco: American Academy of Ophthalmology; 2001.

Hoffer KJ. Personal history in bifocal intraocular lenses. In: *Current Concepts of Multifocal Intraocular Lenses*. Maxwell WA, Nordan LT, eds. Thorofare, NJ: Slack, Inc; 1991:chap 12, pp 127–132.

Accommodating IOLs

These lenses are essentially monofocal IOLs designed to allow some degree of improved near vision, which usually involves accommodative effort being linked to an anterior movement of the IOL, thereby increasing its effective power in the eye. This mechanism may be more effective with higher-power IOLs, because their effective powers are more sensitive to small changes in position than are lower-power IOLs. The FDA has approved one design that has shown some degree of accommodation, and other designs are awaiting FDA approval.

Cumming JS, Slade SG, Chayet A; AT-45 Study Group. Clinical evaluation of the model AT-45 silicone accommodating intraocular lens: results of feasibility and the initial phase of a Food and Drug Administration clinical trial. *Ophthalmology*. 2001;108(11):2005–2009.

Findl O, Kiss B, Petternel V, et al. Intraocular lens movement caused by ciliary muscle contraction. *J Cataract Refract Surg*. 2003;29(4):669–676.

Langenbucher A, Huber S, Nguyen NX, Seitz B, Gusek-Schneider GC, Küchle M. Measurement of accommodation after implantation of an accommodating posterior chamber intraocular lens. *J Cataract Refract Surg*. 2003;29(4):677–685.

Matthews MW, Eggleston HC, Hilmas GE. Development of a repeatedly adjustable intraocular lens. *J Cataract Refract Surg*. 2003;29(11):2204–2210.

Matthews MW, Eggleston HC, Pekarek SD, Hilmas GE. Magnetically adjustable intraocular lens. *J Cataract Refract Surg*. 2003;29(11):2211–2216.

IOL Standards

The American National Standards Institute (ANSI) and the International Standards Organization (ISO) set standards for IOLs. Among these standards is one for IOL power labeling, which requires that IOLs with labeled powers less than 25 D be within ±0.40 D of the labeled power and have no axial power variations of more than 0.25 D. IOLs labeled 25–30 D must be within ±0.50 D of the labeled power; those greater than 30 D must be within ±1.0 D. Most ophthalmologists are unaware of this large range for the labeling of high-power IOLs. Though controversial, attempts are being made to reduce this range so that all IOL powers are within ±0.25 D of the labeled powers.

A mislabeled IOL power is quite rare today. In addition, ANSI, the ISO, and the FDA have set various other standards for *optical performance,* a term used to refer roughly to the image quality produced by an IOL. Lenses are also tested for biocompatibility, for the absence of cytotoxicity of their material and any additives (such as UV filters), for genotoxicity, and for photostability as well as safety with YAG lasers. The resolution efficiency of an IOL is tested, relative to the diffraction-limited, cut-off spatial frequency or by testing with the modulation transfer function. There are also standards for spectral transmission. Physical standards exist to ensure adherence to the labeled optic diameter, haptic angulation, strength, and mechanical fatigability of the components, as well as to ensure sterility and safety during injection.

CHAPTER **7**

Optical Considerations in Refractive Surgery

This chapter provides an overview of the issues and optical considerations specific to refractive surgery. Refractive surgical procedures performed with the intent to reduce or eliminate refractive errors can generally be categorized as *corneal* or *lenticular*. Keratorefractive procedures include radial keratotomy (RK), astigmatic keratotomy (AK), photorefractive keratectomy (PRK), laser subepithelial keratomileusis (LASEK), epithelial laser in situ keratomileusis (Epi-LASIK), laser in situ keratomileusis (LASIK), implantation of plastic ring segments (eg, Intacs), laser thermal keratoplasty (LTK), and radiofrequency conductive keratoplasty (CK). Lenticular refractive procedures include cataract and clear lens extraction with intraocular lens implantation, phakic intraocular lens implantation, and piggyback lens implantation. Although all of these refractive surgical techniques alter the optical properties of the eye in some way, keratorefractive surgery (KRS) is generally more likely than lenticular refractive surgery to produce unwanted optical aberrations. This chapter deals only with KRS and its optical considerations.

Various optical considerations are relevant to refractive surgery, in both screening patients for candidacy and evaluating those with visual complaints after surgery. In the following sections, we discuss optical considerations related to the change in corneal shape following KRS, issues related to angle kappa and pupil size, and the various causes of irregular astigmatism.

Corneal Shape

The normal human cornea has a prolate shape (Fig 7-1), similar to the pole of an egg. In the human eye, the central cornea is steepest, and there is a gradual flattening of curvature toward the periphery. In contrast, a simple spherical refracting surface produces a nearer point of focus for marginal rays than for paraxial rays, a refractive condition known as *spherical aberration*. Factor Q is the relative difference between pericentral and central cornea. Note that this is different from the Q factor that characterizes a resonator such as a laser cavity. In an ideal visual system, asphericity factor Q has a value of –0.50, indicating that the center curvature is steeper than the periphery (prolateness). At this value of Q, spherical aberration equals zero. However, in the human eye, this is not anatomically possible because of the junction between the cornea and the sclera. The Q factor for the

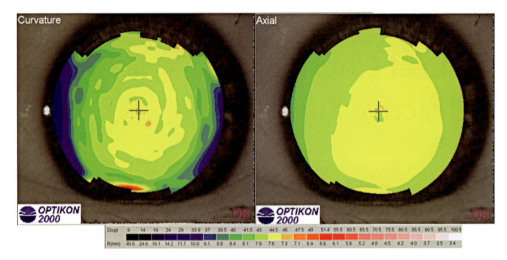

Figure 7-1 An example of the axial *(right)* and meridional (tangential) maps *(left)* of a normal cornea. *(Used with permission from Roberts C. Corneal topography. In: Azar DT, ed. Gatinel D, Hoang-Xuan T, associate eds. Refractive Surgery. 2nd ed. St Louis, MO: Elsevier-Mosby; 2007:103–116.)*

human cornea has an average value of –0.26, allowing for a smooth transition at the limbus. The human visual system, therefore, suffers from a small amount of spherical aberration, which increases with increasing pupil size.

Myopic KRS results in an oblate cornea, which is like an egg on its side. The central cornea becomes flatter than the periphery. This results in an increase in spherical aberration.

To demonstrate this, consider the point spread function produced by all rays from a single object point that traverse the pupil. Generally, KRS reduces spherical refractive error and regular astigmatism, but it does so at the expense of increasing spherical aberration and irregular astigmatism (Fig 7-2). KRS moves the location of the best focus closer to the retina but, at the same time, makes the focus less stigmatic. It is such irregular astigmatism that causes many visual complaints following refractive surgery.

A basic premise of refractive surgery is that the cornea's optical properties are intimately related to its shape. Consequently, manipulating corneal shape changes the eye's refractive status. Although this assumption is true, the relationship between corneal shape and corneal optical properties is more complex than generally appreciated.

Ablative procedures, incisional procedures, and intracorneal rings change the natural shape of the cornea to effect a reduction in refractive error. Keratometry readings in eyes before KRS typically range from 38 D to 48 D. When refractive surgical procedures are being considered, it is important to avoid changes that may result in excessively flat (less than 35 D) or excessively steep (greater than 52 D) corneas. A 0.8 D change in K corresponds to approximately a 1.0 D change of refraction. The following equation is often used to predict corneal curvature after KRS:

$$K_{postop} = K_{preop} + (0.8 \times RE)$$

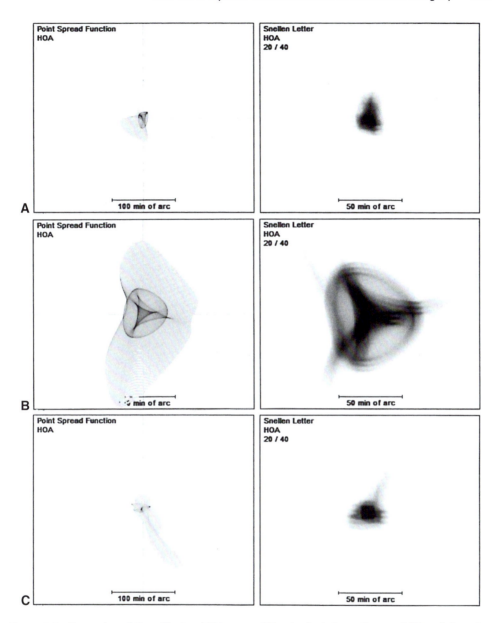

Figure 7-2 Examples of the effects of **(A)** coma, **(B)** spherical aberration, and **(C)** trefoil on the point spread function (PSF) and Snellen letter E. *(Courtesy of Ming Wang, MD.)*

where K_{preop} and K_{postop} are preoperative and postoperative K readings, respectively, and RE is the refractive error to be corrected at the corneal plane. For example, if a patient's preoperative keratometry readings are 45/43, the average K is 44. If the amount of refractive correction at the corneal plane is –8.50 D, the predicted average postoperative K reading is 44 + (–8.50 × 0.8) = 37.2, which is acceptable.

The ratio of dioptric change in refractive error to dioptric change in keratometry approximates 0.8 owing to the change in posterior corneal surface power after excimer ablation. The anterior corneal surface produces most of the eye's refractive power. In Gullstrand's model eye (see Table 3-1 in Chapter 3, Optics of the Human Eye), the anterior corneal surface has a power of +48.8 D and the posterior corneal surface has a power of –5.8 D, for an overall corneal refractive power of +43.0 D. It is important to recognize that standard corneal topography instruments and keratometers do not precisely measure corneal power because they do not assess the back corneal surface. These instruments estimate total corneal power by assuming a constant relationship between the anterior and posterior corneal surfaces. This constancy is disrupted by KRS. For example, after myopic excimer surgery, the anterior corneal curvature is reduced. At the same time, owing to the reduction in corneal pachymetry and weakening of corneal strength, the posterior corneal surface bulges forward, increasing its negative power. The reduction in positive anterior corneal power and the increase in negative posterior corneal power result in an increase in the relative contribution to overall corneal refractive power of the posterior surface. When the change of posterior corneal power is included, the ratio of total corneal power to refractive correction at the corneal plane after KRS is unity.

A small amount of tissue removal (in micrometers, µm) in KRS can result in a significant change in refraction (in diopters) (Fig 7-3). The Munnerlyn formula relates these 2 parameters:

$$t = S^2D/3$$

where t is the central ablation depth in micrometers, S is the diameter of the optical zone in millimeters, and D is the amount of refractive correction.

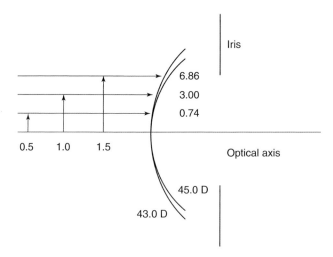

Figure 7-3 Comparison between a 43 D cornea and a 45 D cornea. Numbers below the vertical arrows indicate distance from the optical axis in millimeters; numbers to the right of the horizontal arrows indicate the separation between the corneas in micrometers (µm). A typical pupil size of 3.0 mm is indicated. A typical red blood cell has a diameter of 7 µm. Within the pupillary space (ie, the optical zone of the cornea), the separation between the corneas is less than the diameter of a red blood cell. *(Courtesy of Edmond H. Thall, MD. Modified by C. H. Wooley.)*

An ideal LASIK ablation or PRK removes a convex positive meniscus in myopic corrections (Fig 7-4A). A concave positive meniscus is removed in simple hyperopic corrections (Fig 7-4B). A toric positive meniscus is removed in astigmatic corrections. In toric corrections, the specific shape of the ablation depends on the spherical component of the refractive error.

Azar DT, ed. Gatinel D, Hoang-Xuan T, associate eds. *Refractive Surgery.* 2nd ed. St Louis, MO: Elsevier-Mosby; 2007.

Azar DT, Primack JD. Theoretical analysis of ablation depths and profiles in laser in situ keratomileusis for compound hyperopic and mixed astigmatism. *J Cataract Refract Surg.* 2000;26(8):1123–1136.

Klyce S. Night vision after LASIK: the pupil proclaims innocence. *Ophthalmology.* 2004;111(1): 1–2.

Munnerlyn CR, Koons SJ, Marshall J. Photorefractive keratectomy: a technique for laser refractive surgery. *J Cataract Refract Surg.* 1988;14(1):46–52.

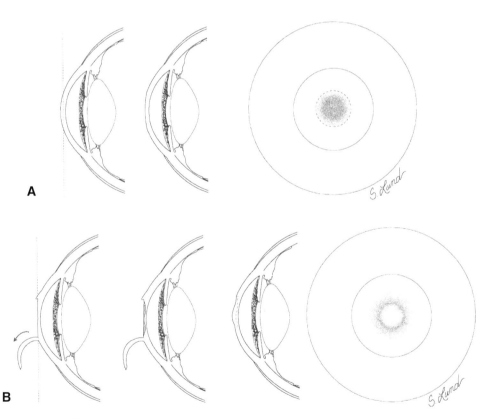

Figure 7-4 **A,** Schematic illustration of myopic photorefractive keratectomy. The shaded area refers to the location of tissue subtraction under the flap. After treatment, the flap is repositioned. **B,** Schematic illustration of hyperopic laser in situ keratomileusis. A superficial corneal flap is raised. The shaded area refers to the location of tissue subtraction under the thin flap. After treatment, the flap is repositioned. *(Used with permission from Poothullil AM, Azar DT. Terminology, classification, and history of refractive surgery. In: Azar DT, ed. Gatinel D, Hoang-Xuan T, associate eds.* Refractive Surgery. *2nd ed. St Louis, MO: Elsevier-Mosby; 2007:1–18.)*

Angle Kappa

As discussed in Chapter 3, the pupillary axis is the imaginary line perpendicular to the corneal surface and passing through the midpoint of the entrance pupil. The visual axis is the line connecting the point of fixation to the fovea. *Angle kappa (κ)* is defined as the angle between the pupillary axis and the visual axis. A large angle kappa results if the pupillary axis differs significantly from the central corneal apex. If angle kappa is large, centering an excimer ablation over the geometric center of the cornea will effectively result in a decentered ablation. This can be particularly problematic in a hyperopic correction, in which a large angle kappa can result in a refractively signifi-cant "second corneal apex," causing monocular diplopia and decreased visual quality. A large angle kappa needs to be identified before surgery so that a poor visual outcome can be avoided.

Freedman KA, Brown SM, Mathews SM, Young RS. Pupil size and the ablation zone in laser refractive surgery: considerations based on geometric optics. *J Cataract Refract Surg.* 2003; 29(10):1924–1931.

Pupil Size

Pupil size measurement became the standard of care in the late 1990s, when it was ob-served that patients with large pupils (greater than 6 mm) had poor night vision after KRS. Typical symptoms included glare, starbursts, halos, decreased contrast sensitivity, and poor overall visual quality. Night-vision problems tend to occur in patients with large pupils and small treatment zones (6 mm or less). The algorithms used in third-generation lasers incorporate larger optical and transition zones, enabling surgeons to perform re-fractive procedures on patients with larger pupils. These algorithms decrease the inci-dence and severity of night-vision problems dramatically.

Many surgeons use default ablation zones during excimer procedures. The accepted standard transition zone between ablated and unablated cornea is 0.5 to 1.0 mm larger than the pupil to minimize night-vision problems. To conserve corneal tissue, smaller op-tical zones are typically used in higher myopic corrections. In these patients, the incidence of night-vision problems increases because of the mismatch between the size of the pupil and that of the optical zone.

Although pupil size does not affect surgical outcome as it once did, pupil size mea-surement continues to be the standard of care in the preoperative evaluation. Patients with extremely large pupils (8 mm or more) should be identified and counseled regard-ing their increased risk of complications. Spherical aberration may be increased in these patients. Clinical management of night-vision problems postoperatively includes the use of miotics such as brimonidine 0.2% or pilocarpine (0.5%–1%).

Freedman KA, Brown SM, Mathews SM, Young RS. Pupil size and the ablation zone in laser refractive surgery: considerations based on geometric optics. *J Cataract Refract Surg.* 2003; 29(10):1924–1931.

Klyce S. Night vision after LASIK: the pupil proclaims innocence. *Ophthalmology.* 2004;111(1): 1–2.

Lee YC, Hu FR, Wang IJ. Quality of vision after laser in situ keratomileusis: influence of dioptric correction and pupil size on visual function. *J Cataract Refract Surg.* 2003;29(4):769–777.

Schallhorn SC, Kaupp SE, Tanzer DJ, Tidwell J, Laurent J, Bourque LB. Pupil size and quality of vision after LASIK. *Ophthalmology.* 2003;110(8):1606–1614.

Irregular Astigmatism

The treatment of postoperative irregular corneal astigmatism is one of the great challenges of refractive surgery today. The diagnosis of irregular astigmatism is made by meeting clinical and imaging criteria: loss of spectacle best-corrected vision but preservation of vision with the use of a gas-permeable contact lens, coupled with topographic corneal irregularity. One important sign of postsurgical irregular astigmatism is a refraction inconsistent with the uncorrected acuity. For example, consider a patient who has –3.50 D myopia with essentially no astigmatism before the operation. Following KRS, the patient has uncorrected acuity of 20/25 but a refraction of +2.00 –3.00 × 060. Ordinarily, this refraction would be inconsistent with an uncorrected acuity of 20/25, but such results can occur in patients who have irregular astigmatism after KRS.

Another important sign is difficulty in determining axis location during manifest refraction in a patient with a large amount of astigmatism. Normally, it is easy to accurately determine the correcting cylinder axis in a patient with significant cylinder. However, a patient with irregular astigmatism following KRS often has difficulty choosing an axis. Automated refractors may identify significant amounts of astigmatism that are rejected by patients on manifest refraction. Because the astigmatism is irregular (and thus has no definite axis), patients may achieve nearly the same acuity with large powers of cylinder at markedly different axes. Streak retinoscopy often demonstrates irregular scissoring in patients with irregular astigmatism.

Astigmatic enhancements (ie, astigmatic keratotomy, LASIK) are unpredictable in patients with irregular astigmatism. Avoid "chasing your tail" in KRS. For instance, it may be tempting to perform an astigmatic enhancement on a patient who had little preexisting astigmatism but has significant postoperative astigmatism. However, if the patient is happy with the uncorrected acuity (despite irregular astigmatism), it may be preferable to avoid further intervention. Astigmatic enhancement in such cases can cause the axis to change dramatically without much reduction in cylinder power.

It is, in fact, possible to quantify irregular astigmatism in much the same way that we quantify regular astigmatism. We think of regular astigmatism as a cylinder superimposed on a sphere. Similarly, irregular astigmatism can be thought of as additional shapes superimposed on cylinders and spheres. This approach is widely used in optical engineering.

Wavefront Analysis

See also BCSC Section 13, *Refractive Surgery,* for a discussion of the topics covered here.

Ophthalmologists should understand irregular astigmatism for 2 important reasons. First, KRS produces visually significant irregular astigmatism in many cases. Second, KRS may also be able to treat it. If irregular astigmatism is to be studied effectively, it needs to be described quantitatively. The most effective method developed to date for describing irregular astigmatism is wavefront analysis.

To understand irregular astigmatism and wavefront analysis, it is best to begin with stigmatic imaging. A stigmatic imaging system brings all rays from a single object point to a perfect point focus. According to the Fermat principle, a stigmatic focus is possible only when the amount of time required for light to travel from an object point to an image point is identical for all possible paths the light might take.

An analogy to a foot race is helpful. Suppose that several runners simultaneously depart from an object point (A). Each runner follows a different path represented by a ray. The runners all travel at the same speed in air and all run at the same (but slower) speed in glass. If all the runners reach the image point (B) simultaneously, the image is stigmatic. If not, the rays do not meet at a single point and the image is astigmatic.

The Fermat principle explains how a lens works. Rays going through the center of a lens travel a short distance in air, but moving through the thickest part of the glass slows them down. Rays going through the edge of the lens travel a longer distance in air but slow down only briefly when they traverse the thin section of glass. The shape of the ideal lens precisely balances each path so that no matter what path the light travels, it reaches point B at the same time. If the lens shape is not ideal, some rays miss point B, and the focus is astigmatic.

Wavefront analysis is based on the Fermat principle. Construct a circular arc centered on the image point with a radius approximately equal to the image distance (Fig 7-5A). This arc is called the *reference sphere*. Again, consider the analogy of a foot race, but now think of the reference sphere as the finish line (instead of point B). If the image is stigmatic, all runners (from point A) will cross the reference sphere simultaneously. If the image is astigmatic, the runners will cross the reference sphere at slightly different times (Fig 7-5B). The *geometric wavefront* is like a photo finish of the race. It represents the position of each runner shortly after the fastest runner crosses the finish line. The *wavefront aberration* is the time each runner finishes minus the time of the fastest runner. In other words, it is the difference between the reference sphere and the wavefront. When the focus is stigmatic, the reference sphere and the wavefront coincide so the wavefront aberration is zero.

Wavefront aberration is a function of pupil position. Figure 7-6 shows some typical wavefront aberrations. Myopia, hyperopia, and regular astigmatism can be expressed as wavefront aberrations. Myopia produces an aberration that optical engineers call *positive defocus*. Hyperopia is called *negative defocus*. Not surprisingly, regular (cylindrical) astigmatism produces a wavefront aberration that looks like a cylinder.

When peripheral rays focus in front of more central rays, the effect is called *spherical aberration*. Clinically, this is the cause of night myopia and is commonly seen after LASIK and PRK.

Another common wavefront aberration is called *coma*. In this case, rays at one edge of the pupil cross the finish line first; rays at the opposite edge of the pupil cross the finish line last. The effect is that the image of each object point resembles a comet with a tail. The word *coma* means "comet." Coma is common in patients with decentered keratorefractive ablation. Coma is commonly seen in the aiming beam during retinal laser

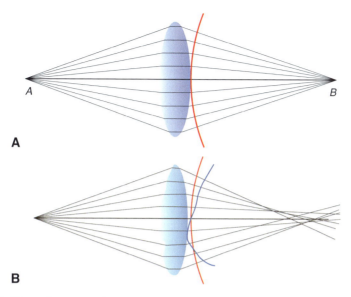

Figure 7-5   A, The reference sphere *(in red)* is represented in 2 dimensions by a circular arc centered on point *B* and drawn through the center of the exit pupil of the lens. If the image is stigmatic, all light from point *A* crosses the reference sphere simultaneously. **B,** When the image is astigmatic, light rays from the object point cross the wavefront *(in blue)*, not the reference sphere, simultaneously. *(Part B modified by C. H. Wooley.)*

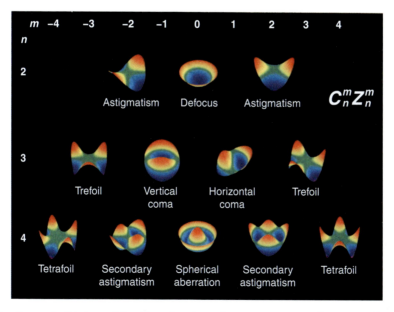

Figure 7-6 Second-, third-, and fourth-order aberrations are most pertinent to refractive surgery. *(Reproduced with permission from Applegate RA. Glenn Fry Award Lecture 2002: wavefront sensing, ideal corrections, and visual performance. Optom Vis Sci. 2004;81(3):169.)*

photocoagulation. If the ophthalmologist tilts the lens too far off-axis, the aiming beam spot becomes coma-shaped.

Higher-order aberrations tend to be less significant than low-order aberrations but may increase in diseased or surgically altered eyes. For example, if interrupted sutures are used to sew in a corneal graft during corneal transplant, they will produce higher-order "clover-shaped" aberrations. Also, in the manufacture of intraocular lenses, the lens blank is sometimes improperly positioned on the lathe; this too can produce higher-order aberrations.

Optical engineers have found about 18 basic types of astigmatism, of which only a few—perhaps as few as 5—are of clinical interest. As you might expect, most patients probably have a combination of all 5.

Wavefront aberrations can be represented in different ways. One approach is to represent them as 3-dimensional shapes. Another is to represent them as contour plots. Irregular astigmatism is a combination of a few basic shapes, just as conventional refractive error is a combination of sphere and cylinder. Our approach does not use graphs or contour plots to represent conventional refractive errors. Instead, we simply specify the amount of sphere and cylinder that make up the refractive error. Similarly, once we are comfortable with the basic forms of irregular astigmatism, there is little need for 3-dimensional graphs or 2-dimensional contour plots. We simply specify the amount of each basic form of astigmatism present in a given patient. The prescription of the future may consist of 8 or so numbers. The first 3 will be sphere, cylinder, and axis. The rest of the numbers will specify the irregular astigmatism as quantitated by higher-order aberration.

Currently, wavefront aberrations are specified by Zernike polynomials, which are the mathematical formulas used to describe wavefront surfaces. Wavefront aberration surfaces are simply graphs generated using Zernike polynomials. There are several techniques for measuring wavefront aberrations clinically, but the most popular is based on the Hartmann-Shack wavefront sensor. In this device, a low-power laser beam is focused on the retina. A point on the retina then acts as a point source. In a perfect eye, all the rays emerge in parallel and the wavefront is a flat plane. In reality, the wavefront is not flat. An array of lenses sample parts of the wavefront and focus light on a detector. The wavefront shape can be determined from the position of the focus on each detector (see Figure 1-6 in BCSC Section 13, *Refractive Surgery*).

Another method of measuring wavefront is a ray-tracing method that projects detecting light beams in a sequential manner rather than simultaneously, as in a Hartmann-Shack device, further improving the resolution of wavefront aberration measurement. Zernike polynomials are less than perfect in their mathematical description of aberrations, however, and alternative methods, such as Fourier transforms, are being considered.

To normalize wavefront and improve postoperative visual quality in KRS, technologies are being developed to improve the accuracy of higher-order aberration measurements and treatment using "flying spot" excimer lasers. Such lasers use small spot sizes (<1 mm diameter) to create smooth ablations, addressing the minute topographic changes associated with aberration errors.

Causes of Irregular Astigmatism

Irregular astigmatism may exist before KRS, it may be caused by surgery, or it may develop postoperatively. Preoperative causes include keratoconus, pellucid marginal degeneration,

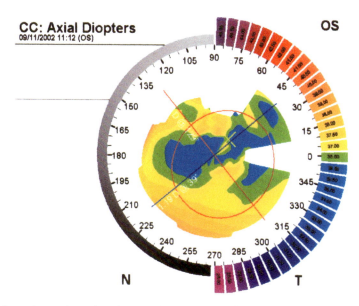

Figure 7-7 Irregular astigmatism in a patient with significant anterior basement membrane dystrophy (ABMD). The patient complained of glare and overall loss of visual quality. *(Courtesy of Ming Wang, MD.)*

contact lens warpage, dry eye, and anterior basement membrane dystrophy (ABMD; Fig 7-7). All these conditions should be identified before surgery. Common intraoperative causes include decentered ablations and central islands, and, less commonly, poor laser optics, nonuniform stromal bed hydration, and flap complications (thin, torn, irregular, incomplete, or buttonhole flaps; folds or striae of the flap; and epithelial defects). Postoperatively, flap displacement, diffuse lamellar keratitis and its sequelae, flap striae, posterior corneal ectasia, dry eye, and flap edema may contribute to irregular astigmatism.

Conclusion

Optical considerations are important in treating patients who undergo KRS. A good understanding of key parameters such as corneal shape, pupil size, the ocular surface, spherical and astigmatic errors, higher-order aberrations, laser centration and angle kappa, and irregular corneal astigmatism can help optimize visual outcomes after KRS. Most patient complaints after surgery are based on subjective loss of visual quality, which can most often be explained by a sound understanding of how refractive surgery changes the optics of the eye.

CHAPTER 8

Telescopes and Optical Instruments

The instruments used in clinical ophthalmology are based on the very optical principles discussed in this book. An understanding of the inner workings of the instruments we use in everyday practice provides a greater degree of proficiency in their use and recognition of their limitations.

Direct Ophthalmoscope

The direct ophthalmoscope (Fig 8-1) allows for a highly magnified, monocular image of the retina and optic disc. The optical principles on which this instrument is based are relatively straightforward (Fig 8-2A). If the retina of an emmetropic patient were self-luminous, an emmetropic observer looking into the patient's eye would see a focused fundus image. This is because light rays from the retina exit the emmetropic patient's eye parallel to one another, and these parallel rays are then focused onto the emmetropic observer's retina.

A series of auxiliary lenses built into the direct ophthalmoscope serves to compensate for the refractive errors of the patient and observer. When a patient is myopic, light rays emanating from the patient's eye are convergent, and a minus "correcting" lens must be dialed in for the clinician to see a sharp image of the retina (Fig 8-2B). When a patient

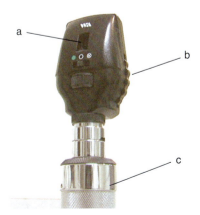

a

b

Figure 8-1 Photograph of a direct ophthalmoscope: *a,* opening for illumination and viewing systems; *b,* dial for "correcting" lenses; *c,* handle and battery supply. *(Courtesy of Neal H. Atebara, MD.)*

c

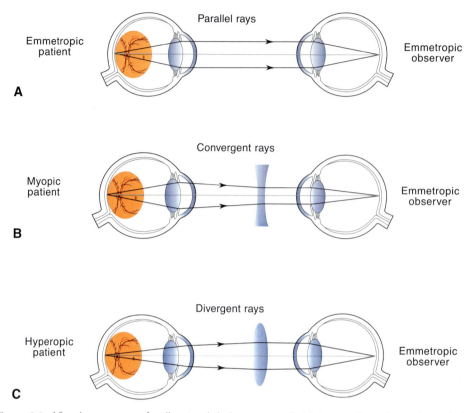

Figure 8-2 Viewing system of a direct ophthalmoscope. **A,** Light rays from the retina exit the eye parallel to one another. **B,** A minus "correcting" lens is used. **C,** A plus lens is used to compensate for the refractive error. *(Courtesy of Neal H. Atebara, MD. Redrawn by C. H. Wooley.)*

is hyperopic, divergent rays emanate from the patient's eye and a plus lens is required (Fig 8-2C).

The patient's fundus can be illuminated in several different ways, but they all require that light be passed through the pupil nearly coaxial to the line of sight of the observer. The light rays cannot be exactly coaxial to the observer's line of sight; otherwise, corneal reflection will interfere with the image. The early direct ophthalmoscopes used a partially reflective mirror. Light rays were reflected by the mirror into the patient's eye. This same mirror allowed some of the returning light rays to pass through it as they traveled from the patient's eye to the observer's eye. This strategy, however, caused light to be lost as it was reflected into the patient's eye and as it passed from the patient's eye to the observer's eye.

Less light is lost when a fully reflective mirror is used. In this case, the observer views the patient's fundus through a circular aperture in the mirror or looks just over the edge of the mirror.

Because an eye acts as a simple magnifier, we can approximate its magnification at a reading distance of 25 cm using the "simple magnifier formula," magnification = power/4. An emmetropic schematic eye has a refractive power of about 60 D, so the magnification is about 15×. If the eye is hyperopic by +10 D, its total refractive power is about 50 D, and the magnification is only 50/4 = 12.5×. If the eye is myopic by −10 D, its total refractive power is about 70 D, and the magnification is 70/4 = 17.5×.

Indirect Ophthalmoscope

The binocular indirect ophthalmoscope (Fig 8-3A) provides a brightly illuminated and wide-angle view of the retina. This instrument, in conjunction with a condensing lens (Fig 8-3B), works on a principle similar to that of the astronomical telescope. A patient's cornea and crystalline lens act as the astronomical telescope's objective lens, and the condensing lens acts as the astronomical telescope's eyepiece lens. As with all images produced by astronomical telescopes, the image produced by the indirect ophthalmoscope is inverted. The principles on which this instrument works can be broken down into 5 aspects.

Optics of Fundus Image Formation

To illuminate the fundus, an intense light is directed through the pupil. The fundus image is projected out, refracted by the crystalline lens and cornea of the patient's eye. An emmetropic eye projects the fundus image to optical infinity (Fig 8-4A). The parallel light bundles emanating from the eye are captured with a handheld condensing lens (eg, +20 D lens), and a new image is created at the lens's posterior focal plane (about 5 cm behind the lens) (Fig 8-4B).

Aerial Image

The image floating above the condensing lens is real and inverted and is called an *aerial image.* This image has depth, representing the depth of the 3-dimensional fundus itself. An observer merely focuses on the aerial image to view the fundus. The only lenses required to view the aerial image are those that correct the observer's refractive error and compensate for the near distance of the image, because the aerial image is usually located within arm's length of the observer (Fig 8-5).

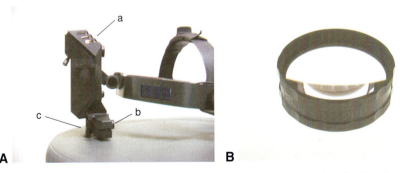

Figure 8-3 **A,** Photograph of an indirect ophthalmoscope: *a,* housing for illumination source; *b,* eyepiece; *c,* mirror complex. **B,** Photograph of a +20 D condensing lens. *(Courtesy of Neal H. Atebara, MD.)*

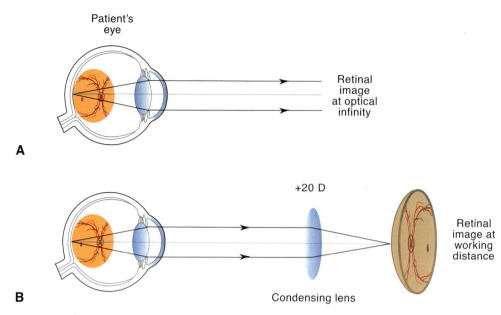

Figure 8-4   Indirect ophthalmoscope: fundus image formation. **A,** A retinal image is formed at optical infinity. **B,** A condensing lens is used to focus light to a comfortable working distance. *(Courtesy of Neal H. Atebara, MD. Redrawn by C. H. Wooley.)*

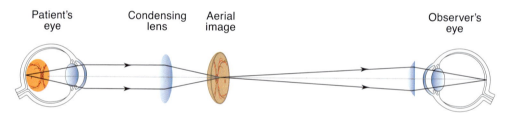

Figure 8-5   Indirect ophthalmoscope: the "aerial" image. *(Courtesy of Neal H. Atebara, MD. Redrawn by C. H. Wooley.)*

Conjugacy of Pupils

In indirect ophthalmoscopy, the pupils of the examiner and patient must be *optically conjugate*—that is, the observer's pupil must project optically to the patient's pupil, and vice versa. When this happens, the maximal amount of light passes from the patient's fundus into the observer's eye (Fig 8-6).

Fundus Illumination

The same condensing lens must also project an image of the illumination source into the patient's eye, and it must do so through an area of the patient's pupil that is not "occupied" by outgoing light; otherwise, reflections will interfere with the observer's view (Fig 8-7).

Binocular Observation

To appreciate the 3-dimensionality of the aerial image, both of the observer's pupils must receive light from the aerial image. This can occur only if both of the observer's pupils are

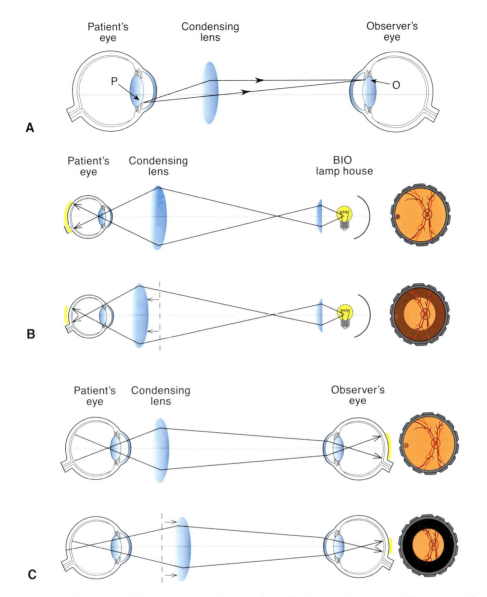

Figure 8-6 Indirect ophthalmoscope: conjugacy of pupils. **A,** In indirect ophthalmoscopy, the pupils must be "in register" with each other—that is, the observer's pupil *(O)* must project optically to the patient's pupil *(P)*. **B,** If the condensing lens is moved too close to the patient's eye, the peripheral fundus will not be illuminated. **C,** If the condensing lens is moved too far from the patient's eye, light from the peripheral retina will not reach the observer's eye. *(Courtesy of Neal H. Atebara, MD. Redrawn by C. H. Wooley.)*

imaged within the patient's pupil. To "fit" both of the observer's pupils in this small space, mirrors must be used to reduce the observer's interpupillary distance (Fig 8-8).

If a patient's pupil does not dilate well, the images of the observer's pupils must be squeezed into an even smaller space. This can be accomplished by retraction of the triangular mirror of the indirect ophthalmoscope, which causes the path of light from the patient's eye to be reflected nearer to the tip of the triangular mirror, resulting in a narrower

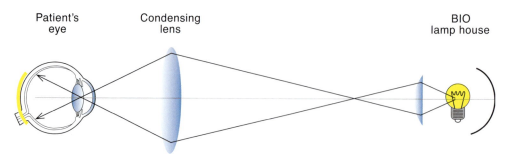

Figure 8-7 Indirect ophthalmoscope: illumination source. *(Courtesy of Neal H. Atebara, MD. Redrawn by C. H. Wooley.)*

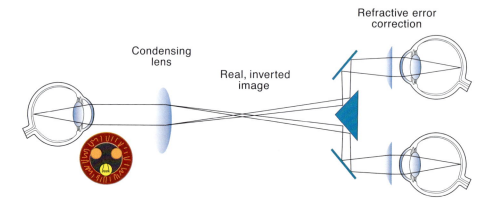

Figure 8-8 Indirect ophthalmoscope: binocular observation. *Orange circles* = observer's pupils; *black circle* = patient's pupil. *(Courtesy of Neal H. Atebara, MD. Redrawn by C. H. Wooley.)*

path of light (Fig 8-9A). Widening the interpupillary distance of the indirect ophthalmoscope produces a similar effect. This causes light from the patient's eye to be reflected nearer to the tip of the triangular mirror, resulting in a narrower path of light (Fig 8-9B).

Fundus Camera

Fundus cameras capture black-and-white, color, fluorescein angiographic, and indocyanine green angiographic images of the fundus. These cameras employ the same optical principles as the indirect ophthalmoscope, except that the condensing lens is fixed within the camera housing and a flash illumination source is required for the photographic exposure. As a result, these cameras are relatively large; their weight is supported on an adjustable platform similar to that of a slit-lamp biomicroscope (Fig 8-10).

As in indirect ophthalmoscopy, the image of the illumination source is projected through a patient's pupil with a series of condensing lenses and mirrors or beam splitters. In addition, a photography flashlamp is folded into the optical pathway via a beam splitter. This allows light from the flash to travel along exactly the same path as that from the illumination source. Optical filters can be positioned within the optical pathway to restrict

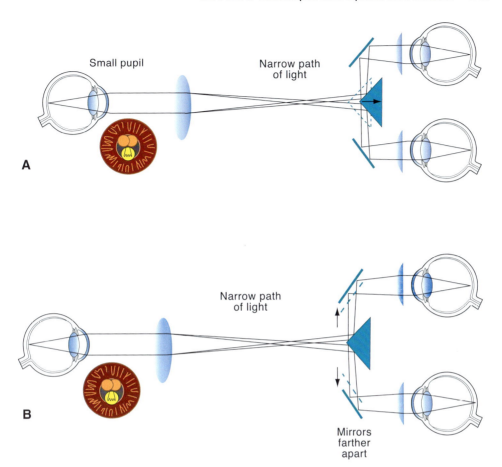

Figure 8-9   A, If a patient's pupil does not dilate well, the observer's interpupillary distance can be narrowed to "squeeze through" a smaller space. Moving the triangular mirror closer to the observer accomplishes this. **B,** Alternatively, the viewing lenses can be moved farther apart. *(Courtesy of Neal H. Atebara, MD. Redrawn by C. H. Wooley.)*

the wavelengths of light used to illuminate the fundus during photography and angiography. A fixation pointer can be placed in the illumination pathway at a position conjugate to the patient's fundus. The patient sees a sharp outline of the pointer, and the shadow of the pointer on the patient's fundus appears on the photographic film.

With the fundus illuminated, an aerial image of the fundus is formed by the camera's objective lens. This image, like the aerial image in indirect ophthalmoscopy, is inverted (Fig 8-11). As in indirect ophthalmoscopy, the optical pathways of illumination and observation/photography must pass through different areas of the patient's pupil; otherwise, reflections from the cornea and crystalline lens will degrade the camera image.

Nonmydriatic cameras have been developed to allow fundus photography without dilation. These cameras use infrared light in conjunction with semiautomatic or automatic focusing systems. Infrared light does not constrict the pupil. After alignment and focusing are completed, a white-light flash is triggered, and the photograph is taken before the pupil has a chance to constrict.

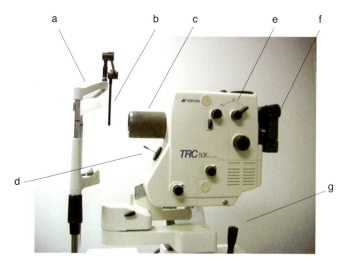

Figure 8-10 Photograph of a fundus and fluorescein angiography camera: *a*, patient forehead rest; *b*, fixation light; *c*, objective lens; *d*, fixation pointer; *e*, magnification lever; *f*, camera housing and eyepiece; *g*, joystick. *(Courtesy of Neal H. Atebara, MD.)*

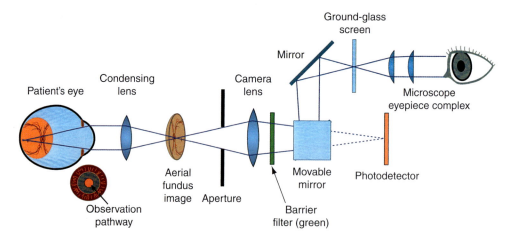

Figure 8-11 Observation system of a fundus camera. The observation system of a fundus camera is similar to that of an indirect ophthalmoscope. The condensing lens takes light rays from the illuminated fundus and creates an "aerial" image. A conventional single-lens reflex camera body, with its microscope eyepiece and ground-glass screen, is then used to focus on the aerial image. When the photograph is taken, a movable mirror flips up, exposing the film or photodetector. *(Courtesy of Neal H. Atebara, MD.)*

Most standard fundus cameras provide a 30° field of view that includes the optic disc and the temporal macula. Special wide-angle fundus cameras have large-diameter, aspheric objective lenses with a field of view of up to 60°. Wide-angle photographs (even up to 148°) are possible, but a contact-type objective lens and a special transscleral illumination source are necessary.

Video ophthalmoscopy has been attempted, but thus far excessive illumination is required and resolution has been poor. Scanning laser ophthalmoscopy is a promising technology. A single spot of laser light is scanned over the fundus, with each point being recorded as it is illuminated. Extremely low levels of total fundus illumination are therefore required.

Slit-Lamp Biomicroscope

A slit-lamp biomicroscope (Figs 8-12, 8-13) is a high-power binocular microscope with a slit-shaped illumination source, specially designed for viewing the different optically

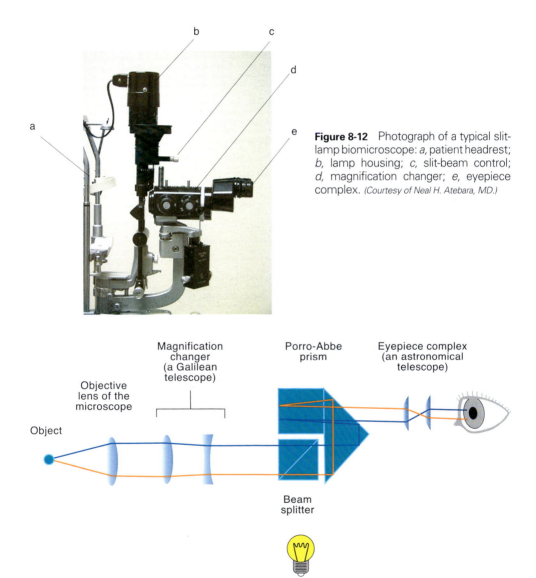

Figure 8-12 Photograph of a typical slit-lamp biomicroscope: *a*, patient headrest; *b*, lamp housing; *c*, slit-beam control; *d*, magnification changer; *e*, eyepiece complex. *(Courtesy of Neal H. Atebara, MD.)*

Figure 8-13 Slit-lamp biomicroscope. *(Courtesy of Neal H. Atebara, MD. Redrawn by C. H. Wooley.)*

transparent layers of the eye. The slit lamp is a compound microscope, meaning that its design employs multiple lenses carefully arranged to form a more magnified and sharper image than a single lens could produce on its own. Other lenses and mirrors are also incorporated into the instrument to ensure an upright image, provide variable magnification, and deliver the brightest image possible. Each manufacturer has its own proprietary refinements, but the basic design includes the following components: (1) astronomical telescope, (2) inverting prism, (3) Galilean telescope, (4) objective lens, (5) illumination system, (6) binocular viewing system.

An *astronomical telescope* is a system of 2 lenses, one in front of the other, both of which are convex (plus-power). The image is more magnified and freer from optical aberrations than that which a single convex lens could produce. The telescope's name derives from the instrument's common usage in astronomy, where observation and photography of the stars and planets are not hampered by the inverted (reversed top-to-bottom and left-to-right) image the telescope produces. The astronomical telescope, when used as a component of a microscope, is often referred to as "the eyepiece."

Because clinicians need to be able to simultaneously observe and manipulate ocular structures, sometimes using fine instruments, an upright image is essential for precise eye–hand coordination. An *inverting prism* takes the upside-down image formed by the astronomical telescope and inverts it to produce an erect image. There are numerous designs for inverting prisms. One of the common ones used in slit-lamp biomicroscopes is the Porro-Abbe prism, which is essentially 2 triangular prisms arranged to reflect light (using the principle of total internal reflection) several times, ultimately resulting in an optically sharp, inverted image with no magnification and little loss of light.

A *Galilean telescope,* in series with an astronomical telescope, is often employed to produce even higher magnifications. The Galilean telescope has a single convex lens and a single concave lens, separated by the difference of their focal lengths. The image produced is upright, so no additional inverting prism is necessary. When the object being studied is in front of the convex lens, the image is magnified. If the telescope is reversed (with the object now closer to the concave lens), the image is minified. Many microscope designs use this optical "trick" to allow variable magnification. A knob or lever rotates the lenses to reverse their positions. This turns the system into a "reverse" Galilean telescope.

The astronomical and Galilean telescope systems just discussed are effective at magnifying the image of a distant object—hence their classification as *telescopes.* The slit-lamp instrument, however, requires a working distance of only a few centimeters—hence its classification as a *biomicroscope.* Just as adult patients sometimes require reading spectacles for up-close work, the slit-lamp biomicroscope needs an "objective lens" to move the working distance from infinity to approximately 10 cm in front of the microscope, a distance close enough to focus on the eye.

The *illumination system* of the slit-lamp biomicroscope is a unique adaptation that greatly increases the amount and quality of information the clinician is able to glean from observing the eye. An aperture can be introduced to restrict the circular light beam to a slit of variable height, width, and rotation, allowing the light beam to cut a cross section through the optically transparent structures of the eye. Furthermore, illumination and observation systems can be pivoted independently around the eye being viewed. This arrangement allows the observer to study the eye from a wide range of angles and vary the angle of incidence of the slit light beam. In this way, a variety of illumination techniques for studying the eye become possible (Fig 8-14).

In ophthalmology, stereoscopic appreciation of the various layers of the eye is vitally important. The slit-lamp biomicroscope uses 2 lens systems of identical design (1 for each eye), each focused on a common point in space, coincident with the point of focus of the slit beam to create a *binocular viewing system*. In this way, the clinician can use both eyes together to get a 3-dimensional appreciation of the magnified eye.

Slit-Lamp Fundus Lenses

Because the cornea has such high refractive power, it is possible to see only about one-third of the way into the eye using a slit-lamp biomicroscope. Special lenses, however, can be placed in front of the slit-lamp objective lens to view the vitreous and posterior pole of the eye. There are 2 approaches to circumventing the high refractive power of the cornea.

The first approach is to nullify the corneal power using a contact lens or a high-power minus lens. Lenses used in this approach include the Goldmann fundus contact lens (Figs 8-15, 8-16), the Hruby lens (Fig 8-17), the Goldmann 3-mirror contact lens (Fig 8-18), and the Zeiss 4-mirror goniolens (Fig 8-19).

The second approach is to use the power of the cornea as a component of an astronomical telescope, in a manner similar to that utilized by the indirect ophthalmoscope. Lenses used in this approach include the 60 D, 78 D, and 90 D funduscopic lenses (Fig 8-20).

In addition, there are lenses that use a combination of both approaches to circumvent high corneal refractive power. This type of lens employs not only a corneal contact lens

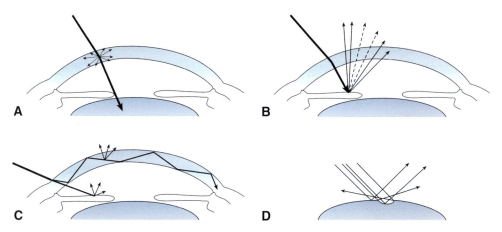

Figure 8-14 Diagram of how light rays interact with the eye in the 4 forms of slit-lamp biomicroscopic examination. **A,** Direct illumination. **B,** Retroillumination. **C,** Sclerotic scatter. **D,** Specular reflection. *(From Tasman W, Jaeger AE, eds. The slit lamp: history, principles, and practice. In: Duane's Clinical Ophthalmology. Philadelphia: Lippincott, 1995–1999:33. Redrawn by C. H. Wooley.)*

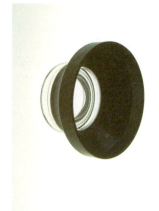

Figure 8-15 Photograph of a Goldmann fundus contact lens. *(Courtesy of Neal H. Atebara, MD.)*

Figure 8-16 A Goldmann fundus contact lens, or any similar planoconcave contact lens, essentially nullifies the refractive power of the cornea, thereby moving the retinal image to a point near the pupillary plane, within the focal range of the slit-lamp biomicroscope. The image formed is virtual, erect, and diminished in size. *I* = image; *O* = object. *(Courtesy of Neal H. Atebara, MD. Redrawn by C. H. Wooley.)*

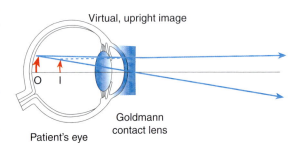

Figure 8-17 A concave Hruby lens, when placed close to a patient's eye, forms a virtual, erect image of the illuminated retina within the focal range of the slit-lamp biomicroscope. *I* = image; *O* = object. *(Courtesy of Neal H. Atebara, MD. Redrawn by C. H. Wooley.)*

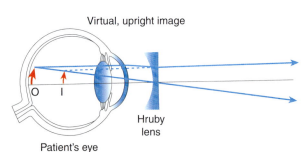

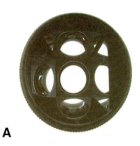

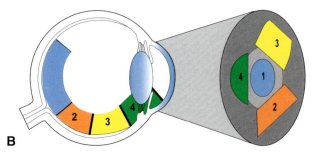

Figure 8-18 **A,** Photograph of a Goldmann 3-mirror contact lens (observer's view). **B,** Schematic diagram of the part of the eye that can be seen with the central contact lens *(1)*, midperipheral fundus mirror *(2)*, peripheral fundus mirror *(3)*, and iridocorneal angle mirror *(4)*. *(Both parts courtesy of Neal H. Atebara, MD. Part B redrawn by C. H. Wooley.)*

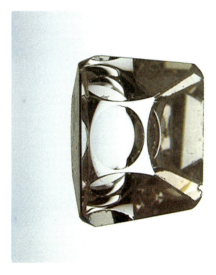

Figure 8-19 Photograph of the Zeiss 4-mirror goniolens. *(Courtesy of Neal H. Atebara, MD.)*

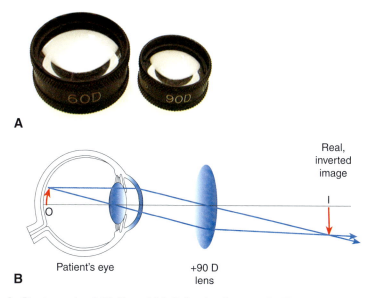

Figure 8-20 **A,** Photograph of 60 D and 90 D fundus lenses. **B,** The 60 D, 78 D, and 90 D lenses produce real, inverted images of the retina within the focal range of a slit-lamp bio-microscope in a fashion similar to that used by an indirect ophthalmoscope. *I* = image; *O* = object. *(Both parts courtesy of Neal H. Atebara, MD. Part B redrawn by C. H. Wooley.)*

but also a high-power spherical condensing lens, within which is created a real, inverted image, resulting in a very wide image of the fundus. Examples of this type of lens are the panfundoscope contact lens and the Rodenstock contact lens (Fig 8-21).

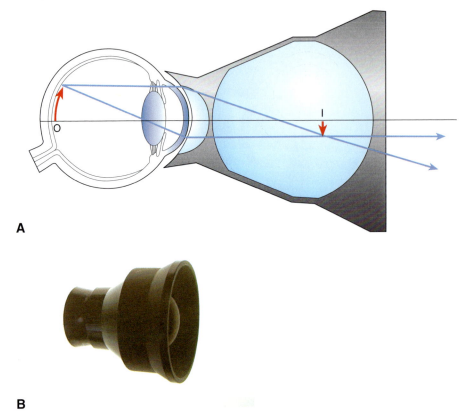

A

B

Figure 8-21 **A,** A panfundoscope lens consists of a corneal contact lens and a high-power, spherical condensing lens. A real, inverted image of the fundus is formed within the spherical glass element, which is within the focal range of a slit-lamp biomicroscope. *I* = image; *O* = object. **B,** Photograph of the panfundoscope lens. *(Both parts courtesy of Neal H. Atebara, MD. Part A redrawn by C. H. Wooley.)*

Goldmann Applanation Tonometer

The applanation tonometer is used to measure intraocular pressure (IOP). This instrument relies on an interesting physical principle: For an ideal, dry, thin-walled sphere, the pressure inside is proportional to the force applied to its surface. Unlike an ideal sphere, however, the human eye is not thin-walled and it is not dry. This produces 2 confounding forces: (1) a force produced by the eye's scleral rigidity (because the eye is not thin-walled), which is directed away from the globe; and (2) a force produced by the surface tension of the tear film (because the eye is not dry), which is directed toward the globe (Fig 8-22). Goldmann determined empirically that if enough force is applied to produce a circular area of flattening 3.06 mm in diameter, the scleral rigidity exactly cancels out the force caused by surface tension. Therefore, the applanating force required to flatten a circular area of cornea exactly 3.06 mm in diameter is directly proportional to the IOP. Specifically, the force (measured in dynes) multiplied by 10 is equal to the IOP (measured in millimeters of mercury).

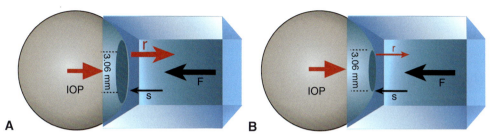

Figure 8-22 **A,** When a flat surface is applied to a cornea with enough force *(F)* to produce a circular area of flattening greater than 3.06 mm in diameter, the force caused by scleral rigidity *(r)* is greater than that caused by the tear film surface tension *(s).* **B,** When the force of the flat surface produces a circular area of flattening exactly 3.06 mm in diameter, the opposing forces of scleral rigidity and tear film surface tension cancel each other out, and the applied force *(F)* then becomes directly proportional to the intraocular pressure *(IOP).* *(Courtesy of Neal H. Atebara, MD.)*

How, then, does an observer know when the area of applanation is exactly 3.06 mm in diameter? First, the applanation tonometer is mounted on a biomicroscope to produce a magnified image. When the cornea is applanated, the tear film—which rims the circular area of applanated cornea—appears as a circle to the observer. The tear film is often stained with fluorescein dye and viewed under a cobalt blue light to enhance the visibility of the tear film ring. Higher pressure from the tonometer head causes the circle to have a larger diameter because a larger area of cornea is applanated. Split prisms—each mounted with its bases in opposite directions—are mounted in the applanation head, and they create 2 images offset by exactly 3.06 mm. The clinician looks through the applanation head and adjusts the applanation pressure until the half circles just overlap one another (Fig 8-23).

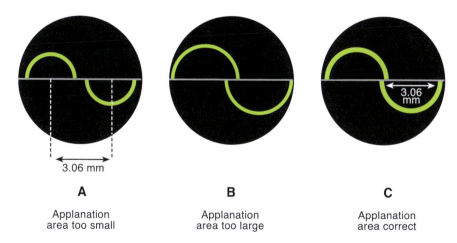

Figure 8-23 The split prism in the applanation head creates 2 images offset by 3.06 mm. This allows greater ease in determining when the circular ring is exactly 3.06 mm in diameter. When the area of applanation is smaller than 3.06 mm, the arms of the inner semicircles do not reach each other **(A).** When the area of applanation is greater than 3.06 mm, the arms of the inner semicircles reach past each other **(B).** When the area of applanation is exactly 3.06 mm, the arms of the inner semicircles just touch each other **(C).** This is the endpoint for measuring IOP. *(Courtesy of Neal H. Atebara, MD. Redrawn by C. H. Wooley.)*

At this point, the circle is exactly 3.06 mm in diameter, and the reading on the tonometer (multiplied by a factor of 10) represents the IOP in millimeters of mercury (Fig 8-24).

Dynamic Contour Tonometry

Although Goldmann applanation tonometry is the current gold standard for clinical measurement of IOP, its accuracy is limited because the instrument is required to deform the

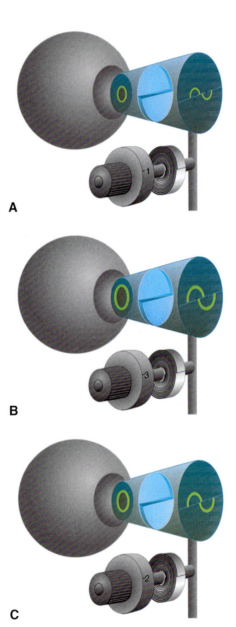

Figure 8-24 When the applanation pressure is **A** too low (1.0 dyne in this illustration), the circular ring is smaller than 3.06 mm in diameter, and the arms of the ring do not reach each other in the split image **(A)**. When the applanation pressure is too high (3.0 dynes in the illustration), the circular ring is larger than 3.06 mm in diameter, and the arms of the ring stretch past each other in the split image **(B)**. When the applanation pressure creates a circular ring exactly 3.06 mm in diameter, the arms of the ring just reach each other in the split image **(C)**. In this illustration, the endpoint is reached at 2.0 dynes of applanation pressure, which corresponds to an IOP of 20 mm Hg. *(Courtesy of Neal H. Atebara, MD. Redrawn by C. H. Wooley.)*

surface of the cornea in order to take each measurement. Many factors, especially central corneal thickness, can substantially affect its accuracy.

Dynamic contour tonometry attempts to minimize these factors by shaping the surface of the probe to accommodate the shape of the human cornea (Fig 8-25). When the concave probe is placed in contact with the cornea, deformation of the cornea is minimized. The IOP is measured by a pressure sensor in the center of the probe surface.

The device can be mounted on a slit lamp and is advanced toward the patient's eye in a fashion similar to that of a Goldmann tonometer. A microprocessor measures IOP continuously, even detecting pulsatile fluctuations.

Pachymeter

Pachymeters are used to measure corneal thickness. These values are especially important in refractive surgery and in monitoring corneal edema. The 3 main methods for measuring corneal thickness are (1) optical doubling, (2) optical focusing, and (3) ultrasonography.

In optical doubling, an image-doubling prism (similar to that used in keratometers and applanation tonometers) is used in conjunction with a slit-lamp biomicroscope. The pachymeter is designed to measure the distance between the Purkinje-Sanson images formed by the anterior and posterior corneal surfaces, a value that represents the corneal thickness. The endpoint is reached when the images are superimposed; a measurement of corneal thickness can then be directly read off a scale (Fig 8-26).

In the optical focusing technique, a specular microscope is calibrated so that when the endothelium is in focus, the corneal thickness measurement is automatically displayed. The zero is established by focusing on the interface between the contact element and the epithelial layer.

Ultrasound techniques can also be used to measure corneal thickness, similar to the way ultrasound is used to measure the axial length of the globe. If the velocity of sound in the cornea is known and if the precise time required for sound waves to pass through the cornea can be measured, the thickness of the cornea can be calculated. Multiple measurements allow construction of a 2-dimensional map of corneal thickness.

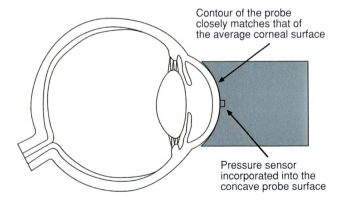

Contour of the probe closely matches that of the average corneal surface

Pressure sensor incorporated into the concave probe surface

Figure 8-25 Dynamic contour tonometry. *(Courtesy of Neal H. Atebara, MD.)*

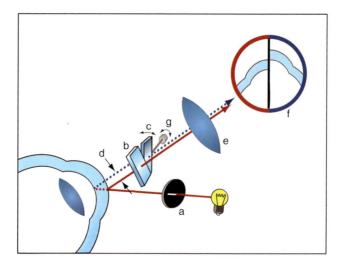

Figure 8-26 In the most common type of optical pachymeter, the cornea is illuminated with a slit beam *(a)*. The image is viewed through a biomicroscope, half through a glass plate orthogonal to the path of light *(b)* and half through a glass plate rotated through an angle *(c)*. The beam path through the plate is displaced laterally for a distance *(d)* that varies depending on the angle of rotation. Through the eyepiece *(e)*, a split image is seen *(f)*, wherein half the image comes from the fixed plate and the other half from the rotatable plate. The endothelial surface of 1 image and the epithelial surface of the other image are aligned by the observer by careful adjustment of the rotatable plate *(c)*, and the corneal thickness measurement is read off a calibrated scale *(g)*. *(Courtesy of Neal H. Atebara, MD.)*

Specular Microscope

Specular microscopy is a modality for examining endothelial cells that uses specular reflection from the interface between the endothelial cells and the aqueous humor. The technique can be performed using contact or noncontact methods. In both methods, the instruments are designed to separate the illumination and viewing paths so that reflections from the anterior corneal surface do not obscure the very weak reflection arising from the endothelial cell surface.

Endothelial cells can also be visualized through a slit-lamp biomicroscope if the illumination and viewing axes are symmetrically displaced on either side of the normal line to the cornea (Fig 8-27). A narrow illumination slit must be used; hence, the field of view is narrow. Photographic recording has been made possible by the addition of a long-working-distance microscope system on the viewing axis and flash capability to the illumination system. Patient eye motion is the chief problem with this technique.

In contact specular microscopy, the illumination and viewing paths are through opposite sides of a special microscope objective, the front element of which touches the cornea. This reduces eye rotation and effectively eliminates longitudinal motion that interferes with focus. Contact specular microscopy allows for higher magnifications than slit-lamp biomicroscopy, making cellular detail and endothelial abnormalities more discernible.

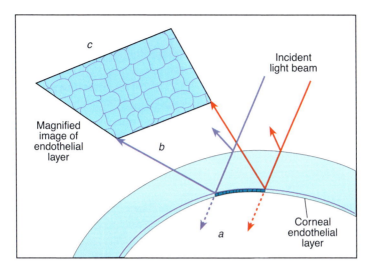

Figure 8-27 Specular reflection microscopy. When a beam of light passes through the transparent corneal structures, most of the light is transmitted *(a)*. However, at each optical interface, such as the corneal endothelium, a proportion of light is reflected *(b)*. This light (called *specular reflection*) can be collected to form a relatively dim image of the corneal endothelium *(c)*, where individual endothelial cells can be counted. *(Courtesy of Neal H. Atebara, MD. Redrawn by C. H. Wooley.)*

Video recording of endothelial layer images makes it possible to document larger, overlapping areas of the endothelial layer. Also, it allows the recording of high-magnification images, despite patient eye motion.

Wide-field specular microscopy employs special techniques to ensure that reflections from the interface between the cornea and contact element do not overlap the image of the endothelial cell layer. Because scattered light from edema in the epithelium and stroma can degrade the endothelial image, variable slit widths are sometimes provided to reduce this problem.

Analysis of specular micrographs may consist simply of assessment of cell appearance together with notation of abnormalities such as guttae or keratic precipitates. Frequently, cell counts are desired; these are often obtained by superimposing a transparent grid of specific dimensions on the endothelial image (photograph or video image) and simply counting the cells in a known area. Cell size distribution can be determined by computer analysis after cell boundaries have been determined digitally. The normal cell density in young people exceeds 3000 cells/mm^2; the average density in the cataract age group is 2250 cells/mm^2, which suggests a gradual decrease with age.

Specular microscopy has been important in studying the morphology of the endothelium and in quantifying damage to the endothelium produced by various surgical procedures and intraocular devices. This in turn has led to refined surgical procedures and new device designs.

Operating Microscope

The operating microscope works on principles similar to those of the slit-lamp biomicroscope. Like the slit-lamp biomicroscope, the operating microscope has the following optical components: (a) an astronomical telescope, (b) an inverting prism, (c) a Galilean telescope, (d) an objective lens, (e) a light source, and (f) a binocular viewing system (Fig 8-28). The illumination source of the operating microscope, unlike that of the slit-lamp biomicroscope, is not slit-shaped, and the working distance for the operating microscope is longer to accommodate the specific requirements of ocular surgery. Also, most operating microscopes contain a zoom lens that smoothly varies magnification without changing focus.

The working distance of the microscope (the distance from the objective lens to the patient's eye) is equal to the focal length of the objective lens. Common focal lengths for objective lenses in ophthalmic surgery are 150, 175, and 200 mm. Use of the proper working distance can greatly lessen surgeon back and neck strain, especially during lengthy operations. A difference as small as 25 mm can affect body comfort and the positioning of the surgeon's arms and hands.

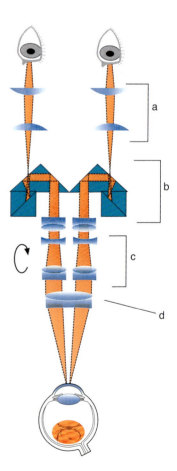

Figure 8-28 Schematic diagram of an operating microscope. The major components include *(a)* an eyepiece, an astronomical telescope, which provides most of the magnification; *(b)* an inverting prism, such as a Porro-Abbe prism, which compensates for the inverted image produced by the eyepiece; *(c)* a magnification changer, such as a Galilean telescope system, in which different lenses can be introduced to change the magnification; and *(d)* an objective lens, which adjusts the working distance. Two parallel optical systems, each a mirror image of the other, provide a stereoptic view of the patient's eye. *(Courtesy of Neal H. Atebara, MD. Redrawn by C. H. Wooley.)*

The total magnification provided by an operating microscope is the product of the magnifications of its various optical components. Because various lenses are available for the objective and eyepiece, magnification can be controlled. Smoothly variable magnification changers (zoom Galilean telescopes) are incorporated into many operating microscopes. The 12.5× eyepiece is the most popular choice for ophthalmic surgery, and the total resultant magnification varies from 6× to 40×.

Various illumination systems are also available, but the most important system for ophthalmic surgery is known as *coaxial illumination*. This type is especially useful for visualization of the posterior capsule and for vitreous surgery. Fiber-optic delivery systems reduce heat near the microscope and allow easier change of bulbs during surgery.

Keratometer

The keratometer is used to approximate the refracting power of the cornea (Fig 8-29). It does this by measuring the radius of curvature of the central cornea (by assuming the cornea to be a convex mirror) and using a mathematical approximation to convert this radius of curvature to corneal refractive power. In essence, a keratometer measures reflecting power and infers refracting power.

The central cornea can be thought of as a convex spherical mirror. If an illuminated object of known size is placed at a fixed distance from the cornea, and we are able to measure the size of the greatly minified reflected image, we can deduce the radius of curvature of the mirror using the following formula: $r = 2u(I/O)$, where r is the radius of curvature

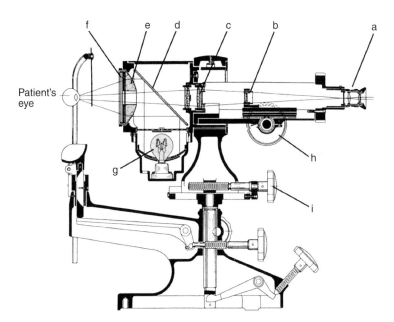

Figure 8-29 Schematic diagram of a keratometer. The major components include *(a)* the eyepiece, *(b)* doubling prisms, *(c)* objective lens, *(d)* mirror, *(e)* condenser lens, *(f)* mire, *(g)* lamp, *(h)* measurement controls, and *(i)* focus control. *(Redrawn by C. H. Wooley.)*

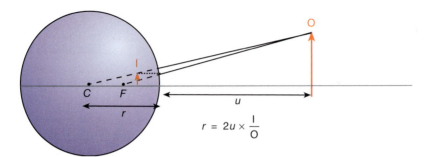

Figure 8-30 Keratometer. The cornea can be thought of as a convex spherical mirror. If an illuminated object *(O)* of known size is placed a known distance *(u)* from the cornea, and the size of the reflected image *(I)* can be measured, then the radius of curvature *(r)* of the sphere can be deduced using the formula $r = 2u(I/O)$. *C* is the center of the sphere, and *F* is the focal point of the convex spherical mirror. *(Courtesy of Neal H. Atebara, MD. Redrawn by C. H. Wooley.)*

of the reflective cornea, *u* is the distance from the object to the cornea, *I* is the size of the image, and *O* is the size of the object (Fig 8-30). Because the cornea is a high-power mirror (approximately 250 D), an object does not have to be very far away to be effectively at optical infinity; that is, the distance *(u)* becomes essentially constant. When this is the case, for all practical purposes, the corneal radius is directly proportional to the size of the reflected image it produces and indirectly proportional to the size of the object (*r* is directly proportional to *I* and indirectly proportional to *O*).

The challenge, then, is to measure the size of the image relative to the object. This is achieved with the use of a microscope to magnify the tiny image. However, because the eye is constantly moving about, it is difficult to measure the image size against a reticule. If we place 2 prisms base to base and position them such that the baseline splits the pupil, the observer will see 2 images separated by a fixed amount (depending on the power of the prisms). Thus, any oscillation of the cornea during measurement will affect both doubled images equally—that is, motion of the eye will not cause the separation between the doubled images to change. This allows the observer to adjust knobs on the keratometer to arrive at the "contact" position despite small eye movements. This technique is commonly employed in other ophthalmic instruments and is called the *doubling principle*.

In practice, keratometers either vary the image size to achieve a known object size (von Helmholtz keratometers, Fig 8-31; also see Fig 8-29) or vary the object size to achieve a known image size (Javal-Schiøtz keratometer, Fig 8-32).

The final step is to convert the radius of curvature into an estimate of the cornea's dioptric refractive power. The following formula can be used for this conversion:

$$P = (n' - n)/r$$

where *P* is the refractive power of the cornea, *n'* is the refractive index of the cornea, *n* is the refractive index of air (which is close to 1.0), and *r* is the measured radius of curvature of the cornea. Because different layers of the cornea have slightly different refractive indices and because the posterior surface of the cornea, which is not measured, contributes −5 to −6 D of power on average, instrument manufacturers and clinicians have adopted an "averaged" corneal refractive index of 1.3375. Therefore, if we measure the corneal

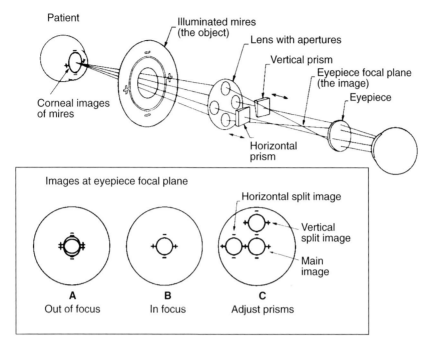

Figure 8-31 von Helmholtz keratometer. In a von Helmholtz keratometer, the object size is fixed and the image size is measured. In one popular design, the object consists of a large, illuminated ring-shaped mire. A vertical prism and a horizontal prism are each adjustable to measure the image size in 2 meridians. The image is formed at the eyepiece focal plane *(inset).* The first step involves focusing the image using the eyepiece (*A* and *B*). Next, the vertical prism is adjusted to bring the vertical split image into alignment with the main image (overlap the minus signs; *C*). The corneal power in this meridian can then be read off the scale. Finally, the horizontal prism is adjusted to bring the horizontal split image into alignment with the main image (overlap the plus signs; *C*). *(Courtesy of Neal H. Atebara, MD. Redrawn by C. H. Wooley.)*

curvature (by using the doubling technique) to be 8.5 mm, we can calculate: $P = (1.3375 - 1.0) \div (0.0085 \text{ m}) = 39.7$ D. In most instruments, this calculation is performed automatically, because the conversion is already built into the reading on the keratometer dial. So all the clinician needs to do is line up the targets to reach their "endpoints" and record the reading on the dial. In this fashion, measurements can be made in each of the 2 major meridians of corneal curvature of an astigmatic eye.

Corneal Topographer

Conventional keratometry measures the curvature of only the central 3 mm of the cornea. This is not representative of the entire surface, however, because corneal curvature generally flattens from apex to limbus. A "map" of corneal curvature can be useful in contact lens fitting and corneal refractive surgery.

Methods for ascertaining the topography of the cornea are commonly based on either a circular mire, similar to a Placido disk (Fig 8-33), which consists of many concentric lighted rings, or a standard keratometer directed to different, off-center areas of the

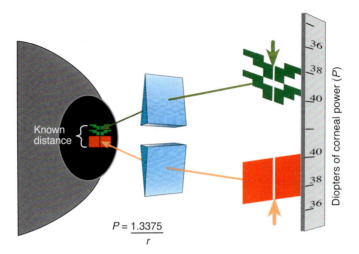

Figure 8-32 Two prisms placed base to base produce doubled images separated by a fixed distance that are not affected by small movements of the eye. The observer varies the object size (ie, the distance between the red and green objects) until the doubled images touch. At this point, the images are a known distance from each other, and the object size can be measured to calculate the corneal radius of curvature. On most Javal-Schiøtz keratometers, the scale that measures the size of the object has already been converted to its corresponding estimates in diopters of corneal refractive power using the formula $P = 1.3375/r$, where P is the refractive power of the cornea, r is the radius of corneal curvature, and 1.3375 is an "averaged" corneal refractive index. *(Courtesy of Neal H. Atebara, MD. Redrawn by C. H. Wooley.)*

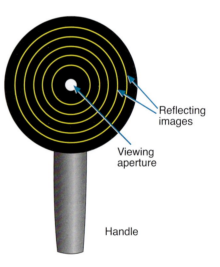

Figure 8-33 A Placido disk. When the disk is placed in front of the cornea, the reflected image can be analyzed to qualitatively assess corneal curvature and corneal surface irregularities. *(Courtesy of Neal H. Atebara, MD. Redrawn by C. H. Wooley.)*

cornea. One may consider a series of concentric lighted rings as a series of many different-sized mires, all in the same plane. Thus, the central ring would function very much like the standard mire on a keratometer and act as a target for the central 3 mm of cornea. The next ring can be considered to subtend the zone surrounding the center and produce a reflected ring representative of the curvature of that zone, and so on.

A flat series of illuminated rings held at the usual distance from the cornea can accurately measure only the central 7 mm of the cornea. To measure corneal curvature closer to the limbus, the concentric rings must be presented in the shape of a concave surface (ie, open bowl) so that the distances from rings to cornea remain similar over the whole cornea. If the series of lighted rings is placed in front of a camera (the camera lens placed at an opening in the center of the ring pattern), the device is called a *photographic keratoscope*, and the picture of the reflected rings may be analyzed. With irregular astigmatism (scars, keratoconus), the irregular pattern of reflected rings can be used as a qualitative representation of the corneal map.

The use of computerized videokeratoscopes (Fig 8-34) has grown rapidly. These devices enable image analysis of multiple rings (often 16 or 32), producing color-coded dioptric maps of the corneal surface. Some of these instruments also calculate the SIM K (simulated keratometry) value, providing the power and location of the steepest and flattest meridians for the 3-mm optical zone (Figs 8-35, 8-36). Other parameters include the surface asymmetry index (SAI) and the surface regularity index (SRI). The SAI is a centrally weighted summation of differences in corneal power between corresponding points 180° apart on 128 meridians that cross the 4 central mires. The SAI can be used to monitor changes caused by contact lens warpage or keratoplasty or by such progressive alterations as keratoconus, keratoglobus, Terrien marginal degeneration, and pellucid degeneration. The SRI is determined from a summation of local fluctuations in power that occur among 256 hemimeridians in the 10 central mires. (See also BCSC Section 8, *External Disease and Cornea*.)

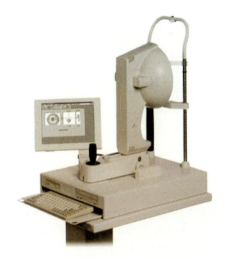

Figure 8-34 Photograph of a computerized corneal topography system. *(Courtesy of Neal H. Atebara, MD.)*

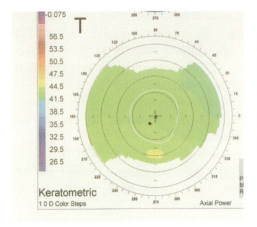

Figure 8-35 In corneal topography, the image produced by a Placido disk is analyzed by a computer. Calculation of the distance between the circular mires in each clock-hour allows for an accurate 2-dimensional map of corneal curvature. The corneal topographic map of a nearly emmetropic eye reveals minute geographic variations in corneal curvature, ranging from 41.5 D *(light green)* to 44.5 D *(yellow)*. *(Courtesy of Neal H. Atebara, MD.)*

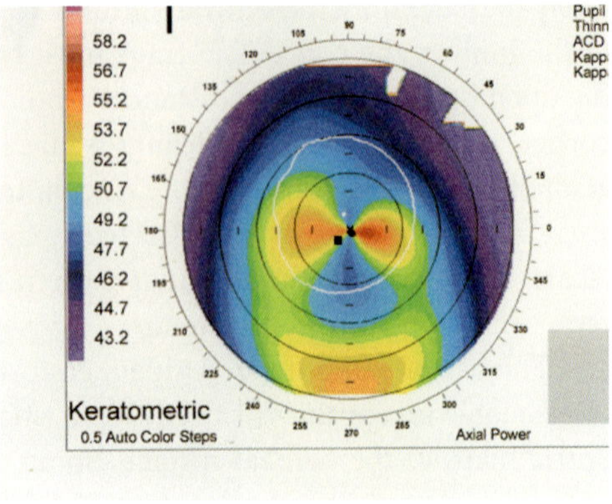

Figure 8-36 Corneal topographic map of an eye with against-the-rule astigmatism. Corneal curvature ranges from relatively flat *(dark blue)* to relatively steep *(orange)*. *(Courtesy of Neal H. Atebara, MD.)*

Manual Lensmeter

The lensmeter (Fig 8-37) (commercially known as a Lensometer, Focimeter, or Vertometer) measures the power of spectacles and contact lenses. This device consists of

- an illuminated target
- a platform for the "unknown" lens (the lens whose power the user intends to measure)
- an eyepiece (an astronomical telescope), which produces a sharp image when parallel light rays enter it
- a standard (or fixed) lens

To understand how a lensmeter works, it is useful to consider first how a simplified version of this instrument works in principle. An illuminated target is moved backward and forward behind the "unknown" lens. At the position where the target is at the unknown lens's focal point, emergent light rays are parallel (by definition of a focal point). These parallel rays, when viewed through the eyepiece, produce a clear image, indicating that the focal length of the unknown lens has been found. Taking the inverse of the focal length gives us the power of the unknown lens (Fig 8-38).

There are 2 major problems with the simple lensmeter. The first is that the instrument would have to be too large to be practical. To measure a +0.25 D lens, the instrument would have to be 4 m long! The second problem is that the scale for measuring the

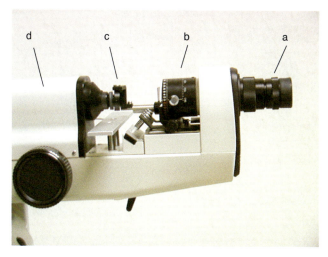

Figure 8-37 Photograph of a manual lensmeter: *a*, eyepiece; *b*, eyepiece graticule; *c*, support for spectacle; *d*, housing for lamp, adjustable target graticule, and standard lens. *(Courtesy of Neal H. Atebara, MD.)*

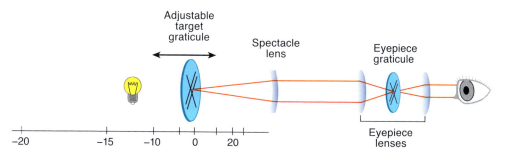

Figure 8-38 Simplified version of a manual lensmeter. *(Courtesy of Neal H. Atebara, MD. Redrawn by C. H. Wooley.)*

lens power would be nonlinear. Therefore, measurements of more powerful lenses would become very inaccurate.

Both of these problems can be solved with the introduction of another lens to the system, called the *standard* (or *field*) *lens*, and the use of an optical trick called the *Badal principle*. If the standard lens is placed so that its focal point coincides with the posterior vertex of the unknown lens, then not only is the length of the instrument shortened considerably, but the dioptric scale of the instrument becomes linear (Fig 8-39).

The target usually has a set of lines that permit the observer to determine whether the lens has cylindrical power. In the measurement of cylindrical power, the target is first rotated, as well as moved forward or backward, until 1 set of lines is sharp. The target is then moved forward or backward until the perpendicular set of lines is sharp. The difference in target settings is the cylindrical power. The cylindrical axis is read from the wheel setting.

It should be kept in mind that a lensmeter measures the back vertex power of a lens (Fig 8-40); therefore, it is important to note which surface of the lens is placed against the

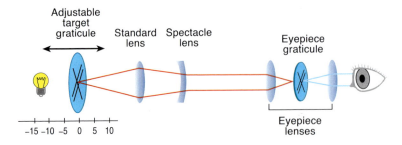

Figure 8-39 Badal principle. *(Courtesy of Neal H. Atebara, MD. Redrawn by C. H. Wooley.)*

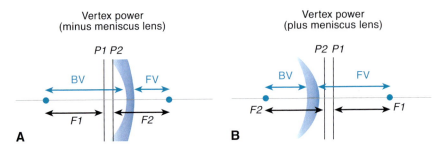

Figure 8-40 The lens power measured by a lensmeter actually represents the back vertex power. With a simple thin lens, a single principal plane goes through the center of the lens perpendicular to the optical axis. Most spectacles, however, are thick, meniscus lenses, which means that there are 2 principal planes (*P1* and *P2*) whose positions are "pushed away" from the concave surface in a minus lens **(A)** and away from the convex surface in a plus lens **(B)**. This makes it difficult to measure the actual focal length (distance from a focal plane to its corresponding focal point) and the actual focal power (inverse of the focal distance). In clinical practice, it is more convenient to measure the back vertex *(BV)* distance of a spectacle, which is the distance from the back surface of the optical center of the lens to the focal point. Taking the inverse of the back vertex distance yields the back vertex power of the lens. In clinical practice, the back vertex power is easier to measure and more clinically relevant than the true lens power. *F1* = primary focal point; *F2* = secondary focal point; *FV* = front vertex distance. *(Courtesy of Neal H. Atebara, MD. Redrawn by C. H. Wooley.)*

holder. The instrument can also detect and determine the amount of prism at any given point in a lens. The procedure is to use a felt-tip pen to mark the point of interest on the test lens, usually the location of the patient's pupil. With the point of interest centered in the lensmeter aperture, the amount and orientation of the prism are read from the reticule scale.

Measuring the Bifocal Add

When determining a patient's distance refraction, the clinician usually measures the required back vertex power of the spectacle lens. Back vertex power would seem, therefore, to be the most relevant optical parameter to consider in the evaluation of spectacle power. However, for a bifocal add, the spectacle is turned around so that the front vertex power is measured.

Parallel light rays from distance enter
lens with zero vergence, which
gives desired back vergence power.

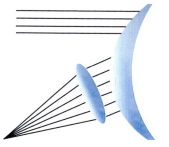

Figure 8-41 The effect of a bifocal add segment in measuring lens power with a lensmeter. *(Courtesy of Neal H. Atebara, MD. Redrawn by C. H. Wooley.)*

Diverging light from   ...enters distance portion of
near hits reading add...   lens with zero vergence

The bifocal add is different from the rest of the spectacle lens. The distance portion is designed to deal with essentially parallel light, and that is the basis on which the lensmeter is calculated. The bifocal add, however, is designed to work on diverging light, originating, for example, at 40 cm from a +2.50 bifocal add. If one imagines the bifocal add as being an additional lens placed an infinitesimal distance in front of the distance lens, the principle becomes clearer. Diverging light rays from the near object pass through the bifocal lens and are made parallel. The parallel light rays then enter the distance lens from its anterior surface and are refracted with the expected optical effect, yielding the back vertex vergence required to give the patient clear vision. In a sense, the bifocal add exerts its effect on the light *before* it passes through the rest of the lens (Fig 8-41).

Thus, the add segment should be measured from the front. The front vertex power of the distance portion is measured, and the difference in front vertex power between the distance and near portions specifies the add. The spectacle power itself is still the back vertex power of the distance portion. With a distance lens of strong plus power, there will be a significant difference in the front and back vertex measurements of the add, which will cause errors if the add is not measured from the front. In cases other than a distance lens with strong plus power, there is usually little or no clinically significant difference in the measurements.

Automatic Lensmeter

The principles underlying automatic electronic lensmeters are different from those of manual lensmeters. A lens bends or reflects a beam of light passing through it (except at its optical center), and automatic lensmeters use this effect to calculate a lens's power. The deviation of a beam of light passing through a lens is based on 2 factors: the power of the lens and the prismatic effect related to the distance from the lens center (the Prentice rule). Consider the number of variables we need to measure. For the calculation of the lens's power, 3 variables must be ascertained: spherical power, cylindrical power, and axis. Because the lens may be placed on the instrument off-center, we must be prepared to determine 2 more variables: the x and y displacements from lens center. Thus, the automatic lensmeter must somehow obtain at least 5 independent pieces of information to characterize the lens being measured.

By examining a single light beam passing through a test lens, a lensmeter can determine the light beam's displacement from a straight path (ie, its x and y displacement). Most commercial lensmeters actually shine 4 beams (in an approximately square pattern, 5×5 mm) through the lens and thus obtain measurements of 4 pairs of x and y displacements. The 4 light beams are projected either simultaneously or sequentially. They pass through various optical devices so that they are made parallel as they approach the test lens. After passing through the test lens, the light beams fall on a detector that determines their respective displacements. Thus, each of the 4 beams produces 2 variables—its x displacement and its y displacement. From these 8 independent variables (3 more than actually needed), lens power and decentration/prism can be determined. The 3 extra variables allow confirmation of the accuracy of the measured power and toricity of the lens—that is, this built-in redundancy confirms that the lens is of a legitimate spherocylindrical form and that the measurements are consistent. Note that with this system, no gross movement of the optical elements is necessary.

Diagnostic Ultrasonography

Ophthalmic ultrasonography is an invaluable diagnostic tool. Its primary uses in ophthalmology include detection and differentiation of intraocular and orbital lesions, location of intraocular foreign bodies, biomicroscopy, and biometry (for intraocular lens power calculations and tissue thickness measurements). A brief discussion of specific clinical applications of ultrasonography may be found in BCSC Section 4, *Ophthalmic Pathology and Intraocular Tumors,* and Section 7, *Orbit, Eyelids, and Lacrimal System.* It is appropriate to discuss the basic principles of ultrasonography in this section, as sound waves behave in many respects as light waves, obeying many similar laws of physics.

Sound is produced as an oscillating particle collides with a neighboring particle, causing that particle to oscillate at the same frequency. Ultrasound has a frequency greater than 20,000 cycles per second (20 kHz), which is beyond the range of audible sound. Most ophthalmic ultrasonography is performed in the range of 8–15 MHz (8–15 million cycles per second). Ultrasound is produced in the ultrasonographic probe by the oscillation of a piezoelectric crystal, which converts electrical energy into mechanical energy. Ultrasound spreads in advancing wavefronts from the emitting crystal and is attenuated (reduced in amplitude) by 3 factors:

- distance from the probe head
- differential absorption by different media
- acoustic interfaces within a given medium causing reflection, refraction, or scattering of sound

After modification by scattering and differential absorption, the emitted sound waves are reflected to the probe as ultrasonographic signals. These are electronically processed and displayed as ultrasonograms on a display screen. The echoes themselves are produced by acoustic interfaces that reflect sound in characteristic patterns. An acoustic interface occurs where 2 substances with different sonic densities are juxtaposed. The strength of the returned (reflected) signal is greatest when the beam is perpendicular to the reflecting surface. Therefore, to sonically characterize an interface, the probe must be perpendicular to it in order to maximize the signal. Interfaces that are smooth and characterized by significant acoustic differences (in density and in sound velocity) are said to be highly reflective. Both corneal surfaces, both lens surfaces, and the inner scleral surface are all examples of highly reflective interfaces. Irregular interfaces between acoustically similar tissues do not reflect effectively; rather, they weakly scatter sound waves.

The major differences between the 2 most commonly used ultrasound modes (A and B) depend on probe design and mode of signal processing and display. Standardized A-scan ultrasonography uses a parallel nonfocused beam emanating from a stationary 8-MHz piezoelectric crystal that emits and receives pulsed signals. Reflectivity versus time is displayed for the single direction in which the probe is pointing, as shown in Figure 8-42. Biometric determination may be performed using A-scan, measuring the time delay (in microseconds) before a particular signal is displayed (Fig 8-43). This value may then be converted to millimeters. A-scan biometry is used in calculating intraocular lens power, determining extraocular muscle thickness (in thyroid eye disease), and measuring tumor height (in choroidal melanomas).

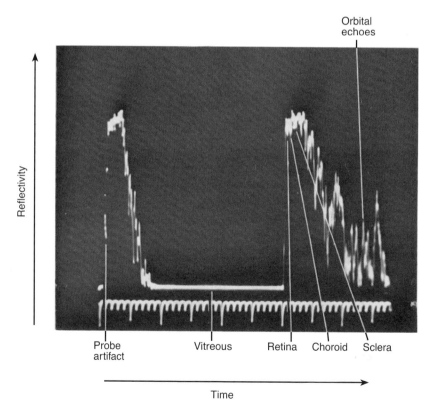

Figure 8-42 Normal A-scan ultrasonogram.

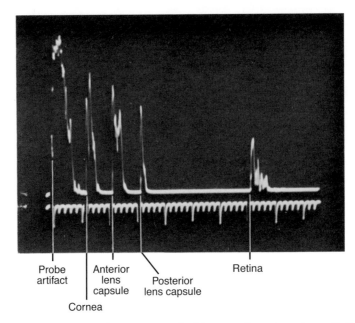

Probe artifact Anterior lens capsule Posterior lens capsule Retina

Cornea

Figure 8-43 A-scan ultrasonogram for biometry (at reduced sensitivity).

B-scan, on the other hand, uses a focused crystal in an oscillating probe that scans a chosen acoustic section. The image is displayed as a 2-dimensional slice, similar in gross appearance to computed tomography, as shown in Figure 8-44. B-scan ultrasonography of the globe can be performed by immersion or contact techniques. Immersion scanners are

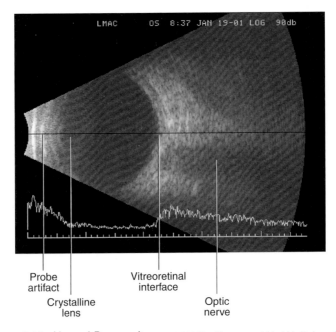

Probe artifact Crystalline lens Vitreoretinal interface Optic nerve

Figure 8-44 Normal B-scan ultrasonogram. *(Courtesy of Neal H. Atebara, MD.)*

of particular value in scanning the anterior segment, an area to which the contact scanner is blind (because of superimposition of the probe artifact on anterior segment echoes). Disadvantages of immersion scanners include the cumbersome water-bath setup and the inability to perform kinetic, real-time ultrasonography. Contact B-scan ultrasonography allows kinetic studies and is easier to perform in infants and in patients with ruptured globes. In contact scanning, the probe head is placed on the eyelids or on the globe itself, with methylcellulose as a coupling medium.

Standardized A-scan ultrasonography is much less aesthetically attractive to the beginner and is more difficult to perform. However, it potentially conveys much more diagnostic information than the B-scan. (Note that the A-scan displayed on many B-scan instruments is not standardized and has less value in judging reflectivity.) For instance, in evaluation of a choroidal mass lesion, B-scan ultrasonography demonstrates gross topography of the lesion, such as secondary overlying membranes and choroidal excavation. However, A-scan ultrasonography can measure elevation to within 0.5 mm, quantify overlying membranes, and identify the presence of large vascular channels. Most important, based on the lesion's internal reflectivity (acoustic density), it can help differentiate a melanoma from a metastatic lesion, from a choroidal hemangioma, from a choroidal osteoma, and from a disciform lesion.

In practice, the 2 ultrasonographic modes are complementary: the B-scan for general topography and gross reflectivity of the lesion and the A-scan for detailed information regarding measurement, internal structure, and intrinsic vascularity. Ultrasonography may be a useful tool in the following clinical settings:

- opaque media
- previtrectomy evaluation
- choroidal mass lesions
- intraorbital or intraocular foreign bodies
- proptosis
- optic nerve abnormalities
- abnormalities of the extraocular muscles

Automated Refraction

More than 100 automated refractors have been devised during the past century. Most have been based on the optometer principle, providing smoothly variable change in vergence for the neutralization of refractive error. Variations of the Scheiner double-pinhole principle (Fig 8-45) have frequently been used to achieve an alignment endpoint of measurement rather than a focus endpoint. The Scheiner principle, however, provides refractive measurement through only small portions of the eye's optics, and alignment of the various measuring apertures with the patient's pupil becomes critical. Furthermore, in the presence of even minor optical irregularities (found in almost all eyes), the refraction obtained through small portions of the eye's optics may not represent the eye's refractive state as a whole. Experience has shown that automatic objective measurements using infrared light must usually be refined subjectively for best results, using the entire pupil.

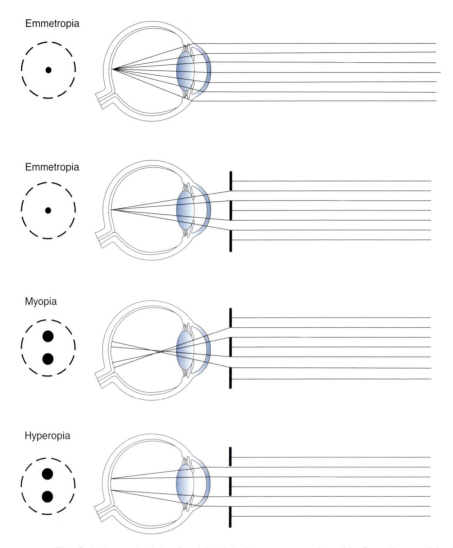

Figure 8-45 The Scheiner principle. Double-pinhole apertures placed before the pupil isolate 2 small bundles of light. An object not conjugate to the retina appears doubled instead of blurred. *(From Tasman W, Jaeger AE, eds.* Duane's Clinical Ophthalmology. *vol 1, chap 67. Hagerstown, MD: Harper & Row; 1983:2.)*

So-called *instrument myopia*, the tendency to accommodate when looking into instruments, has caused major problems with automated refractors in the past. Various methods of fogging and automatic tracking have been developed to overcome this problem, with some success.

Automated refractors generally fall into 5 categories:

- manual objective refractors
- automatic objective refractors (automatic retinoscopes) without visual acuity capability

- automatic objective refractors with visual acuity capability
- automated subjective refractors
- remote-controlled conventional refractors

Manual objective refractors require the operator to align mires formed with infrared light on a patient's retina. Automatic objective refractors obtain the refractive measurements automatically using infrared light, requiring 0.2–10 seconds for the actual measurement. Most of the automatic objective refractors are purely objective, with no visual acuity capability. Some, however, have built-in spherocylindrical optics and visual acuity charts. Most of these same instruments also have subjective refinement capability.

Automated subjective refractors use subjective responses from the patient to arrive at the refractive correction. Instruments with subjective capability require more patient cooperation than the strictly objective instruments but have the advantage of providing subjective refinement and visual acuity as part of the refracting procedure.

Remote-controlled conventional refractors have been introduced. Some are impressive and they ease back strain, but they require the same skill in refracting as a conventional phoropter.

Overrefraction techniques (see Chapter 4, Clinical Refraction) are possible with some instruments. Such techniques are particularly recommended for patients with high refractive errors to avoid problems from vertex distance and pantoscopic tilt.

Macular Function Testing

Laser Interferometer

Several instruments are available for evaluating the functional status of the macula in the presence of a visually significant cataract. All are based on the principle that even a cataractous lens may have small, relatively clear regions, which allow a narrow beam of light to reach the retina relatively unaffected by the cataract.

Of these devices, perhaps the simplest to understand is the laser interferometer. A beam, usually from a helium-neon laser, is optically split. The 2 beams are then projected at a small angle relative to one another through separate clear areas of the lens. Inside the eye they overlap, and because the laser light is coherent, the beams interfere, forming interference fringes on the retina. Changing the relative angle between the 2 beams varies the spacing of the fringes. Retinal function is estimated by the finest fringes that can be identified by the patient.

The laser interferometer has disadvantages, one being that it requires 2 somewhat separated clear areas of lens. Another is that the fringes may be difficult for some patients to recognize. In addition, fringe spacing does not correlate directly with visual acuity.

Potential Acuity Meter

The Guyton-Minkowski Potential Acuity Meter (PAM) (Fig 8-46) avoids these problems by imaging a Snellen chart on the retina. From our discussion on image movement (see Chapter 2, Geometric Optics), we know that if the Snellen screen is imaged onto the

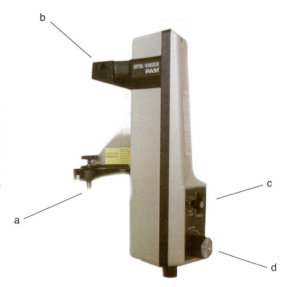

Figure 8-46 Photograph of a Potential Acuity Meter (PAM): *a*, point of attachment to slit-lamp biomicroscope; *b*, small-aperture view projector for imaging a Snellen chart on the retina; *c*, dial for changing the projected image; *d*, dial for adjusting illumination intensity. *(Courtesy of Neal H. Atebara, MD.)*

patient's retina, and if there is a real image of the aperture, the aperture, which is anterior to the screen, must be imaged anterior to the patient's retina. By appropriate selection of optical parameters, we can arrange for the image of the aperture to be located within the patient's lens. What this means is that all the light reaching the retina passes through a very small aerial opening, approximately 0.1 mm in diameter, somewhere at the antero-posterior position of the patient's lens. By appropriate positioning, we try to select a small clear area of the patient's lens to "shoot through."

Glare Testing

As discussed in the section on visual function (see Chapter 3, Optics of the Human Eye), Snellen acuity does not completely characterize the quality of a patient's visual optical system. Some patients may have a disabling media opacity with reduced contrast sensitivity and still have otherwise good Snellen acuity. Modulation transfer function testing (contrast grating) is one approach to testing these patients.

Another approach is to simulate the clinical situations that patients find most disabling. Most of these patients notice that extraneous light markedly degrades their visual performance. For example, headlights from oncoming cars at night may render an individual unable to see any detail of the road ahead. Various instruments have been devised to simulate this situation, including the Brightness Acuity Tester (BAT; Fig 8-47). They all shine a bright light into the eye at an angle or at many angles away from the visual axis. With normal media, the glare source is imaged away from the macula and does not affect central acuity. In the presence of a scattering lesion such as cataract, light from the glare

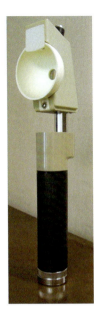

Figure 8-47 Photograph of a brightness acuity tester (BAT). *(Courtesy of Kenneth J. Hoffer, MD.)*

source reaches the macula, reducing the image contrast of an on-axis target and making it harder to discern.

The major limitation of the various glare testers is that results are qualitative, not quantitative, and not very reproducible. Nevertheless, they do document the problem of glare and alert the physician to problems not detectable with routine Snellen testing.

Wavefront Aberrometers

Corneal topography is able to measure the shape of the surface of an irregular cornea, but it is not able to measure the actual refractive topography of the entire lens–cornea optical system. For such measurements, instruments traditionally used in astronomy to reduce the complex and continually changing refractive effects of the earth's atmosphere have been applied to the examination of the human eye. These instruments are called *wavefront aberrometers.*

In *Hartmann-Shack aberrometry,* a low-intensity laser beam is directed onto the retina, and this is used as the object for the aberrometer. Light rays from the laser spot diverge as they leave the retina (Fig 8-48A), thereby creating convex spherical wavefronts (blue lines in the figure). The wavefront created at a specific point in time is represented by "moment 1." These wavefronts travel toward the front of the eye (moments 1–3 in the figure). In an ideal eye, the lens and cornea would transform the spherical wavefronts into plano wavefronts. A lens array in the aberrometer focuses these light rays onto a photodetector (CCD [charge-coupled device]). An ideal eye produces Hartmann-Shack

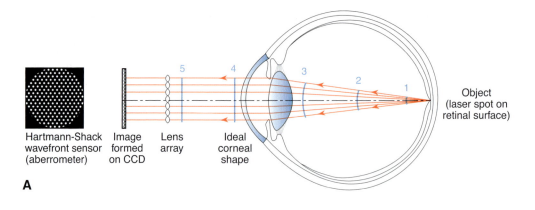

Hartmann-Shack wavefront sensor (aberrometer) | Image formed on CCD | Lens array | Ideal corneal shape | Object (laser spot on retinal surface)

A

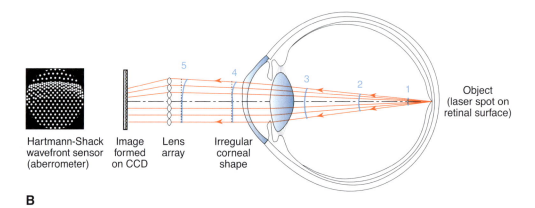

Hartmann-Shack wavefront sensor (aberrometer) | Image formed on CCD | Lens array | Irregular corneal shape | Object (laser spot on retinal surface)

B

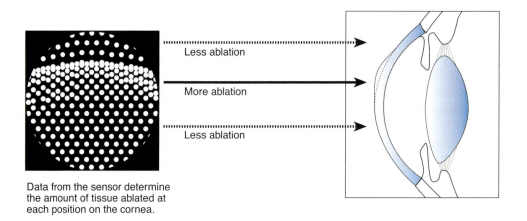

Less ablation

More ablation

Less ablation

Data from the sensor determine the amount of tissue ablated at each position on the cornea.

C

Figure 8-48 Hartmann-Shack image produced by an ideal optical system **(A)** and by an aberrated optical system **(B)**. The Hartmann-Shack image is used to perform corrective corneal ablation **(C)**. *(Courtesy of Neal H. Atebara, MD. Redrawn by C. H. Wooley.)*

images with dots of light that are equally spaced from each other. Because the measured wavefronts are those *exiting* the eye, this is considered *outgoing aberrometry.*

In an aberrated eye, the wavefronts are not entirely planar. In Figure 8-48B, the dashed black lines represent ideal planar wavefronts, whereas the solid blue lines represent the aberrated wavefronts. The images captured by the photodetector show areas where the spots of light are more closely spaced; these represent areas where the eye's optical aberration of the system is greatest.

The data from the photodetector are then processed in a manner similar to those from an automated lensmeter to arrive at a correction that includes low- and higher-order aberrations. The data further define the amount of photoablation performed at each position on the cornea using a wavefront-guided excimer laser (Fig 8-48C).

See BCSC Section 13, *Refractive Surgery,* for further discussion.

Optical Coherence Tomography

Optical coherence tomography (OCT) is used to create a cross-sectional image of the living retina at a resolution of 10 μm or less. This technology is increasingly useful in the diagnosis and management of many different macular conditions, such as macular edema and vitreomacular traction. OCT is based on the Michelson interferometer, which takes advantage of the interference properties of temporally coherent light.

When 2 coherent light waves that are fully "in phase" with one another overlap, their superposition results in a doubling of light intensity. When they are precisely "out of phase," they cancel each other out, resulting in darkness. Between the 2 extremes, the intensity varies as a function of how closely in phase the waves are.

The major components of an OCT include a light source (usually a superluminescent diode), a light detector, a beam splitter, and a movable mirror, arranged as in Figure 8-49. Light from the diode is split by the beam splitter, with half the light directed to the movable mirror (called the *reference beam* [blue waves]) and half to the retina (called the *object beam* [red waves]). These 2 beams are superimposed by the beam splitter and transmitted together to the light detector.

The principle of the Michelson interferometer tells us that light reflected from the movable mirror (reference beam) will cancel out almost all light from the retina (objective beam) except light from the level of the retina corresponding to the position of the movable mirror. That is, if the movable mirror is positioned "6 units" from the beam splitter, only light from the retina at a distance of "6 units" from the beam splitter will be seen by the light detector; light from all other layers of the retina will be canceled out by destructive interference. Likewise, when the mirror is moved up and down, it will allow only light from the corresponding retinal distance.

The various layers of the retina reflect light to different degrees, with the highest reflection occurring in layers with cell surfaces and membranes, such as the RPE layer, the inner and outer nuclear layers, and the internal limiting membrane. If light intensity as measured by the detector is plotted against the position of the movable mirror, an "A-scan"

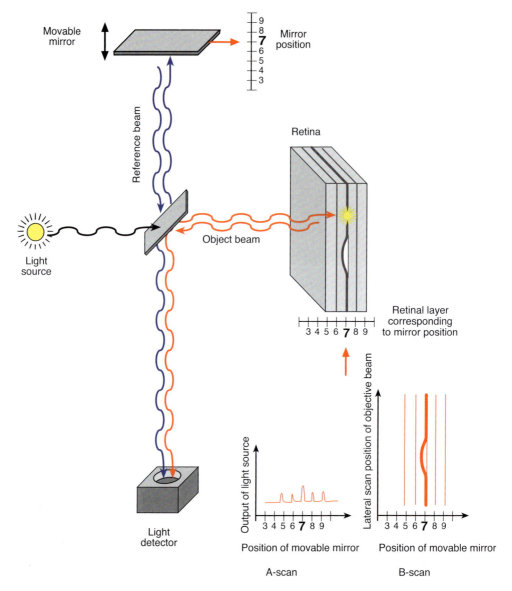

Figure 8-49 Optical coherence tomography (OCT). Based on the principle of the Michelson interferometer, the OCT analyzes the interference patterns between a reference beam and the object beam to create a precise cross-sectional reflectivity map of the internal retina. *(Courtesy of Neal H. Atebara, MD. Redrawn by C. H. Wooley.)*

image of the retina cross section can be generated (see Fig 8-49). A tilting mirror positioned between the beam splitter and the retina can be used to scan the retina to generate a 2-dimensional B-scan cross-sectional image of the retina (see Fig 8-49).

See BCSC Section 12, *Retina and Vitreous,* for additional discussion.

CHAPTER 9

Vision Rehabilitation

The goal of examining and treating patients in ophthalmology is twofold. The first goal is to prevent, recognize, and treat disease in order to preserve ocular and adnexal function. The second goal is to alleviate the functional consequences of impaired vision. A thorough understanding of the principles and practice of vision rehabilitation allows the ophthalmologist to address a patient's visual deficits more effectively and to recognize when appropriate referral to a vision rehabilitation specialist is required.

Patients present for help if their visual *function* is impaired, not their visual acuity, and even minimal vision loss can have a great impact on patient functioning. The goal of helping patients who have *functional* deficits can be accomplished by employment of a *functional* approach to patient assessment and treatment in order to improve performance and function.

Any patient with a loss of visual function that cannot be remedied by standard optical, medical, or surgical means is a "low vision" patient who requires "rehabilitation." Vision rehabilitation seeks to reduce the functional impact of visual impairment so that patients can effectively maintain their customary activities, their independence, and their quality of life. It should not be thought of as a separate entity from comprehensive ophthalmologic care. All ophthalmologists treat glaucoma patients, retina patients, and external disease patients even if they may not be subspecialists in those fields. Vision rehabilitation is the same.

Vision rehabilitation is not a domain limited to improving reading but rather comprises a number of rehabilitative interventions pertaining to nearly every part of a person's life. It may be as simple as completing an accurate refraction and prescribing single-vision reading spectacles or as complicated as prescribing spectacle-mounted telescopes, eccentric viewing training, or high-tech electronic devices.

However, the most important contribution the ophthalmologist can make to ensure a patient's rehabilitation is to offer information that encourages patients to seek comprehensive vision rehabilitation. The ophthalmologist is in a unique position to support the vision rehabilitation of his or her patients.

Figure 9-1 presents a useful framework that demonstrates both the overlapping areas of low vision management and how anatomical changes lead ultimately to socioeconomic consequences. For example, a patient with macular degeneration (disorder) who has decreased visual acuity (impairment) may not be able to read road signs (disability) and may ultimately lose his or her driver's license (handicap).

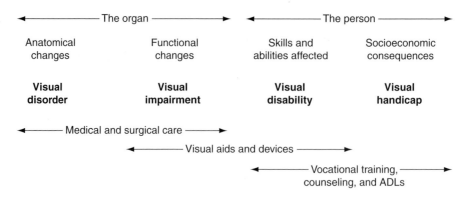

Figure 9-1 Overlapping areas of management for patients with ocular disease. ADLs = activities of daily living. *(Courtesy of Mathias Fellenz, MD.)*

Epidemiology of Vision Impairment

It is estimated that 13.5 million Americans older than 45 years have visual impairments, and more than two-thirds of them are older than 65 years. The number of Americans older than 65 years is expected to increase from 33.2 million in 1994 to 80 million by 2050. Thus, the percentage of individuals with vision impairment will increase as well. Vision loss is ranked third after arthritis and heart disease as the most common chronic condition requiring aid in activities of daily living (ADLs) among people older than 70 years.

Age-related macular degeneration (AMD) accounts for 45% of low vision patients in the United States, and every year 200,000 Americans lose significant vision from AMD, requiring rehabilitation assistance. Glaucoma and diabetic retinopathy are the next most frequent causes. These patients may cope with significant functional visual impairment for many years. Identifying patients who remain impaired after medical or surgical treatment and then offering them vision rehabilitation constitute a logical progression of appropriate treatment.

Important Definitions in Low Vision

Legal Blindness

The World Health Organization (WHO) defines legal blindness as best-corrected Snellen visual acuity of 20/200 or worse in the better eye or a visual field of 20° or worse in the better eye. Although this definition is not clinically appropriate, it is widely quoted and in 1932 was adopted by the federal government to determine eligibility for income tax benefits and federal and state assistance in the United States. It is interesting to note that, because visual field testing is not required in all states to obtain a driver's license, one can be "legally blind" by virtue of visual field constriction yet still hold a valid license to drive in some states.

Low Vision

The traditional definitions of low vision also rely on quantitative measures of visual acuity and visual field. For example, the WHO defined *low vision* in 1992 as follows:

> A person with low vision is one who has an impairment of visual functioning even after treatment and/or standard refractive correction, and has a visual acuity of less than 6/18 (20/60) to light perception or a visual field of less than 10° from the point of fixation, but who uses or is potentially able to use, vision for the planning and/or execution of a task.

The International Classification of Diseases, Ninth Revision, Clinical Modification (ICD-9-CM) divides low vision into 5 categories, as follows:

1. *Moderate visual impairment.* Best-corrected visual acuity of less than 20/60 to 20/160
2. *Severe visual impairment.* Best-corrected visual acuity of less than 20/160 to 20/400, or visual field diameter of 20° or less (largest field diameter for Goldmann isopter III-4e, 3/100 white test object or equivalent)
3. *Profound visual impairment.* Best-corrected visual acuity of less than 20/400 to 20/1000, or visual field diameter of 10° or less (largest field diameter for Goldmann isopter III-4e, 3/100 white test object or equivalent)
4. *Near-total vision loss.* Best-corrected visual acuity of 20/1250 or less
5. *Total blindness.* No light perception

More recent definitions of low vision include measures of contrast sensitivity and central or paracentral scotomata. The trend to include measures of visual function in addition to visual acuity and visual field reflects an evolving understanding of the complex nature of vision and the factors that lead to functional visual impairment as opposed to visual impairment alone.

The weakness inherent in all definitions of legal blindness and low vision is that the emphasis is placed on only a few objective, quantitative measures that do not fully express the visual system's capabilities and do not directly address patients' difficulties.

Visual Function

The term *visual function* is defined simply as the ability to perform important tasks that require vision. It is not synonymous with *visual acuity.* In fact, visual acuity is only 1 measure of visual function. Other measures of visual function include visual field, contrast sensitivity, electroretinography (ERG), glare sensitivity, preferred retinal locus ability, color vision, binocularity, eye dominance, and stereopsis. In order to improve visual performance and patient function, an organized approach to patient assessment and treatment is required.

Low vision can be better defined as *reduced visual function resulting from any disorder of the eye or visual system.*

Classification of Visual Function Deficits

An important classification of visual deficits was pioneered by Eleanor E. Faye, MD, and allows a better understanding of the way in which various eye diseases affect visual performance. From this classification, 3 predictable patterns of visual deficits emerge that clearly relate the pathologic process to the patient's functional status: cloudy media, central visual field deficit, and peripheral visual field deficit. These categories help predict patient difficulties and complaints and help the practitioner choose and implement rehabilitation strategies.

Cloudy Media

For a clear overall image to be formed on the retina, light rays must travel through the refractive media: tear film, cornea, anterior chamber, pupil, lens, and vitreous. Diseases affecting these structures usually impair overall image clarity, causing blurred vision, decreased detailed vision, and significant glare. Contrast sensitivity is typically reduced uniformly at all spatial frequencies. Performance on visual function tests often depends on illumination; this is reflected by patient complaints of poor function in too much light (glare) or too little light.

Examples of conditions in this category include uncorrected refractive errors, corneal epithelial and stromal disease (dry eyes, dystrophies, keratoconus, scarring from herpes simplex), traumatic mydriasis, cataracts, complications from LASIK surgery, vitreous hemorrhage, and posterior uveitis.

Central Visual Field Deficit

A clear central image depends on an intact macula and the nerve pathways subserving central vision. Diseases affecting these structures cause relative or absolute scotomata (blind spots) at or near fixation and/or decreased retinal contrast sensitivity.

Symptoms depend on the number, size, location, and density of the scotomata and on the ability of the patient to reliably use an alternate (eccentric) point of fixation, called a *preferred retinal locus (PRL).* In the same way that normally sighted people do not perceive their own blind spot as a dark area in their visual field, patients with central and paracentral scotomata usually do not complain of black spots or missing areas in their visual field. This is due to the extraretinal phenomenon of *perceptual completion,* in which the brain fills in the missing information using surround information from the edges of the scotoma.

If available, the scanning laser ophthalmoscope (SLO) can be used to map the size, location, and depth of scotomata in the macular region, while directly observing and quantifying patient fixation and eye movement patterns. A great deal of information regarding patient function can be learned from the results of SLO testing and studies (Fig 9-2).

Usual symptoms in patients include difficulties with reading, recognizing people's faces, or performing any task that requires detail vision. Common descriptions of reading difficulties include blurred or distorted vision, missing letters in words, or the need for more light. Because the highest concentration of cones is found in the macula, color vision deficits can also occur.

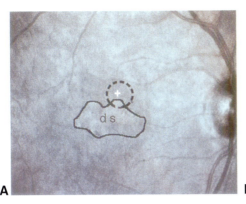
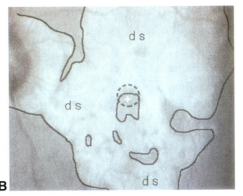

A   B

Figure 9-2   Patient with a complex scotoma. The *cross* and *circle* indicate preferred retinal locus (PRL) location; *ds,* dense scotoma. **A,** Right eye with a small inferior retinal (superior field) scotoma. **B,** Left eye with a ring scotoma. Even though these eyes have the same acuity, the right eye functions better. For reading, the right eye will not encounter scotomata (which would slow reading speed) to the right or left of fixation. The left eye has only a small functioning central island surrounded by large dense scotomata. *(From Colenbrander A, Schuchard RA, Fletcher DC. Evaluating visual function. In: Fletcher DC, ed.* Low Vision Rehabilitation: Caring for the Whole Person. Ophthalmology Monograph 12. *San Francisco: American Academy of Ophthalmology; 1999:45.)*

These patients may be legally blind but usually are not visibly disabled. Further, mobility is not affected because the peripheral visual field is spared. It is for this reason that patients with central vision loss are often overly protected by their family and friends. For although these patients may not be able to recognize a friend or read a bus number, they can navigate with ease in their environment and do not require a white cane. They can spot small items in their normal peripheral visual field and often continue to drive despite not meeting legal visual requirements, because good visual acuity is usually required only to read street signs in unfamiliar areas.

Visual acuity tests that use single letters or numbers (Snellen, ETDRS) should be administered at a distance of 10 ft (3 m). Tests that use continuous text are used to estimate reading skill and to determine the strength of the optical magnifying device needed by the patient.

Contrast sensitivity is a more significant indicator of visual function than are high-contrast acuity tests. Performance for tasks such as reading can be greatly diminished in the presence of a reduction in contrast sensitivity. One of the benefits of vascular endothelial growth factor (VEGF) treatment of neovascular (wet) macular disease has been the dramatic improvement not only in acuity, but also in contrast sensitivity.

Examples of conditions in this category include wet or dry macular degeneration, macular hole, diabetic macular edema, myopic degeneration, toxoplasmosis and histoplasmosis, phototoxicity, toxic reaction to drugs, and cecocentral scotomata. Focal and grid laser treatment of macular edema and photocoagulation of choroidal neovascular membranes, which may cause iatrogenic central and paracentral scotomata, have been supplanted by recently introduced anti-VEGF drugs. Diet and carotenoid supplements are under investigation for the treatment of atrophic macular disease.

Peripheral Visual Field Deficit

The peripheral visual field is crucial for mobility and orientation. Variable patterns of visual field loss can result from diseases of the retina, optic nerve, and central nervous system. The functional implications for the patient are very different from those of the other 2 categories of deficits and, as such, require different rehabilitation strategies.

Typical symptoms caused by a peripheral visual field defect include bumping into objects or people and difficulty navigating through unfamiliar territory, particularly in poor illumination or at night, as well as difficulty reading if there is a constricted residual central visual field.

Visual acuity is not affected until very advanced stages; therefore, acuity testing may completely miss early evidence of constricted visual fields. Visual field testing is necessary to quantify deficits in this category. Central contrast sensitivity testing should be performed but will usually be normal until late in the disease.

Examples of conditions in this category include retinitis pigmentosa, retinal dystrophies, retinal detachment, proliferative diabetic retinopathy, glaucoma, ischemic optic neuropathy, stroke, trauma, and tumor. Panretinal laser photocoagulation causes iatrogenic peripheral visual field loss and reduced contrast sensitivity function that can significantly limit a patient's performance at night.

Patient Assessment

Taking a functional history and measuring visual function are essential to effective assessment.

Functional History

The goal of taking a medical history is to collect information from the patient that guides the investigation and leads to a diagnosis and treatment plan. This same approach is used for patients who require vision rehabilitation. A shift in emphasis to the patient's functional deficits is required, but a few specific questions can easily elicit this information. Patients welcome this approach because, from their point of view, only function matters—how can they more easily accomplish the task they are having difficulty with? The following information is a useful guide to completing a functional history.

Ocular history

Correlate the patient's functional complaints to progression of the disease and to any medical and surgical interventions. Miotic therapy and panretinal photocoagulation are 2 examples of treatments that may adversely affect visual function while having a positive effect on ocular disease.

General medical history

Systemic diseases indirectly affect patient functioning in the completion of visual tasks, in addition to their direct effects on the visual system. Orthopedic conditions, arthritis, tremors, or paralysis from a stroke can impair a patient's ability to hold a book or a handheld magnifier and thus interfere with reading.

Task analysis

The goal of the task analysis is to determine which tasks the patient values and finds difficult or impossible to perform. Enabling the patient to perform these tasks will be the goal of rehabilitation. Questions may address near tasks (eg, reading books, medication labels, or newspapers), intermediate tasks (eg, shopping, cooking, dialing a phone number, seeing a computer screen, or shaving), or distance tasks (eg, seeing signs or watching television or sporting events). Questions about difficulty with independent travel, such as seeing steps and curbs, as well as driving, are important to ask. In addition, it is useful to ask general questions about the adaptations that the patient has already made and to note the patient's observations about lighting requirements.

Well-Being

As the history is obtained, most patients will describe the impact that vision loss has had on their lifestyle, family, vocation, and hobbies. It is important to determine whether patients have experienced falls, because fall prevention can be addressed. Patients who have Charles Bonnet Syndrome, in which they see images of objects that are not real and which affects one-third of visually impaired persons, are relieved to discuss their hallucinations. When asked directly, many patients with vision loss will report being depressed, and this can prompt referral to appropriate professionals.

Measuring Visual Function

The following tests are useful in quantifying functional losses and gathering important information to guide clinical decisions. One should not endeavor to perform all tests on all patients in a clinical ophthalmology setting. However, knowledge of their use, application, and common patterns of deficit allows one to selectively employ the appropriate test and enhance the understanding of the patient's functional deficits.

Distance visual acuity

Obtaining an accurate measure of visual acuity is important for the following reasons:

- to follow disease progression and the effects of treatment
- to measure improvement during refraction
- to determine the power of spectacles or optical aids needed for reading and near work
- to estimate a person's ability to perform specific tasks such as reading and driving
- to categorize patients so that they can obtain Social Security, insurance, and other benefits or exemptions

The single-letter Snellen visual acuity chart is the most commonly used test of visual acuity. Although Snellen acuity provides useful information, it measures only a narrow range of the visual system's capabilities (see Chapter 3, Optics of the Human Eye). It consists of high-contrast black letters on a white background under near-ideal illumination conditions. A patient's performance on this test does not characterize typical function, especially under low light or poor-contrast conditions. The effects of glare from extraneous light sources, the presence of retinal scotomata, and the status of the peripheral visual field are also not taken into account.

Standard projection charts are not ideal for obtaining accurate visual acuity measurements at 20 ft (6 m) for patients with reduced vision. Most charts were designed to measure vision for purposes of refracting patients with normal or near-normal vision. There are too few lines and too few letters per line on most charts below acuities of 20/70. This can underestimate a patient's functional capability and makes an accurate refraction almost impossible for the low vision patient. Consequently, there is a serious underestimation of not only true acuity but also the effect of illumination and contrast.

The Lighthouse Distance Visual Acuity Test (a modified ETDRS chart) overcomes many of these disadvantages and is widely used to assess patients with reduced visual acuity (see Fig 3-6 in Chapter 3, Optics of the Human Eye). It uses metric notation and has equal line difficulty, proportional interletter and interline spacing, and geometric progression of optotype sizes from line to line. There are more lines at lower levels of acuity (eg, a 160 line and a 125 line between the 100 and 200 lines) and 5 letters on each line, making assessment and measurement of change more accurate. This is especially important during refraction. There are 3 charts (one each for OD, OS, and OU, with all 3 used in research studies), but for clinical application, 1 chart is commonly selected and a test distance of 10 ft used (equivalent to a test distance of 3 m), which covers visual acuities to 20/400 (10/200). At 5 ft (a 1.5-m equivalent), it covers visual acuities to 20/800 (5/200).

If only standard visual acuity charts are available, the examiner can move the patient or the chart to 10 ft (3 m) or 5 ft (1.5 m) and annotate the resulting acuity using the shorter distance from the patient to the chart.

Near visual acuity

The task of reading words and sentences is more complex than recognizing single letters. Testing near "reading" ability with text samples better estimates a patient's functional reading ability than doing so with single-letter acuity charts. Reading speed is also of practical importance to the reader, who might find it frustrating or even pointless if information cannot be acquired at a reasonable rate.

When the clinician is recording near visual acuity, using metric notation is simpler and more informative than using Snellen equivalents, Jaeger numbers (J), or points (p). The metric unit for letter size is the M unit. A 1-M symbol subtends 5 minutes of arc at 1 m. It is roughly equal in size to regular newsprint, which can be read with a visual acuity of approximately 20/50. Any visual acuity result can be recorded simply as the distance of the chart or reading material (in meters) over the letter size (in M units). For example, reading 2-M letters at 40 cm would result in a visual acuity of 0.4 meter/2 M, or 0.4/2. This can be easily converted to Snellen acuity: $0.4/2 = 20/x$ ($x = 100$); therefore, the Snellen acuity is 20/100.

Several commercial reading tests are available, including the Lighthouse Continuous Text Cards, the Minnesota Low Vision Reading Test (MNRead), the Colenbrander 1-m chart, and the Pepper Visual Skills for Reading Test. Before reading glasses are prescribed, the patient should demonstrate proficiency with actual print material.

Many patients wish that new glasses could take away the poor vision associated with their eye disease. Their disappointment is compounded when further loss of vision occurs after they have made expenditures for glasses. Clinicians must be careful to manage patients' unrealistic expectation that glasses will improve their vision.

Contrast sensitivity

The visual system's ability to resolve detail depends not only on the size or separation of the objects in question but also on the contrast or luminance difference between the object and its surroundings. Research has demonstrated that visual spatial processing is organized as a series of independent, parallel channels. Each channel is sensitive to different frequencies or separations between lines, and each channel has a different threshold or contrast level at which it functions. A contrast sensitivity function curve can be constructed that, like an audiogram, records a wider range of visual sensitivity than can visual acuity testing (see Chapter 3, Optics of the Human Eye).

Many activities are difficult for patients with reduced contrast sensitivity. Reading low-contrast print, or colored text on a colored background; walking in foggy or cloudy conditions or in dim light, and pouring milk into a white cup are just a few examples.

When the ophthalmologist evaluates patients with reduced visual function, contrast sensitivity testing can reveal important information about the following:

- *Magnification need.* Patients who have poor contrast sensitivity usually require more magnification than would otherwise be anticipated for their level of visual acuity. Knowing this saves time, allows for realistic recommendations to be made regarding device prescription, and helps explain why patients may not be functioning as well as expected.
- *Ability to use optical aids.* Patients with extremely poor contrast sensitivity may require additional contrast enhancement to be able to read using magnification. These patients may require a closed-circuit television (CCTV), which can significantly enhance contrast and enlarge the field of view so that they will be able to see more than 1 or 2 letters at a time.
- *Lighting.* Patients with poor contrast sensitivity often benefit from better illumination for certain tasks. Although this can be determined clinically, confirmation is helpful.
- *Dominant eye.* By testing contrast sensitivity monocularly and binocularly, the ophthalmologist can determine whether the patient will perform better or worse with binocular optical aids (glasses, CCTV). Superior monocular performance suggests potential interference from a poorer functioning dominant eye and supports the use of monocular aids such as magnifiers and monocular spectacles, as well as occlusion of the poorer eye.
- *Overall function.* Keeping all the preceding in mind, we see how contrast sensitivity testing can better characterize a patient's functional ability and guide rehabilitative strategies in a directed manner. Specific measures to improve contrast can be employed when a significant deficit is revealed through testing.
- *Longitudinal projection.* Following contrast sensitivity over time may reveal deterioration in function that might not otherwise have been detected by visual acuity testing alone. This can often corroborate a patient's subjective report of deterioration in function.

Several contrast sensitivity charts are available commercially, with different features and advantages, including the Functional Acuity Contrast Test (FACT), the Pelli-Robson chart, the LEA Low-Contrast Test, and the Mars Letter Contrast Sensitivity Test. The Vision Contrast Test System (VCTS) is another contrast sensitivity chart; although it is no longer available, many ophthalmology offices have the test stored away. It is not necessary to test contrast sensitivity in all patients; however, it is especially useful in patients who appear to be functioning at a lower level than expected and in patients with deteriorating vision despite stable acuity.

Contrast sensitivity tests are clinically accessible and the most informative for predicting the ultimate visual function of the low vision patient. If tests are not available, there are other ways to assess contrast sensitivity function (Clinical Pearl 9-1).

> Arditi A. Improving the design of the letter contrast sensitivity test. *Invest Ophthalmol Vis Sci.* 2005;46(6):2225–2229.

Peripheral visual field

Kinetic (Goldmann) and static (Humphrey, Octopus) perimetry are the standard tests for peripheral visual field assessment. Early peripheral visual field loss is usually asymptomatic, and even moderate to advanced loss in the periphery does not affect function for tasks such as reading. Patients who experience peripheral scotomata generally present with orientation and mobility difficulties, which usually occur in unfamiliar surroundings. Severe loss (as in advanced glaucoma or retinitis pigmentosa) that leaves a residual central visual field of less than 20° is one of the criteria for *legal blindness* in the United States and Canada.

Central visual field

Goldmann kinetic perimetry and static macular perimetry (eg, 10-2 test on the Humphrey Field Analyzer) depend on stable fixation at the fovea and have no way of accurately monitoring or compensating for small eye movements. Central tangent screening and Amsler grid testing also depend on foveal fixation and are inadequate for detecting small scotomata. Some of these methods work well for peripheral visual field testing but present problems for accurate central visual field testing in the presence of macular disease, where fixation is often unstable or extrafoveal. In fact, both problems often coexist.

CLINICAL PEARL 9-1

The ophthalmologist can often assess contrast sensitivity function by asking a few relevant questions. For example, patients are usually aware that their reading ability is greatly enhanced under better illumination. If a contrast sensitivity chart is unavailable, visual acuity can be retested under low room illumination. Patients with poor contrast sensitivity function will have a greater reduction in visual acuity under these circumstances. However, this works only with nonilluminated and nonprojector charts.

If fixation is unstable, the patient will show significant eye movement, and the size of measured scotomata will be inaccurate. If fixation is extrafoveal, then all points will be shifted with respect to their true foveal location, and a correct map of the defects will be impossible. In addition, perceptual filling in of scotomata may render some tests, such as the Amsler grid, useless because the patient may not perceive the scotomata at all.

Macular perimetry is best accomplished with a scanning laser ophthalmoscope (SLO), a diagnostic tool. The SLO is a fundus perimeter that allows simultaneous visualization of the retina and stimulus presentation so that one can observe the exact retinal site being tested. This permits a precise correlation between visual field defects and their true retinal location. Simpler methods to map scotomata also exist, such as performing a tangent field at near using a laser pointer as a stimulus on a white sheet of paper.

Most patients with central scotomata reliably develop an eccentric "pseudofovea" called the *preferred retinal locus (PRL)*. The PRL may change over time as the disease progresses, and there may be multiple loci of eccentric fixation. Knowing the location and ability of the PRL in a patient with a scotoma helps the clinician understand the specific difficulties the patient has in carrying out visual tasks.

The presence of central and paracentral scotomata in diseases that affect macular function, such as macular degeneration and macular edema, is more common than once thought. In addition, the presence of scotomata may not correlate with the visible retinal changes of atrophy, scarring, or pigment alteration. There may be a single scotoma or multiple scotomata, which may be irregularly shaped or ring-shaped surrounding the macula. They greatly affect visual acuity and contrast sensitivity (see Fig 9-2).

Eccentric fixation training can sometimes help patients improve coordination, tracking, and scanning and thereby facilitate function for tasks such as reading.

In some cases a prism, with base in the direction of the PRL, can be introduced, preferably binocularly, to determine whether the patient appreciates a shift of the image to a more viable retinal area.

Glare

Many patients suffer from glare or light sensitivity, which interferes with visual performance under certain lighting conditions. Common conditions resulting in glare include corneal edema and scarring, iris defects and abnormalities, posterior subcapsular cataracts, and retinal diseases such as retinitis pigmentosa, cone–rod dystrophy, and albinism. The simplest way to assess glare is by getting the history or performing visual acuity and contrast sensitivity testing with and without a direct source of light pointed toward the patient. Commercially available tests include the Brightness Acuity Test (BAT) and the Miller-Nadler Glare Tester, which reflect light into the patient's eye off a diffusing surface. (Both of these tests are difficult to obtain.)

Because many patients with reduced visual function require increased illumination in the face of poor contrast sensitivity function, determining whether patients experience glare is important. The patient's actual light source should be evaluated. A halogen or fluorescent light may be a source of glare, or the patient may have the light in an inefficient position. Light-emitting diodes (LEDs) in magnifiers may also be a glare source, particularly for the patient with corneal or lens pathology.

Color vision

Acquired color vision deficits may occur in patients with reduced visual function. Poor color vision can affect performance in tasks involving color identification or matching at work, home, or school. It is important to ask patients whether they are having any color perception problems that need to be addressed.

Most acquired color vision defects in low vision patients are blue-yellow defects. However, the commonly used pseudoisochromatic plate tests (Ishihara) do not allow assessment of blue-yellow defects; rather, they detect hereditary color vision deficits.

The Farnsworth Dichotomous Test for Color Blindness (Panel D-15) jumbo version is probably the most convenient color vision test for low vision patients, although it can miss mild deficits.

Helping Patients Function Better

Ophthalmologists can help patients function better through a careful refraction and by providing them with the appropriate optical or nonoptical aid.

Refraction

An accurate refraction is particularly important for patients with vision loss. A careful refraction helps determine not only the correct reading add but also the appropriate best spectacle prescription for optimizing distance vision. In addition, it helps ophthalmologists advise patients properly in the use of optical and electronic aids with respect to their spectacles and incorporate accurate cylindrical and/or asymmetric corrections into glasses or optical devices.

The following key points will help in obtaining a quick and accurate refraction:

- Use an appropriate acuity chart with sufficient lines and optotypes at the low acuity range.
- Use a radical refraction technique if the reflex is dull or the motion of the reflex difficult to see. For example, use the retinoscope at half the customary distance to the eye, which requires doubling the power of the working-distance lens. If the reflex is still difficult to see, move the retinoscope half the remaining distance, using the appropriate add for that working distance.
- Use a trial frame instead of a phoropter to allow for an atypical head position, nystagmus, and maximal light transmittance during retinoscopy, and to allow for a sufficiently large dioptric interval, or *just noticeable difference,* to be displayed during subjective refraction. In order for patients with reduced visual function to perceive a change between the 2 choices shown during manifest refraction, the dioptric interval between the lenses must be increased. As a starting point, increase the interval from the usual 0.50 D (+0.25 D/−0.25 D) to 1.00 D (+0.50 D/−0.50 D) for patients with visual acuity from 20/50 to 20/100 and to 2.00 D (+1.00 D/−1.00 D) for patients with visual acuity worse than 20/100.
- Use a keratometer to measure exceptional astigmatic errors, as occurs in keratoconus. Occasionally, an automatic refractor will detect a cylinder that is difficult to see with a retinoscope.

Distance Spectacles

New distance glasses should be prescribed if a patient perceives an improvement in distance vision with the new manifest refraction compared to his or her current glasses.

Optical Aids Providing Magnification

Optical aids include spectacles, handheld and stand magnifiers, and telescopes.

Spectacles

A number of lens types are available in spectacles.

Near (reading) spectacles The simplest way to obtain a larger retinal image is to bring the object closer to the eye. This requires either accommodation or a lens (add) that focuses at the appropriate, shortened distance. The amount of add needed depends on the patient's accommodative amplitude (which decreases with age) and the required reading distance.

The clinician can predict the reading add by using the *Kestenbaum rule* (Clinical Pearl 9-2). The result is, however, only a starting point. Patients with poor contrast sensitivity or macular scotomata or those who must read print that is smaller than 1 M invariably require greater magnification than predicted by the Kestenbaum rule.

How to prescribe low vision reading spectacles:

1. Determine the best distance refraction and resulting best distance acuity.
2. Place this prescription in a trial frame and add to it the predicted add (determined using the Kestenbaum Rule). Increase the near addition until the patient can comfortably read the target size print (at least 1 M letter size) at a reasonable reading speed. Be sure to reduce the reading distance (1/add, in meters) as you increase the add. Since the patient's typical reading material (newspapers, bills, magazines, and so on) may be of poorer contrast and quality than standard text reading cards, use the patient's own reading material when making the final decision about the strength of the reading add.
3. Adjust the lighting to determine both the type of lamp and the lamp position that will help the patient with reading.

CLINICAL PEARL 9-2

The Kestenbaum Rule. The add required to read 1 M print can be quickly estimated from the measured visual acuity. This *predicted add* in diopters is simply the inverse of the visual acuity fraction. For example, a 20/200 patient (200/20 = 10) would benefit from a +10 D lens, with the material held at the focal point of the lens, 1/10 m (ie, 10 cm, or 4 inches). This, however, is only a starting point, and a stronger addition may be needed for some patients, especially those with reduced contrast sensitivity function.

4. When binocular function is better than monocular function, determine whether the patient requires base-in prism glasses (available in +4.00 to +12.00 D). This may easily be determined clinically and does not always require the 2 eyes to have identical visual acuity (Clinical Pearl 9-3).

5. If the patient is functionally monocular, try occluding the poorer eye to determine whether reading improves. Consider frosting the fellow lens or occluding if this helps performance.

The near (reading) add may be provided in several ways, depending on the strength of the add and the patient's visual needs.

Progressive addition lenses   Although progressive adds up to +3.50 D are available, patients have difficulty with the small bifocal area of these lenses, particularly if they use a head tilt or have an eccentric eye position. If the distance prescription is significant, and the intermediate add useful, it may be practical (after taking cost into account) to prescribe a separate pair of single-vision readers in addition to the progressive lenses. As a rule, patients need to wear a separate pair of low vision reading glasses to see small print.

Bifocals   Bifocals can be prescribed in strengths greater than +3.00 D as long as the shortened working distance is explained to the patient. Such adds are usually well tolerated binocularly up to the +4.50 D range, and up to +16.00 D monocularly for the better-seeing eye. In binocular patients, the optical centers of the high-power segments should be decentered more than required by the near pupillary distance, as this will induce base-in prism and assist accommodative convergence for patients with binocular function.

Single-vision readers   A separate pair of reading glasses affords several advantages over bifocals or progressive lenses for patients who are already having difficulty at near.

- The wider field of view facilitates eccentric viewing, atypical head positions, and the positioning of the illumination source.
- There is full lens power throughout the spectacle lens.
- A separate, less powerful add may also be prescribed as a wide-segment flat-top bifocal for intermediate tasks.
- Task-specific glasses can be purchased less expensively than a single pair of bifocals or progressive lenses and used for more than 1 activity. For example, a patient may have a pair of glasses for reading small print, a stronger pair for loading insulin syringes, and a weaker pair for writing, looking at photographs, or reading large-print books.

In patients with predominantly monocular function, always consider prescribing the correct spectacle lens power rather than just a balance lens for the poorer eye, because a balance lens may create an optical "imbalance" (Clinical Pearl 9-4). In patients with mild visual impairment, an accurate refraction and the prescription of single-vision readers may be the only intervention required to improve reading performance and function.

High-plus prismatic half-eye glasses   Prismatic half-eye glasses are commercially available from +4 D to +14 D with the appropriate base-in prism already incorporated with the spheres. If fusion is difficult for a patient, prescribe custom-made lenses with more base-in prism. Commercial prism glasses are inexpensive and suitable for patients with ametropia, with minimal astigmatism and better binocular than monocular function. High-index "thin lenses" with fashionable frames address past cosmetic concerns but are more expensive. Custom-made glasses with astigmatic correction for each eye can also be fabricated (see Clinical Pearl 9-3). Half-eye spectacle frames are convenient for patients with ametropia, as patients can look above the frames to see at a distance and use their reading glasses to see at near (Fig 9-3).

High-plus aspheric lenses   Aspheric spectacles reduce lenticular distortion when a higher-power addition is required for near tasks. They are commercially available from +6 D to +20 D and are essentially a monocular aid. The short working distance of these lenses makes them more difficult to use, requiring patients to receive proper instruction and training.

ADVANTAGES   Spectacle aids are familiar and cosmetically acceptable, and they provide hands-free functioning for a wide range of tasks. They provide the largest field of vision and allow for greater reading speed than devices from other categories. Binocular vision is possible up to approximately +12 D of add with base-in prism.

CLINICAL PEARL 9-3

Base-in prism should be incorporated into high-plus, single-vision reading spectacles for patients who function better binocularly. The ideal range for the use of such prisms is usually between +4 and +10 add. The amount of prism required is 2Δ more base-in than the add, in each eye. For example, if the distance prescription is plano OU and the appropriate add for reading is 8 D, then the prescription should read as follows: OD +8 with 10Δ BI; OS +8 with 10Δ BI. If additional prism is needed, the lenses must be custom-made.

CLINICAL PEARL 9-4

Patients with greatly asymmetric visual acuity and/or function are often prescribed a balance lens in the poorly seeing eye, because it is thought that they "will not use this eye." This logic and practice are flawed. If a central visual field defect exists, the entire peripheral field image will be out of focus without the correct prescription. If the eye with the more advanced disease is the patient's dominant eye, interference with the current "better" eye may be increased by the blurred image. In the latter case, frosting the lens or occluding may be necessary.

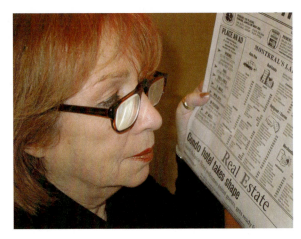

Figure 9-3 Prismatic, half-eye glasses allow binocular, hands-free function at a shortened working distance. *(Courtesy of Darren L. Albert, MD.)*

DISADVANTAGES   High-add spectacles require a shortened working distance that can obstruct lighting and make tasks such as writing difficult. They are inconvenient for spot reading tasks (eg, seeing price tags when shopping) because they must be put on and taken off and they cannot be worn for ambulation unless they are in half-eye frames.

Magnifiers

One can think of a magnifier as simply the add-on lens in a spectacle that is moved away from the eye (spectacle plane). As the object and add-on lens are moved as a unit (constant lens-to-object distance), the virtual image also moves. As the lens and object are moved away, the working distance (eye to object) is increased by the eye-to-lens distance. Because the virtual image moves away also, the retinal image becomes smaller. The effective (retinal) magnification of a magnifier is less than that of the corresponding reading add. With handheld magnifiers, the lens-to-object distance can be changed to bring the plane of the virtual image to the posterior focal plane of the eye. Thus, a patient with emmetropic presbyopia can use a +4 magnifier in lieu of reading glasses.

Because the effective field of view is limited by the rim of the lens, the field of view decreases as the lens is moved away from the eye. Hence, a spectacle correction may provide the most effective use of magnification for a patient.

Continuous text reading is possible with magnifiers for patients with mild to moderate vision loss. When function is more severely affected, magnifiers may allow for shorter reading periods or for spot reading because of the reduced reading speed associated with a smaller field of view.

Handheld magnifiers   The handheld magnifier is a familiar optical "aid." The low-power variety found in most optical stores and pharmacies has a high incidence of lens aberrations. Higher-quality lenses, including aspheric models, greatly enhance image quality and function. Once the magnification need is calculated for a specific task, several models, including illuminated lenses, should be demonstrated to the patient. The most commonly prescribed powers usually fall between +5 D and +20 D. Above +20 D, the higher magnification and reduced field of view make it more difficult for the patient to maintain a steady focus.

ADVANTAGES   Handheld magnifiers are readily accepted, as they are familiar devices that allow a greater working distance than high-plus spectacles. They are relatively inexpensive and portable, and patients can use them with their regular spectacles in place. Illuminated models are available that enhance contrast, if needed, while limiting glare. Some models use LEDs, which allow prolonged battery life—an important consideration, as battery life is often a factor in the use of illuminated magnifiers by older persons.

DISADVANTAGES   Patients with tremors, arthritis, paralysis, or poor hand–eye coordination have difficulty holding handheld magnifiers steady as they scan along lines of continuous text. Prolonged reading can be tedious because of the reduced field of view, especially with higher-power magnifiers. To obtain the maximum effect, patients must hold the magnifiers at the correct working distance.

Stand magnifiers   Resting on a flat surface with perfect stability, stand magnifiers maintain the correct lens-to-object distance. They can be moved along a page to read or used for other near tasks. They are useful for patients who are unable to hold a handheld magnifier steady or for those who need greater magnification than is practical to provide in a handheld magnifier or spectacle. Illuminated stand magnifiers are one of the most useful devices for patients with macular degeneration who have poor contrast sensitivity (Fig 9-4). The added illumination improves contrast and reduces the amount of magnification needed, usually resulting in faster reading speeds.

ADVANTAGES   It is easy to maintain a stabilized image at higher magnifications. For those with hand tremors, these magnifiers are easier to maneuver than the handheld ones.

DISADVANTAGES   Stand magnifiers may be bulky to carry and difficult to use on uneven surfaces. They require proper positioning of reading material and tend to elicit poor posture. The design of stand magnifiers often blocks good lighting unless they are self-illuminated.

Telescopes

Tasks that require magnification for distance viewing are far less common than those for near viewing, especially in older patients. Clear distance vision for a normally sighted person is usually appreciated for reading street signs while driving, reading a blackboard in school, or reading text or subtitles on television or at the movies. For the low vision patient, a distance prescription may result in only minor improvement; nevertheless, it may be worthwhile. This patient may also benefit from using (when possible) "approach magnification"—sitting closer to the television or the blackboard, for example.

Telescopic devices can be prescribed to improve function for specific tasks. For example, monocular, handheld telescopes fastened to a cord can be worn around the neck and used for intermittent distance viewing. The patient stops walking or moving, holds the telescope up to the better-seeing eye, views the material, and then puts down the telescope

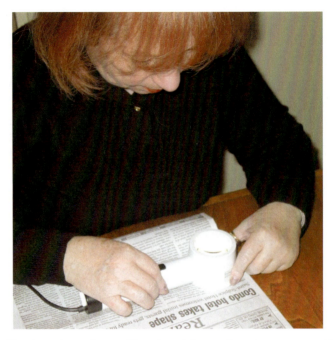

Figure 9-4 An illuminated stand magnifier placed flat against the page combines magnification, illumination, and stability. As with all optical magnifiers, the field of view decreases with increased magnification. *(Courtesy of Darren L. Albert, MD.)*

to resume activities. Binoculars are familiar devices that are available in different powers and can be used at sporting events and theaters (Fig 9-5).

Monocular or binocular spectacle-mounted full-field telescopes can allow hands-free use for continuous distance or near viewing, but patients cannot use them while ambulating or driving, because of the limited field of view and magnified motion. Self-contained, autofocus models are also available. Bioptic telescopes mounted in the top of distance spectacles can be used for driving in many states. The telescopic portion of the spectacles is positioned superiorly and temporally to the line of sight and used only briefly to read signs. If these telescopes are to be used for driving, proper prescription and training are required on an individual basis.

ADVANTAGES   Models are available that focus from near through intermediate and distance for a wide range of tasks. Most are lightweight and portable and can be mounted on spectacles in some cases.

DISADVANTAGES   Because telescopes have a restricted field of view and a narrow depth of field, they are somewhat more difficult to use than other optical devices. Luminance and contrast are reduced by the multiple-lens system, and the device must be held very steady—especially as magnification power increases. In addition, they are relatively expensive.

Prisms

Suppose a patient has a dense or complete left homonymous hemianopia that makes visualization of the left visual field a matter of deliberate attention and action. If 10Δ base-left

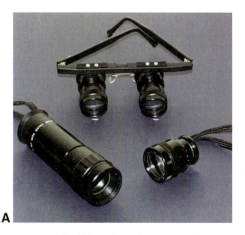
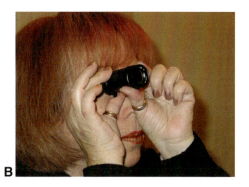

Figure 9-5 **A,** *Top:* Binocular, spectacle-mounted telescopes are available for prolonged distance tasks such as watching a play in a theater and/or near tasks such as reading. *Bottom left:* A high-power (6×), monocular, handheld Keplerian telescope may be difficult to hold steady and on target because of magnified motion and a narrow field of view. *Bottom right:* A low-power (2.8×) monocular, handheld Galilean telescope is ideal for intermittent distance tasks such as reading a street sign or bus number. **B,** Both hand–eye coordination and training are required for successful use of telescopic and other visual aids. *(Courtesy of Darren L. Albert, MD.)*

prisms are placed over the spectacle lenses, the patient will be able to see 5° more of the obscured left visual field, which is shifted to the right by the prisms. This provides a simple method of visual field enhancement for a patient who has had a stroke. Bilateral prisms are used, with both bases in the direction of the defect, for any hemianopic visual field defect.

Nonoptical Aids

Many devices are available to facilitate the daily activities of patients with vision loss. It is helpful to provide patients and/or their family members with a catalog or a list of stores where these items can be seen and purchased. Many vision rehabilitation programs or centers can identify specific patient needs via a home visit.

Large-print books are printed in a font size 2 to 3 times that of normal newsprint. Patients with moderate vision loss benefit from books, newspapers, magazines, playing cards, and bank checks with larger-than-normal letters. Also useful for these patients are extra-large numbers on digital clocks, wristwatches, telephones, remote controls, and thermostats. Patients should be made aware of useful aids such as needle threaders, dark-lined writing paper, felt-tip pens in black ink, and reverse-contrast keyboard stickers.

Nonvisual assistance

As visual loss becomes more profound, vision enhancement may become less effective, and the importance of "visual substitution skills" such as tactile and auditory aids increases.

Tactile aids range from raised dots on a kitchen dial to a white cane for mobility to the use of braille for reading. Scanners that convert standard print directly into braille are available for blind students.

Auditory aids include such information sources as radio and television, talking books, and reader services. Talking wristwatches and voice output computers are also available.

Optical character recognition (OCR) and screen-reading software, coupled with a voice synthesizer, are employed to help blind or severely visually impaired people read.

Electronic magnification

Closed-circuit television (CCTV) systems consist of a camera to capture an image of the object to be viewed (eg, written text, photograph) and a monitor to display the material to the person with a visual impairment. The image can be processed to enlarge it, increase the brightness, improve the contrast, or change the color, in much the same way that the image on a television can be adjusted.

Thanks to the revolution in display technology, a clear image can be rendered on a television or a portable liquid crystal display (LCD) or on goggles that were developed for the computer game industry. Flexible organic light-emitting diode (OLED) displays and retinal scanning technology, which projects an image pixel by pixel directly onto the retina, will greatly improve the design possibilities for electronic magnification systems in the coming years.

Improvements in video camera technology and control systems have allowed for CCTVs with autofocus or focus-free zoom lenses, voice-activated controls, automatic scrolling, and simple lightweight designs that make these devices accessible to a greater audience (Fig 9-6).

Miniaturization of electronics allows complete systems that provide magnification for intermediate and near viewing in a small, portable viewing system (Amigo, Enhanced Vision, Huntington Beach, CA) that rests on the page and offers a choice of magnifications. The development of handheld cameras that use a patient's own television monitor has lowered prices significantly.

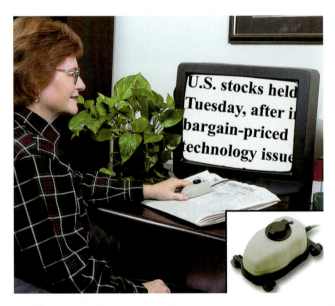

Figure 9-6 A portable, handheld closed-circuit television can be plugged into any monitor or television. It provides magnification as well as contrast enhancement. *(Courtesy of Enhanced Vision.)*

Whereas optical magnifying systems suffer from numerous problems with increasing magnification—such as a smaller field of view, closer working distance, critical depth of field, decreased contrast, increased aberrations, and problems with lighting and glare—CCTVs allow for very high magnification without any of these drawbacks. Patients can view objects and text at a comfortable distance, using variable magnification, and, with practice, attain sufficient reading speeds to allow for useful continuous text reading. Bright, even illumination and contrast enhancement greatly improve function in patients with poor contrast sensitivity. Most systems allow text to be viewed with reverse contrast (white letters on a black background), which offers excellent contrast with reduced glare because the normally bright white background of a page is eliminated. Traditional CCTV models and those with a writing stand allow for a sufficient camera-to-object distance such that writing and other tasks can be performed with these devices.

Computers as low vision devices

Years ago, access to computers by people with visual impairment was difficult, if not impossible. Today, not only is computer access easier, but computers allow people with visual impairment to access a world of information in ways that were previously impossible. For someone to use a computer, he or she needs to input information and access information.

Inputting information is made easier by improved keyboard access due to keys with large, reverse-contrast characters or *tactile-key* labels placed on a regular keyboard. Special *large-key* keyboards and alternative input devices also exist, including voice recognition systems.

There are several ways that screen access can be improved: moving the monitor closer, using a larger monitor, fitting an optical magnifier over the screen, or using alternative displays such as those just described. Microsoft Windows and Apple Macintosh operating systems incorporate several accessibility features, including a magnifier, narrator, and on-screen keyboard; these can be very useful for people with mild to moderate visual impairment. Several vendors (eg, Ai Squared, Manchester Center, VT [ZoomText, www.aisquared.com] and Freedom Scientific, St Petersburg, FL [JAWS for Windows, www.freedomscientific.com]) sell excellent screen enlargement software and screen readers that convert information on-screen to audible speech. These third-party software packages have more flexibility and are helpful for people with moderate to severe dysfunction.

Electronic magnification systems and computer technology are merging and will likely provide the most useful and flexible low vision aids in the near future. However, they will not replace optical devices completely, as optical devices offer portability, ease of use, and convenience for short-term reading tasks.

Reading device A computer can be thought of as a reading device for people with low vision, because any material that can be scanned or photographed or retrieved from a compact disc or the Internet can be enlarged on-screen or printed using a larger, darker font. As with CCTVs, the color and contrast can be enhanced at the same time. Conversion to speech and braille output allows those with severe vision loss and blindness to benefit as well.

Writing device   A computer is also a writing device, allowing one to record information using a variety of font sizes for later access without the difficulties inherent in writing and reading handwritten text. A laptop computer can be used as a portable electronic note-book, with all the possibilities for access just described.

Contrast Enhancement

Contrast enhancement strategies have already been discussed, but several different approaches can be used simultaneously, such as

- increasing the contrast of the material by reprinting the material via a computer, photocopying it with darker print, or enlarging it on a photocopier
- using electronic magnification, with its inherent contrast enhancement
- enhancing color contrast between objects and their background—light object on dark background and vice versa
- using contrast-enhancing yellow- or orange-tinted lenses, which have an effect similar to that of lenses in ski goggles

Lighting and Glare Control

Proper lighting is important for patients with reduced visual function, especially when contrast sensitivity is affected. Depending on the disease process and patient preferences, lighting recommendations can be made that will help patients perform better.

In the absence of glare, patients with macular degeneration who have poor contrast sensitivity perform better, read faster, and require less magnification when adequate illumination is provided. Patients should be shown how to position light sources, such as lamps and overhead lighting, so that glare is not produced by a direct light shining toward the patient's face or reflecting from the page. Illuminated handheld and stand magnifiers often provide the additional boost in function that patients need.

Too much light can also be a problem for some patients. Patients may suffer from glare, both indoors and outdoors. Glare may be controlled via nonoptical solutions such as wearing a hat, visor, sunglasses, and/or tinted lenses of varying color and density; or by reducing indoor lights. Wraparound and fit-over glasses provide additional protection from overhead and side glare sources. Polarizing lenses (eg, Drivewear, Younger Optics USA, Torrance, CA) can be especially useful for reducing reflected light from water or roads.

Instruction and Training

Some instruction, training, and practice are required for patients to be successful at using any of the devices or techniques described. The use of magnifiers, high-add spectacles, and adaptations for activities of daily living is not intuitive, and either the physician or a qualified vision rehabilitation therapist must provide explanations. Training sessions should be given to the patient and, preferably, also to a significant other, who can later reinforce the training.

Counseling and Support Groups

Vision loss has an impact on patients' quality of life and emotional well-being, as well as on their family. Patients with vision loss experience fear, isolation, anger, and depression when dealing with loss of their independence. Seniors with vision loss are at high risk for falls, injuries, medication errors, nutritional decline, social isolation, and depression at far higher rates than reported for any other disease process.

Psychological counseling and support groups may be part of the rehabilitation team's approach to helping patients and their families cope and adapt. Social workers and other counselors may be called upon to contribute to this rehabilitation process.

Vision Rehabilitation Professionals and Services

A number of rehabilitation professionals provide services for low vision patients, including ophthalmologists, optometrists, occupational therapists, *orientation and mobility (O&M) specialists*, vision rehabilitation teachers, assistants in low vision, psychologists, and social workers. The ophthalmologist should know of the availability of local services and must be able to initiate an appropriate referral.

O&M specialists help patients whose ability to move about safely is compromised by vision loss. Through skill training, independent movement (aided by a long cane, remaining visual cues, or a telescope if residual vision is adequate) is encouraged and maintained.

Resource materials should be provided to all patients. Such materials may include information about alternative transportation, free local and national services (like the Library of Congress Talking Books Program and radio reading services), sources of large-print books and music, telephone information and dialing services, and support groups.

Levels of Vision Rehabilitation Services

Vision rehabilitation services span a continuum from a simple refraction and prescription of high-add single-vision readers to a complex bundle of services provided through several rehabilitation professionals. Many of the principles and techniques described in this chapter can easily be incorporated into the armamentarium of the comprehensive ophthalmologist and must become part of everyday practice.

Patients will benefit if ophthalmologists offer an appropriate level of vision rehabilitation service directly or by referral. The American Academy of Ophthalmology SmartSight initiative in vision rehabilitation recommends a 3-level model of incorporating rehabilitation into the continuum of ophthalmic care. For patients with decreased visual acuity, scotomata, visual field loss, or reduced contrast sensitivity, all ophthalmologists can recommend the SmartSight patient handout (http://one.aao.org/CE/EducationalContent/Smartsight.aspx), which directs patients to vision rehabilitation services in their community. See also the Academy's Preferred Practice Pattern entitled *Vision Rehabilitation for Adults.*

A directory of rehabilitation services, *Directory of Services for the Blind and Visually Impaired Persons in the United States and Canada* (27th ed.), is available from the American Foundation for the Blind, 11 Penn Plaza, New York, NY 10001 (www.afb.org/services.asp).

> Preferred Practice Patterns Committee, Vision Rehabilitation Panel. *Vision Rehabilitation for Adults.* San Francisco: American Academy of Ophthalmology; 2007.

Pediatric Low Vision Issues

Most adults with low vision have lost vision because of an ocular disease. As such, they have already acquired many of the vision-aided skills (eg, reading) that are important for functioning in our society. Children with low vision, however, need to learn these skills despite poor or no vision. Most of these children have coexisting physical and/or mental disabilities that create further challenges to successful integration into society. In addition, skill acquisition is developmentally linked to vision, thus requiring different interventions at different ages. It is important to be aware of the needs of each age group and then to tailor the assistance to those needs. Rehabilitation of infants and children requires a team approach involving occupational and physical therapists, special educators, and physicians working together with the child and family from the earliest possible moments. Ophthalmologists are the most consistent contact for the parent of a visually impaired child and, as such, need to be aware of and involved in the rehabilitation process. (See BCSC Section 6, *Pediatric Ophthalmology and Strabismus.*)

> Fletcher DC. *Low Vision Rehabilitation: Caring for the Whole Person.* Ophthalmology Monograph 12. San Francisco: American Academy of Ophthalmology, 1999:chap 7.

Infants

The ophthalmologist plays a key role in the examination and assessment of an infant with suspected low vision. A definite diagnosis, together with a realistic prognosis, helps guide the rehabilitation plan. Early intervention by a skilled multidisciplinary team is critical during this stage of development. Vision is the primary means by which infants interact with their world, and vision drives motor development as well. Interventions must be individualized, as each child has different capabilities and challenges.

Preschool Children

For preschool children, more sophisticated low vision testing and more precise evaluation are possible. Near visual aids are usually not necessary due to a child's high accommodative amplitude and the relatively large size of toys and images or text in printed books. In order for accommodation to be used effectively, large astigmatic errors, hyperopic errors, and anisometropia must be treated. As children grow, their interests and needs change rapidly; the rehabilitation plan must be adjusted accordingly.

Kindergartners to Preadolescents

The whole spectrum of low vision aids should be made available to school-aged children. The introduction of a dome-type magnifier for near tasks may be well accepted. A hand-held monocular telescope can be used for viewing the blackboard. It is a good idea to introduce new devices at home, so the child becomes comfortable with their use before using them among his or her peers. The child with low vision should acquire typing skills and learn to use the computer early, because the computer will likely become his or her main portal to the world of information, and many adaptations are possible through its use.

As each child matures, he or she will begin to formulate and express personal goals. Parents and the vision rehabilitation team need to be sensitive to these goals, because the ultimate success of the rehabilitation program depends on the child's continued active participation.

A catalog listing vision testing equipment for infants and preschool and school-aged children is available from the Good-Lite Company, 1155 Jansen Farm Drive, Elgin, IL 60123 (www.good-lite.com).

Teenagers

Low vision aids that were used at a younger age may be rejected by teenagers concerned about peer acceptance. Peer pressure, real or perceived, may influence adolescents so much that they may choose to compromise their visual functioning in order to appear "normal." Good communication and sensitivity to these issues allow the rehabilitation specialist to provide aids that maximize visual function but minimize the cosmetic unacceptability.

Faye E, Albert D, Freed B, et al. *The Lighthouse Ophthalmology Resident Training Manual: A New Look at Low Vision Care.* New York: Lighthouse International; 2001.

Fletcher DC. *Low Vision Rehabilitation: Caring for the Whole Person.* Ophthalmology Monograph 12. San Francisco: American Academy of Ophthalmology; 1999.

Common Guidelines for Prescribing Cylinders

[The material in this appendix is reprinted from Guyton DL. Prescribing cylinders: the problem of distortion. *Surv Ophthalmol.* 1977;22(3):177–188. Copyright © 1977, *Survey of Ophthalmology.*]

Commonly taught guidelines are the following:

1. Children accept the full astigmatic correction.
2. If an adult cannot tolerate the full astigmatic correction, rotate the cylinder axis toward 90° or 180° and/or reduce the cylinder power to decrease distortion. When reducing the cylinder power, keep the spherical equivalent constant by appropriate adjustment of sphere.
3. With older patients, beware of changing the cylinder axis.

The Problem: Distortion

Why have such guidelines developed? Why can some patients not tolerate the full astigmatic correction in the first place? One text on clinical refraction states that full correction of a high astigmatic error may initially result in considerable blurring of vision. Another teaching is that with the full astigmatic correction the image is too sharp—the patient is not used to seeing so clearly. Statements such as these are not only misleading; they are incorrect.

The reason for intolerance of astigmatic spectacle corrections is distortion caused by meridional magnification. Unequal magnification of the retinal image in the various meridians produces monocular distortion manifested by tilting lines or altered shapes of objects (Fig A-1). But monocular distortion by itself is rarely a problem; the effect is too small. Maximum tilting of vertical lines (declination error) in the retinal image will occur when the correcting cylinder axis is at 45° or 135°, but even under these conditions each diopter of correcting cylinder power produces only about 0.4° of tilt.

The clinically significant problem occurs only under binocular conditions. Minor degrees of monocular distortion can produce major alterations in binocular spatial perception. Consider, for example, a patient with symmetrical oblique astigmatism wearing a +1.00 diopter cylinder, axis 135° before the right eye and a +1.00 diopter cylinder, axis 45° before the left eye. If the patient looks at a vertical rod 3 meters away, the retinal images of the rod will be tilted toward each other at the top (declination error) approximately

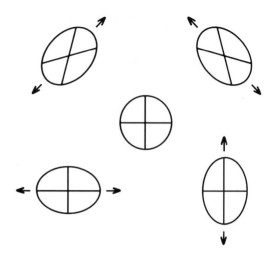

Figure A-1 Monocular distortion caused by meridional magnification. If the retinal image is magnified more in one direction than the other (as indicated by the arrows), vertical lines may become slanted, horizontal lines may become tilted, and objects may appear taller or shorter.

0.4° each, a barely perceptible amount under monocular conditions. But under binocular conditions, the vertical rod will theoretically appear tilted toward the patient (inclination) approximately 35°! Such large errors in stereoscopic spatial localization are clearly intolerable, seemingly out of proportion to the amount of monocular distortion that produces them. Oblique distortion in one or both eyes causes more distressing binocular symptoms than vertical or horizontal distortion, and movement accentuates the symptoms.

Fortunately, errors in stereoscopic spatial localization are usually compensated for in most patients by experiential factors: perspective clues, the known size and shape of familiar objects, the knowledge of what is level and what is perpendicular, etc. The possibility of permanent adaptation to binocular distortion will be discussed later, but the fact remains that some patients cannot or will not tolerate binocular spatial distortion, and herein lies our problem.

We have no effective means of treating binocular spatial distortion except by altering or eliminating the monocular distortion that produces it. Complete understanding of the causes and management of monocular distortion is difficult, involving several areas of physiological optics that the average practitioner would prefer to avoid: blur theory, spectacle lens design, obliquely crossed cylinders, and theory of the Jackson cross cylinder. However, with a few key facts from each of these areas, we can suddenly gain a working understanding of astigmatic spectacle corrections.

Sources of Monocular Distortion

As illustrated in Figure A-1, monocular distortion is caused by meridional magnification. We can identify two basic sources of meridional magnification, one involving the design of the spectacle lens, and the other involving the location of the spectacle lens with respect to the entrance pupil of the eye.

"Shape Factor" of the Spectacle Lens

All spectacle lenses having curved front surfaces produce a magnification inherent to the lens itself. The more convex the front surface and the thicker the lens, the greater will be this "shape factor" magnification. If the front surface of the lens is spherical, the shape factor magnification will be the same in all meridians, producing only an overall size change in the retinal image. On the other hand, if the front surface of the lens is cylindrical or toric, the shape factor magnification will vary from one meridian to another, producing distortion of the retinal image. Again, this only occurs with lenses having the cylinder ground on the front surface of the lens, the so-called *plus cylinder form* or anterior toric spectacle lens. Lenses having the cylinder ground on the back surface (minus cylinder lenses, posterior toric lenses, "iseikonoid" lenses) do not produce differential meridional magnification due to the shape factor, because the front surface power is the same in all meridians. The lens clock may be used to check the front and back curves.

Meridional magnification arising from the shape factor of plus cylinder spectacle lenses is rarely more than 1% to 2%. Many patients can perceive this difference, however, and for this reason and others, since the mid-1960s, minus cylinder spectacle lenses have become the preferred form for routine dispensing.

Distance of the Spectacle Lens From the Entrance Pupil

More important than the shape factor of the spectacle lens in producing distortion is the location of the spectacle lens relative to the entrance pupil of the eye. We shall consider both the conventional method and the general method of analyzing the magnification produced.

The Conventional Analysis: A Special Case

The conventional method of calculating the total magnification produced by a spectacle lens is to multiply the shape factor magnification times the "power factor" magnification. The power factor magnification is a function of the dioptric power of the correcting lens and the distance of the correcting lens from the "seat of ametropia." For example, consider a +4.00 D cylindrical lens placed at a vertex distance of 12 mm from an eye with simple hyperopic astigmatism. Assume that the eye's astigmatism arises in the cornea and that the +4.00 D cylindrical lens fully corrects the astigmatic error. This lens will produce a power factor magnification of 0% in the axis meridian and 5% in the meridian perpendicular to the axis meridian, for a differential meridional magnification of 5%. Figure A-2 shows the (differential) meridional magnification to be expected for this lens as a function of vertex distance. The shorter the vertex distance, the less will be the meridional magnification, an important point to remember when trying to minimize distortion.

The conventional analysis is only valid, though, when the spectacle lens actually *corrects* the corneal astigmatism. What sort of meridional magnification and resulting distortion can we expect with *uncorrected* astigmatism, or with astigmatism that is only partially, or inappropriately, corrected?

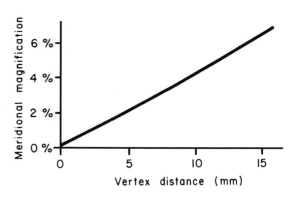

Figure A-2 Meridional magnification as a function of vertex distance for a +4.00 diopter cylindrical spectacle lens.

The General Case: Blurred Retinal Images

To investigate the general nature of meridional magnification, we must consider what happens in the case of blurred retinal images. The size of a blurred retinal image is defined as the distance between the centers of those blur circles which represent the extremities of the object.[1] Each blur circle is formed by a bundle of rays limited by the entrance pupil of the eye with the chief ray of the bundle passing toward the center of the entrance pupil and forming the center of the blur circle on the retina. Therefore, the chief rays from the extremities of the object determine the size of the retinal image, and because the chief rays pass toward the center of the entrance pupil, the angle subtended by the object *at the entrance pupil* is proportional to the size of the retinal image.[2]

We need not be concerned here with *computing* meridional magnification of blurred retinal images; we simply need to examine the relationship of the entrance pupil to meridional magnification in a qualitative sense. The entrance pupil of the eye (Fig A-3) is the pupil we see when we look at a patient's eye. It is actually the image formed by the cornea of the real pupil and is located about 0.5 mm in front of, and is about 14% larger than, the real pupil.

Figure A-3 The entrance pupil of the eye. Note the approximate location of the entrance pupil with respect to the cornea, to the crystalline lens, and to the corrective spectacle lens.

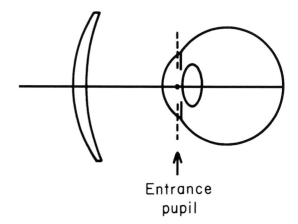

Entrance pupil

Illustrating the Location Effect of Cylindrical Lenses

Figure A-4 illustrates the general case of distortion of the retinal image produced by a cylindrical lens placed before a nonastigmatic eye. In Figure A-4, rays *ef* and *gh* represent the chief rays from the vertical extremities of the object. These chief rays cross at the center of the entrance pupil and continue on to form the vertical extremities of the retinal image.[3] No distortion of the retinal image is present in Figure A-4a.

In Figure A-4b, a cylindrical lens is placed before the eye in the usual spectacle plane with its axis *xy* oriented in the 45° meridian. Chief rays *ijk* and *lmn* pass through the cylindrical lens at points away from the axis *xy* and are therefore bent by the lens. Chief ray *ijk* undergoes a small prismatic deviation down and to the patient's left, while chief ray *lmn* undergoes a small prismatic deviation up and to the patient's right. The chief rays continue on through the center of the entrance pupil to the retina, but the ray segments *jk* and *mn* lie in a tilted plane because of the prismatic deviations that occurred in opposite horizontal directions at the cylindrical lens. (Note that ray segments *i* and *I* do not lie in the same common plane as the segments *jk* and *mn*, and neither do they follow the same paths as ray segments *e* and *g* in Figure A-4a.) Because ray segments *jk* and *mn* lie in a tilted plane, the vertical arrow in the retinal image of Figure A-4b is tilted. In fact, the entire retinal image in Figure A-4b is distorted. In the case of this retinal image as a whole, we may speak of the distortion as arising from meridional magnification caused by the cylindrical lens—a meridional magnification in the direction of the double arrows, perpendicular to axis *xy* of the cylindrical lens.

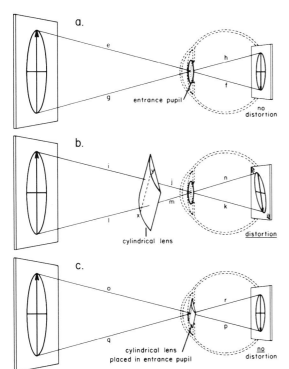

Figure A-4 The relationship between the position of a cylindrical lens relative to the entrance pupil of a nonastigmatic eye and the distortion of the retinal image produced. *a*, No distortion in the absence of the cylindrical lens. *b*, Distortion produced by the cylindrical lens located in the usual spectacle plane. *c*, No distortion when the cylindrical lens is placed hypothetically in the entrance pupil of the eye.

In Figure A-4c the cylindrical lens has been moved toward the eye until it is located hypothetically within the entrance pupil. Chief rays *op* and *qr* pass to the center of the entrance pupil where they now pass *undeviated* through the cylindrical lens because they strike the lens along its axis. Chief rays *op* and *qr* continue on to the retina and may be seen to be identical with rays *ef* and *gh* of Figure A-4a, causing no distortion of the retinal image.

Summary of the General Case

To summarize the lesson of Figure A-4, astigmatic refracting surfaces located away from the entrance pupil of the eye cause meridional magnification and distortion of the retinal image. The direction of meridional magnification is determined by the axis orientation of the astigmatic refracting surface, and the amount of meridional magnification increases not only with the power of the astigmatic refracting surface but also with increased distance of the astigmatic refracting surface from the entrance pupil of the eye.[4]

Distortion With Uncorrected and Inappropriately Corrected Astigmatism

We can now predict what sort of meridional magnification and resultant distortion to expect in the case of uncorrected astigmatism or inappropriately corrected astigmatism. In uncorrected astigmatism the astigmatic refracting surfaces are those of the cornea or lens. Because these surfaces are located near the entrance pupil (see Fig A-3), meridional magnification and distortion will be minimal. The meridional magnification produced by uncorrected corneal astigmatism is approximately 0.3% per diopter of astigmatism, which is a rather small amount.

The situation with inappropriately corrected astigmatism is much the same as the situation with properly corrected astigmatism. Whenever an astigmatic spectacle lens is placed before an eye, whether it is the correct lens or not, significant meridional magnification is likely to occur because of the relatively remote location of the spectacle lens from the entrance pupil (see Fig A-3). Even though the eye may be astigmatic, the effect of astigmatic surfaces located near the entrance pupil is so small that the direction and amount of meridional magnification are primarily determined not by the astigmatism of the eye itself, but by the axis and power of the astigmatic spectacle lens—whatever the axis and power may be, correct or not.

Common Misconceptions

It is time to correct some common misconceptions in clinical teaching. It is almost universally taught in clinical ophthalmology, with a rare exception, that retinal images slant in uncorrected oblique astigmatism and are straightened by the proper astigmatic spectacle correction. The opposite, of course, is closer to the truth. Undoubtedly, this misconception has arisen from the simple experiment of holding a cylindrical lens before one's emmetropic eye to "simulate" astigmatism, and noting the distortion produced. The fallacy, of course, is that the trial lens simulates the effect of a *spectacle* lens and not the effect of an astigmatic cornea. It is easily confirmed that as the trial lens is brought closer and closer to the entrance pupil of the eye, the observed distortion progressively decreases.

A second misconception in clinical teaching, again with only a rare exception, deals with the effect of residual astigmatism on distortion. When an axis error is made in correcting an astigmatic eye with a spectacle lens, the general rules for combination of cylinders having obliquely crossed axes may be used to calculate the axis and power of the residual astigmatism. It is taught that the axis and power of this residual astigmatism determine the direction and amount of distortion that will be present. From the preceding discussion it should be evident that the axis and power of the residual astigmatism are only coincidental and that the primary determinants of distortion are simply the axis and power of the spectacle lens itself. For example, if a correcting cylindrical lens is rotated to produce an axis error, the amount of distortion will remain substantially the same, but the direction of distortion will rotate an amount corresponding to the rotation of the cylindrical lens.

Relative Contributions From Sources of Distortion

The various sources of meridional magnification do not make equal contributions to the amount of magnification produced. The relative contributions may be appreciated more easily from the graphs in Figure A-5. These graphs show the meridional magnification to be expected with various degrees of astigmatism, both in the uncorrected state and in the corrected state, using for correction a common form of astigmatic spectacle lens. Note that with uncorrected astigmatism, the meridional magnification that occurs is much less than, and in the opposite direction to, the meridional magnification produced by the correcting spectacle lens. Also note that the shape factor of the spectacle lens, if a plus cylinder lens is used, increases the meridional magnification only about 2%.

Photographic Simulation of Distortion

Figure A-6 illustrates by exaggerated photographs the monocular distortion that is produced by spectacle correction of oblique astigmatism. Note that despite the presence of

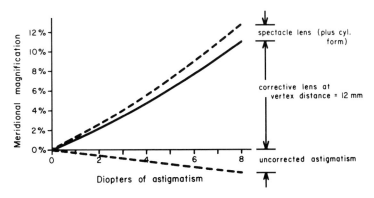

Figure A-5 Contributing factors to meridional magnification in uncorrected and corrected astigmatism. Calculations are for a positive cylindrical spectacle lens having no spherical power, with base curve of 6 D, thickness of 3 mm, and vertex distance of 12 mm.

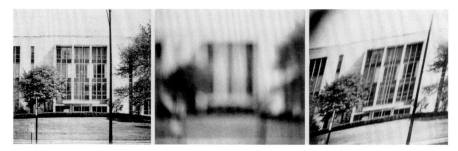

Figure A-6 Photographic simulation of distortion with oblique astigmatism. *Left,* no astigmatism. *Center,* uncorrected oblique astigmatism with the circle of least confusion on the retina. No significant distortion is present. *Right,* spectacle-corrected oblique astigmatism producing significant distortion.

blur in the uncorrected state, no significant distortion is present. With spectacle correction of the astigmatism, the distortion becomes painfully apparent.

Minimizing Monocular Distortion

Having discussed the sources of monocular distortion, we can now explore various ways to minimize meridional magnification and, with it, monocular distortion. This will be necessary in patients who cannot tolerate their present spectacles or in those whose new refractions demand a change in prescription such that we might anticipate problems with distortion. How can we minimize meridional magnification? We can specify minus cylinder spectacle lenses, minimize vertex distance, and sometimes alter the astigmatic correction by rotating the axis or reducing the power of the correcting cylinder.

Specifying Minus Cylinder (Posterior Toric) Spectacle Lenses

The small amount of meridional magnification caused by plus cylinder (anterior toric) spectacle lenses is avoided simply by specifying minus cylinder lenses in the prescriptions. In practice, this distinction is rarely necessary, for minus cylinder lenses have become the preferred form for routine dispensing. Most dispensers will choose the minus cylinder form automatically and reserve the plus cylinder form only for duplication of an old pair of plus cylinder lenses.

Minimizing Vertex Distance

As previously discussed, meridional magnification decreases as the correcting spectacle lens is placed closer and closer to the eye (see Fig A-2). There is often little room for manipulation of vertex distance with common styles of frames, but when distortion is anticipated, we can at least avoid the so-called fashionable glasses that sit at the end of the patient's nose.

With contact lenses, the vertex distance is reduced to zero and distortion is practically eliminated. Contact lenses should always be considered as an alternative to spectacle correction if the patient remains unsatisfied with other attempts to reduce distortion. In fact, contact lenses may be the only means available (other than iseikonic corrections) to reduce distortion while maintaining clear imagery, for further attempts to reduce distortion by manipulating the spectacle lens correction, as we shall see in the next section, involve a certain sacrifice in the sharpness of the retinal image.

Altering the Astigmatic Correction

Rotating the cylinder axis

Clinical experience suggests that new astigmatic spectacle corrections in adults are better tolerated if the axis of the cylinder is at 90° or 180° rather than in an oblique meridian. In fact, it has long been taught that oblique axes should be rotated toward 90° or 180°, if visual acuity does not suffer too much, to avoid problems from oblique distortion. This makes sense, for the *direction* of meridional magnification is determined principally by the axis orientation of the correcting cylinder, whether or not the axis is correct, and vertical or horizontal aniseikonia is known to be more tolerable than oblique aniseikonia.

There have been recurrent arguments in the literature regarding why cylinder axes should not be rotated away from the correct position, but these arguments are primarily based on the misconception stated earlier that the axis and power of the *residual* astigmatism determine the direction and amount of distortion. As we have seen, it is the axis and power of the spectacle lens itself, correct or not, that principally determine the direction and amount of distortion. With this concept understood, and on the basis of clinical experience, we may thus state that the *direction* of distortion may be made more tolerable, if necessary, by rotating the cylinder axis toward 90° or 180°.

There is another situation in which the cylinder axis should sometimes be rotated away from the correct position. An older patient may have *adapted* to an incorrect axis position in his or her previous spectacles, and may not tolerate the change in direction of distortion produced by rotating the cylinder axis to the correct position. The nature of such adaptation will be discussed later, but there is no question that it occurs and can cause problems. In this case, the cylinder axis should be rotated toward the position of the *old* cylinder axis, even if the old cylinder axis is oblique. This maneuver does not *reduce* distortion but does change the *direction* of distortion back toward the position of adaptation.

Reducing the cylinder power

The other method that is commonly used to lessen distortion is reduction of the power of the correcting cylinder. This makes sense, for we have seen that the *amount* of meridional magnification is largely determined by the power of the correcting cylinder—the less the cylinder power, the less the meridional magnification.

Photographic simulation

Figure A-7 illustrates by exaggerated photographs the reduction of distortion by altering the astigmatic correction. In each case when the cylinder power is altered, the spherical correction is changed the appropriate amount to keep the circle of least confusion on the retina, as will be discussed later. Note that distortion may be decreased by reducing the cylinder power or changed in direction by rotating the cylinder axis, but either of these manipulations causes blurring of the image. We have decreased distortion, but at the expense of visual acuity. What produces the blur? Residual astigmatism.

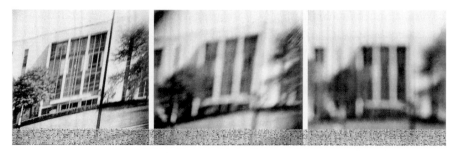

Figure A-7 Photographic simulation of altering the astigmatic correction to reduce distortion. *Left,* distorted image resulting from full spectacle correction of oblique astigmatism. *Center,* decreased amount of distortion obtained by reducing the cylinder power. *Right,* improved direction of distortion (vertical) as well as decreased amount of distortion obtained by rotating the plus cylinder axis to 180° and reducing the cylinder power.

Residual astigmatism

Whenever the cylinder power is reduced from its correct value, or the cylinder axis is rotated away from its correct position, residual astigmatism appears. The residual astigmatism does not produce distortion, but it does produce blur of the retinal image, limiting the amount that the cylinder power may be reduced or the amount that the cylinder axis may be rotated away from its correct position. If we must minimize distortion, we must be careful at the same time not to create excessive blur from residual astigmatism.

It is the *amount* of residual astigmatism that produces the blur, not the axis[5] of the residual astigmatism. It is easy to judge the amount of residual astigmatism when reducing the cylinder power of a spectacle correction, for the residual astigmatism is simply equal to the amount the cylinder power is reduced. It is more difficult, however, to judge the amount of residual astigmatism induced by rotating the cylinder axis away from the correct position. The resulting residual astigmatism may always be calculated using the rules for combination of obliquely crossed cylinders, but this calculation requires considerable mental gymnastics. A simple graph may be easier to remember. Figure A-8 should provide a working knowledge of the amount of residual astigmatism induced by rotating the cylinder axis.

As indicated by the graphs in Figure A-8, when we rotate the cylinder axis away from its correct position and keep the cylinder at its full value, we rapidly introduce residual astigmatism.[6] If the cylinder axis is rotated 30° from its correct position, the residual astigmatism becomes equal to the original uncorrected astigmatism. If the cylinder axis is rotated 90° from its correct position, the residual astigmatism becomes *twice* the value of the original uncorrected astigmatism!

From the mathematics of obliquely crossed cylinders, it may be shown[7] that as the cylinder axis is rotated away from its correct position, the power of the cylinder should be reduced in order to minimize residual astigmatism. For each position of the cylinder axis, there exists an optimal value for the cylinder power that minimizes residual astigmatism as indicated by the graphs in Figure A-8.

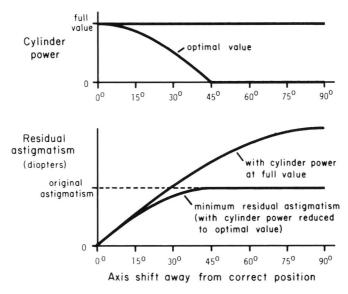

Figure A-8   Residual astigmatism produced when a cylinder axis is shifted away from its correct position. Graphs illustrate how reducing the cylinder power to an optimal value can minimize residual astigmatism.

Optimal value for cylinder power

Thus, if we choose to shift the cylinder axis to make the direction of meridional magnification more tolerable, we should also reduce the cylinder power slightly to minimize residual astigmatism. But how can we know the optimal value for cylinder power without performing complicated trigonometric calculations? Here we are lucky, for we may simply use the Jackson cross cylinder test for cylinder power. It may be shown from cross cylinder theory that for *any* setting, this test automatically gives us the optimal cylinder power to result in minimum residual astigmatism. The axes of the cross cylinder are simply aligned with the principal meridians of the correcting lens, and the patient is asked, "Which is better, one or two?" as the cross cylinder is flipped. From the patient's responses, the refractionist adjusts the cylinder power until both flipped positions of the cross cylinder appear equally clear.

It is generally known that the cylinder axis should be refined first with cross cylinder testing, for the correct axis will be found even if the cylinder power is incorrect. The cylinder power is generally refined *after* the axis is refined, for the correct cylinder cannot be found if an axis error is present. It has never been pointed out, however, that the cylinder power which *is* found in the presence of an axis error is truly the optimal cylinder power for that axis error, resulting in the least residual astigmatism possible for that axis error.[8]

This is a profound coincidence—a coincidence which, as previously explained, greatly simplifies our task of reducing distortion while maintaining acceptable visual acuity.

Optimal value for sphere power

When reducing the cylinder power by *any* method, we must take care to maintain the proper spherical correction for best visual acuity. The usual teaching is that the spherical equivalent of the refractive correction must be kept constant when reducing the cylinder power, a concept based on the conoid of Sturm and the supposition that visual acuity is best when the circle of least confusion falls on the retina. Although this is probably true in many cases, it is certainly not true in every case. For example, a patient with residual astigmatism with the rule may obtain best visual acuity with the vertical focal line of the conoid of Sturm falling on the retina—simply because more of our customary test letters are recognizable when the vertical strokes are clear. Thus, the spherical equivalent concept is not always strictly applicable when reducing the power of the cylinder.

When refining the cylinder power by cross cylinder testing, the sphere should be adjusted for best visual acuity during the refinement and also as the final step. When *empirically* reducing the cylinder power, the spherical equivalent concept provides a useful estimate for adjusting the sphere, but it should not be relied upon without a final subjective check.

Adaptation to Distortion

It is a common clinical observation that children adapt readily to induced distortion from astigmatic spectacle corrections. Adults adapt less readily. Little is known of the actual mechanism of adaptation. Experiments in adults with induced aniseikonia for periods of up to two weeks have suggested that adaptation to spatial distortion is primarily an interpretive process rather than a physiological process. In these adult subjects, the sense of distortion usually disappeared completely in several days, but in unfamiliar surroundings, where there were few monocular perspective cues, the spatial disturbance returned. In these experiments, however, there appeared to be some physiological adaptation to distortion. A physiological component was measured as being responsible for 20%–60% of the total adaptation, and there was an aftereffect of aniseikonia in the opposite direction when the distorting lenses were discontinued.

There is evidence that physiological adaptation to distortion is age-dependent. In a large study at the Dartmouth Eye Institute in 1945, adults with astigmatism at oblique axes tended to show a larger physiological component of adaptation to distortion if their astigmatism had been corrected at an early age.

Physiological adaptation to distortion appears to involve a reordering of the retinal meridians and may therefore be thought of as a form of rotational anomalous retinal correspondence. Indeed, the ability to physiologically adapt to distortion appears to parallel in patient age the ability to develop conventional anomalous retinal correspondence. The ability is well developed in children and decreases rapidly with advancing age.

The ability to reorder the retinal meridians on a permanent basis is further evidenced by patients having oblique extraocular muscle dysfunction with large anatomical cyclodeviations (5°–15°) of the eyes. Patients having these cyclodeviations since birth or since early childhood experience no spatial distortion and have no measurable cyclophoria. Acute cyclodeviations in older patients (for example, after bilateral oblique muscle surgery) produce both measurable cyclophorias and spatial distortion. This spatial distortion disappears in a few days, but the measurable cyclophoria remains much longer—months to possibly years—indicating the poor ability of the older patient to develop a rotational type of anomalous retinal correspondence. Physiological adaptation to cyclodeviations requires a pure rotational reordering of the retinal meridians, while adaptation to astigmatic distortion requires a scissors-type of reordering of the retinal meridians, but the neurological mechanisms are probably quite similar.

Regardless of the mechanism and extent of physiological adaptation to distortion, the greater portion of adaptation to astigmatic distortion appears to be the interpretive type of adaptation. Monocular perspective cues, if they are abundant enough, prevail over the altered binocular stereoscopic cues. Usually in a few days the distorted spatial frame of reference comes to be interpreted in view of the known monocular cues, and the sense of spatial distortion disappears—to reappear only if the monocular cues are removed.

Occasional older patients cannot even adapt to distortion by the interpretive mechanism, and it is for these patients that we must be able to reduce or minimize distortion by manipulating the astigmatic spectacle correction.

Revised Guidelines for Prescribing Cylinders

We can now formulate a revised set of guidelines for prescribing cylinders.

1. In *children,* give the full astigmatic correction.
2. In *adults,* try the full astigmatic correction first. Give warning and encouragement. If problems are anticipated, try a walking-around trial with trial frames before prescribing.
3. To minimize distortion, use minus cylinder lenses and minimize vertex distances.
4. Spatial distortion from astigmatic spectacle corrections is a *binocular* phenomenon. Occlude one eye to verify that this is indeed the cause of the patient's complaints.
5. If necessary, reduce distortion still further by rotating the cylinder axis toward 180° or 90° (or toward the *old* axis) and/or by reducing the cylinder power. Balance the resulting blur with the remaining distortion, using careful adjustment of cylinder power and sphere. Residual astigmatism at *any* position of the cylinder axis may be minimized with the Jackson cross cylinder test for cylinder power. Adjust the sphere using the spherical equivalent concept as a guide, but rely on a final subjective check to obtain best visual acuity.
6. If distortion cannot be reduced sufficiently by altering the astigmatic spectacle correction, consider contact lenses (which cause no appreciable distortion) or iseikonic corrections.

Special cases occasionally arise. If a patient's sense of spatial distortion seems out of proportion to his astigmatic correction, consider the possibility of spherical aniseikonia as the cause of his symptoms, and prescribe accordingly.

If the patient with moderate to high astigmatism has no complaints about distance spectacle correction but has difficulty reading at near, remember that changes in the astigmatic axes of the eyes (from cyclorotations) and changes in the effectivity of astigmatic corrections may cause problems at near. Such patients may require separate reading glasses.

Finally, patients who desire spectacles only for part-time wear may not be able to adapt to distortion during short periods of wear. In such cases, the astigmatic correction should be altered to reduce distortion according to the principles outlined above.

The revised set of guidelines for prescribing cylinders is now complete. With a rational basis for these guidelines, we should be able to place our confidence in them and prescribe cylinders more from knowledge and less from empirical rumors.

For a complete list of references see the original article: Guyton DL. Prescribing cylinders: The problem of distortion. *Surv Ophthalmol.* 1977;22(3):177–188.

NOTES

1. In the case of astigmatism, the blur patches on the retina may be ellipses or lines instead of blur circles, and the size of the blurred retinal image may appear somewhat altered by the effect of the *shape* of the blur patches on the outline of the image. This effect, however, only affects the *outline* of the retinal image and does not cause the type of monocular distortion (tilting of lines, etc) which concerns us here.

2. The size of the retinal image is usually computed as being proportional to the angle subtended by the object at the first nodal point of the eye (which is approximately 4 mm posterior to the center of the entrance pupil), but this is true only for sharp retinal images. The nodal point cannot be used to compute the size of blurred retinal images.

3. Chief rays such as those in Figure A-4, although they initially pass *toward* the center of the entrance pupil, are actually refracted by the cornea, pass through the center of the *real* pupil, and are further refracted by the crystalline lens before continuing on to the retina. However, each pair of chief rays such as *ef* and *gh,* or *jk* and *mn,* because of the axial symmetry of the ocular media, remain *in the same plane* with each other as they pass through the eye's optics. Therefore, while the retinal images in Figure A-4 are not exactly the proper size because of the simplified representation of the chief rays, the presence or absence of distortion is accurately represented.

4. An alternate way to analyze the effect of a cylindrical lens is to consider the lens as an integral part of the eye's optical system and calculate the position of the entrance pupil for the system as a whole in each principal meridian. The pairs of chief rays in the two principal meridians would then cross the optical axis at different points, producing the same differential meridional magnification as obtained with the present analysis.

5. The axis of residual astigmatism is of no consequence in the consideration of blur except perhaps as it may affect the reading of letters that have predominantly vertical strokes. If the axis of the residual astigmatism is vertical or horizontal, and if the patient is able to clear the vertical strokes of the letters by accommodating, his reading ability may be somewhat better than would otherwise be predicted.

6. The residual astigmatism in this case is approximately equal to $2C \sin \theta$, where C is the dioptric value of the cylinder and θ is the angle that the cylinder axis has been rotated away from its correct position.

7. By differentiating the trigonometric expression for residual astigmatism with respect to the correcting cylinder power and setting the expression equal to zero, the optimal cylinder power for minimal residual astigmatism may be shown to be equal to $C \cos 2\theta$, where C is the original full dioptric power of the correcting cylinder and θ is the angle the cylinder axis has been rotated away from its correct position. With this "optimal value" for the cylinder power, the residual astigmatism is equal to $C \sin 2\theta$.

8. Other methods of determining cylinder power may also be used for determining the optimal cylinder power for a given axis error. For example, the rotating types of astigmatic dials, if aligned with the correcting cylinder at *any* axis setting, will measure the "optimal" power at that axis setting.

Basic Texts

Clinical Optics

Albert DM, Miller JW, Azar DT, Blodi BA, eds. *Albert and Jakobiec's Principles and Practice of Ophthalmology.* 3rd ed. Philadelphia: Saunders; 2008.

Campbell CJ. *Physiological Optics.* Hagerstown, MD: Harper & Row; 1974.

Corboy JM. *The Retinoscopy Book: An Introductory Manual for Eye Care Professionals.* 5th ed. Thorofare, NJ: Slack; 2003.

Duke-Elder S, Abrams D. *System of Ophthalmology.* Volume V, *Ophthalmic Optics and Refraction.* St Louis: Mosby; 1970.

Michaels DD. *Visual Optics and Refraction: A Clinical Approach.* 3rd ed. St Louis: Mosby; 1985.

Milder B, Rubin ML. *The Fine Art of Prescribing Glasses Without Making a Spectacle of Yourself.* 3rd ed. Gainesville, FL: Triad; 2004.

Rubin ML. *Optics for Clinicians.* Gainesville, FL: Triad; 1993.

Stein HA, Slatt BJ, Stein RM. *Fitting Guide for Rigid and Soft Contact Lenses: A Practical Approach.* 4th ed. St Louis: Mosby; 2002.

Tasman W, Jaeger EA, eds. *Duane's Clinical Ophthalmology.* Philadelphia: Lippincott-Raven; 1995.

Yanoff M, Duker J. *Ophthalmology.* 2nd ed. St Louis: Mosby; 2004.

Related Academy Materials

Focal Points: Clinical Modules for Ophthalmologists

For information on Focal Points modules, go to http://one.aao.org/CE/Educational Products/FocalPoints.aspx.

Arbisser LB. Anterior vitrectomy for the anterior segment surgeon (Module 2, 2009).

Hill WE, Byrne SF. Complex axial length measurements and unusual IOL power calculations (Module 9, 2004).

Liegner JT. Rehabilitation of the low vision patient (Module 5, 2002).

McMahon TT, Guinn TG. Pearls for fitting contact lenses (Module 4, 2006).

Monica ML, Campbell RC. Managing the dissatisfied optical patient (Module 10, 2006).

Rubenstein JB, Yeu E. Management of astigmatism in lens-based surgery (Module 2, 2008).

Strauss L. Spectacle lens materials, coatings, tints, and designs (Module 11, 2005).

Print Publications

Arnold AC, ed. *Basic Principles of Ophthalmic Surgery* (2006).

Fletcher DC, ed. *Low Vision Rehabilitation: Caring for the Whole Person.* Ophthalmology Monograph 12 (1999).

Rockwood EJ, ed. *ProVision: Preferred Responses in Ophthalmology.* Series 4. Self-Assessment Program, 2-vol set (2007).

Wilson FM II, ed. *Practical Ophthalmology: A Manual for Beginning Residents.* 5th ed. (2005).

Online Materials

For Preferred Practice Patterns, Ophthalmic Technology Assessments, and Complementary Therapy Assessments, go to http://one.aao.org/CE/PracticeGuidelines/default.aspx.

Basic and Clinical Science Course (Sections 1–13); http://one.aao.org/CE/Educational Products/BCSC.aspx

Clinical Education Cases; http://one.aao.org/CE/EducationalContent/Cases.aspx

Clinical Education and Ethics Courses; http://one.aao.org/CE/EducationalContent/ Courses.aspx

Focal Points modules; http://one.aao.org/CE/EducationalProducts/FocalPoints.aspx

Maintenance of Certification Exam Study Kit, version 2.0 (2007); http://one.aao.org/CE/ MOC/default.aspx

Rockwood EJ, ed. *ProVision: Preferred Responses in Ophthalmology.* Series 4. Self-Assessment Program, 2-vol set (2007); http://one.aao.org/CE/EducationalProducts/ Provision.aspx

Preferred Practice Patterns

Preferred Practice Patterns are available at http://one.aao.org/CE/PracticeGuidelines/PPP.aspx.

Preferred Practice Patterns Committee, Refractive Management/Intervention Panel. *Refractive Errors and Refractive Surgery* (2007).

Preferred Practice Patterns Committee, Vision Rehabilitation Panel. *Visual Rehabilitation for Adults* (2007).

Ophthalmic Technology Assessments

Ophthalmic Technology Assessments are available at http://one.aao.org/CE/Practice Guidelines/Ophthalmic.aspx and are published in the Academy's journal, *Ophthalmology*. Individual reprints may be ordered at http://www.aao.org/store.

Ophthalmic Technology Assessment Committee, Refractive Surgery Panel. *Excimer Laser Photorefractive Keratectomy (PRK) for Myopia and Astigmatism* (1999).

Ophthalmic Technology Assessment Committee, Refractive Surgery Panel. *Intrastromal Corneal Ring Segments for Low Myopia* (2001).

Ophthalmic Technology Assessment Committee, Refractive Surgery Panel. *Laser In Situ Keratomileusis for Myopia and Astigmatism: Safety and Efficacy* (2002).

Ophthalmic Technology Assessment Committee, Refractive Surgery Panel. *LASIK for Hyperopia, Hyperopic Astigmatism, and Mixed Astigmatism* (2004).

Ophthalmic Technology Assessment Committee, Cornea and Anterior Segment Disorders Panel. *Safety of Overnight Orthokeratology for Myopia* (2008).

Ophthalmic Technology Assessment Committee, Refractive Management/Intervention Panel. *Wavefront-Guided LASIK for the Correction of Primary Myopia and Astigmatism* (2008).

Complementary Therapy Assessments

Complementary Therapy Assessments are available at http://one.aao.org/CE/Practice Guidelines/Therapy.aspx.

Complementary Therapy Task Force. *Visual Training for Refractive Errors* (2004).

CDs/DVDs

Basic and Clinical Science Course (Sections 1–13) (CD-ROM; 2009).

Farrell TA, Alward WLM, Verdick RE. *Fundamentals of Slit-Lamp Biomicroscopy*. From *The Eye Exam and Basic Ophthalmic Instruments* (DVD; reviewed for currency 2007).

Guyton DL. *Retinoscopy and Subjective Refraction* (DVD; reviewed for currency 2007).

To order any of these materials, please order online at www.aao.org/store or call the Academy's Customer Service toll-free number 866-561-8558 in the U.S. If outside the U.S., call 415-561-8540 between 8:00 AM and 5:00 PM PST.

Credit Reporting Form

Basic and Clinical Science Course, 2012–2013
Section 3

The American Academy of Ophthalmology is accredited by the Accreditation Council for Continuing Medical Education to provide continuing medical education for physicians.

The American Academy of Ophthalmology designates this enduring material for a maximum of 15 *AMA PRA Category 1 Credits™*. Physicians should claim only the credit commensurate with the extent of their participation in the activity.

If you wish to claim continuing medical education credit for your study of this Section, you may claim your credit online or fill in the required forms and mail or fax them to the Academy.

To use the forms:

1. Complete the study questions and mark your answers on the Section Completion Form.
2. Complete the CME Activity Evaluation.
3. Fill in and sign the statement below.
4. Return this page and the required forms by mail or fax to the CME Registrar (see below).

To claim credit online:

1. Log on to the Academy website (www.aao.org/cme).
2. Select Review/Claim CME.
3. Follow the instructions.

Important: These completed forms or the online claim must be received at the Academy by June 1, 2013.

I hereby certify that I have spent _____ (up to 15) hours of study on the curriculum of this Section and that I have completed the study questions.

Signature: _____
                                                                      Date

Name: _____

Address: _____

City and State: _____   Zip: _____

Telephone: (_____) _____   Academy Member ID# _____
            area code

Please return completed forms to: **Or you may fax them to:** 415-561-8575
American Academy of Ophthalmology
P.O. Box 7424
San Francisco, CA 94120-7424
Attn: CME Registrar, Customer Service

2012–2013
Section Completion Form

Basic and Clinical Science Course

Answer Sheet for Section 3

Question	Answer	Question	Answer
1	a b c d e	26	a b c d
2	a b c d e	27	a b c d
3	a b c d e	28	a b c d
4	a b c d	29	a b c d
5	a b c d	30	a b c d
6	a b c d	31	a b c d
7	a b c d	32	a b c d
8	a b c d	33	a b c d
9	a b c d e	34	a b c d
10	a b c d e	35	a b c d
11	a b c d e	36	a b c d
12	a b c d e	37	a b c d
13	a b c d e	38	a b c d
14	a b c d e	39	a b c d
15	a b c d	40	a b c d e
16	a b c d e	41	a b c d
17	a b c d	42	a b c d
18	a b c d e	43	a b c d
19	a b c d e	44	a b c d
20	a b c d e	45	a b c d e
21	a b c d e	46	a b c d e
22	a b c d	47	a b c d e
23	a b c d e	48	a b c d
24	a b c d	49	a b c d
25	a b c d e	50	a b c d

CME Activity Evaluation

To comply with guidelines from the Accreditation Council for Continuing Medical Education and the American Medical Association and to assist us in planning future activities, please provide us accurate and important feedback as requested below.

1. Has this activity enhanced your professional abilities?

    ☐ Yes

    ☐ No

2. Because of my participation in this activity, I will make the following change to my practice:

3. How effective was the activity at meeting the stated objectives?

    ☐ All objectives were met.

    ☐ Most objectives were met.

    ☐ Few objectives were met.

    ☐ No objectives were met.

    ☐ I do not recall the objectives for this activity.

4. To what degree is this activity likely to have a positive impact on health outcomes of your patients?

    ☐ Extremely likely

    ☐ Highly likely

    ☐ Somewhat likely

    ☐ Not at all likely

    ☐ Not applicable

5. Was this activity free of commercial bias?

    ☐ Yes

    ☐ No

    If you selected "No," please comment:

6. How might we improve this activity to make it more relevant to your practice?

Study Questions

Although a concerted effort has been made to avoid ambiguity and redundancy in these questions, the authors recognize that differences of opinion may occur regarding the "best" answer. The discussions are provided to demonstrate the rationale used to derive the answer. They may also be helpful in confirming that your approach to the problem was correct or, if necessary, in fixing the principle in your memory.

1. The ability of a light wave from a laser to form interference fringes with another wave from the same beam, separated in time, is a measure of its

   a. temporal coherence

   b. spatial coherence

   c. polarization

   d. directionality

   e. intensity

2. Which of the following properties of a laser is least clinically important in ophthalmic applications?

   a. energy level

   b. power level

   c. pulse duration

   d. polarity

   e. focal spot size

3. All the following pairs are matched correctly *except:*

   a. diopter—reciprocal meter

   b. prism diopter—centimeters per meter

   c. refractive index—dimensionless

   d. wavelength—nanometers

   e. frequency—cycles per degree

4. When a lens material has a higher index of refraction, all of the following are true *except:*

   a. The velocity of light is increased in this material.

   b. The spectacle lens made from this material can be thinner.

   c. Its value of n is higher.

   d. It has a greater ability to refract light.

5. The Airy disk image on the retina is larger when

   a. the wavelength of light is shortened

   b. the focal length of the eye is shorter

   c. the pupil size decreases

   d. macular degeneration is present

6. Corneal haze secondary to corneal edema is primarily caused by
   a. reflection
   b. light scattering
   c. refraction
   d. diffraction

7. *Candela* is a unit of measure for which of the following?
   a. luminous intensity
   b. luminous flux
   c. illuminance
   d. luminance

8. All ophthalmic lasers require each of the following basic elements *except:*
   a. an active medium
   b. energy input (pumping source)
   c. optical feedback
   d. plasma

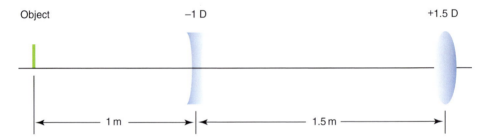

Object   −1 D   +1.5 D

1 m   1.5 m

Questions 9–14 concern the figure above. An object is placed 1 m in front of a −1 D spherical lens.
The −1 D lens, in turn, is positioned 1.5 m in front of a +1.5 D spherical lens.

9. Where does the −1 D lens form an intermediate image?
   a. at optical infinity
   b. 2 m in front of the lens
   c. 1 m in front of the lens
   d. 0.5 m in front of the lens
   e. 2 m behind the lens

10. Describe the intermediate image.
    a. upright, real, magnified
    b. upright, real, minified
    c. upright, virtual, magnified
    d. upright, virtual, minified
    e. inverted, virtual, minified

11. What is the size of the intermediate image as compared to the object?
    a. indeterminate
    b. one-fourth the size

    c. half the size

    d. same size

    e. twice the size

12. What is the location of the final image?

    a. 1 m in front of the second lens

    b. 1 m behind the second lens

    c. 4 m behind the second lens

    d. 10 m behind the second lens

    e. at optical infinity

13. Describe the final image.

    a. upright, real, magnified

    b. upright, real, minified

    c. inverted, real, magnified

    d. inverted, real, minified

    e. inverted, virtual, minified

14. What is the size of the final image as compared to the object?

    a. indeterminate

    b. one-fourth the size

    c. half the size

    d. same size

    e. twice the size

15. An object is placed 25 cm in front of a concave spherical mirror with a radius of curvature of 1 m (see the following figure). The image is

    a. virtual with a transverse magnification of 1.77

    b. virtual with a transverse magnification of −0.56

    c. real with a transverse magnification of −1.77

    d. real with a transverse magnification of 0.56

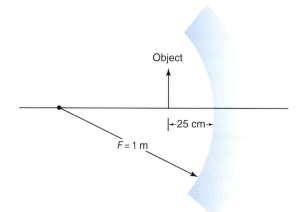

16. Which of the following statements regarding dispersion and chromatic aberration is false?

a. In the human eye, blue rays focus in front of red rays.

b. Blue print appears nearer than red print when both are displayed against a black background.

c. Image sharpness is reduced by chromatic aberration in the eyes of patients with achromatopsia.

d. Retinal image quality is limited by chromatic aberration and diffraction even if all monochromatic refractive errors are eliminated by wavefront-guided LASIK.

e. Blue-blocking and red-blocking sunglasses improve image sharpness by eliminating part of the chromatic interval, thereby reducing chromatic aberration.

17. The far point of the nonaccommodated myopic eye

a. and the fovea are corresponding points

b. is posterior to the eye, optically speaking

c. is nearer to the eye than the point of focus of the fully accommodated eye

d. cannot be moved by placing a lens in front of the eye

18. The near point of the fully accommodated hyperopic eye

a. is beyond infinity, optically speaking

b. is between infinity and the cornea

c. is behind the eye

d. is beyond minus infinity, optically speaking

e. cannot be determined without additional information

19. Which of the following is a recognized notation of visual acuity?

a. Snellen fraction

b. minimum angle of resolution

c. logMAR

d. 4-m standard fraction

e. all of the above

20. In which type of astigmatism do the focal lines straddle the retina?

a. mixed astigmatism

b. compound myopic astigmatism

c. compound hyperopic astigmatism

d. simple myopic astigmatism

e. simple hyperopic astigmatism

21. The nodal point of the reduced schematic eye

a. represents a point through which light rays enter or leave the eye undeviated

b. is equivalent to the posterior focal point of the cornea

c. allows the size of a retinal image to be calculated if the object height and object distance are known

d. a and c

e. all of the above

22. You are about to write the postoperative spectacle prescription for a cataract surgery pa-
    tient with macular degeneration. The best choice for a reading add for the patient with
    20/70 best-corrected vision is

    a. +3.00 D

    b. +3.50 D

    c. +7.00 D

    d. a 3.5× magnifier

23. In bifocal design, image jump may be minimized by

    a. placing the optical center of the segment as close as possible to the top of the segment

    b. placing the top of the segment as close as possible to the distance optical center

    c. using a smaller bifocal segment

    d. using a blended bifocal segment having no visible line of separation

    e. lowering the bifocal segments by 3 mm

24. An angle of 45° corresponds to how many prism diopters (Δ)?

    a. 45

    b. 22.5

    c. 90

    d. 100

25. When bifocal lenses are prescribed for a patient with myopia,

    a. the practitioner should leave the choice of the segment type to the optician

    b. a round-top segment is preferred because of its thin upper edge, which causes less
       prismatic effect

    c. a flat-top segment is preferred because it lessens image jump

    d. the 1-piece shape is indicated for adds greater than +2.00 D

    e. a split bifocal should be used because patients with myopia do not accept bifocals
       easily

26. Following are the results of a streak retinoscopy performed at a testing distance of 0.67 m
    on a 5-year-old with an accommodative esotropia. In the right eye, a +5 D sphere neutral-
    izes the 180° meridian and a +3.5 D sphere neutralizes the 90° meridian. In the left eye, a
    +7 D sphere neutralizes the 180° meridian and a +6 D sphere neutralizes the 90° meridian.
    Which of the following statements is false?

    a. The spherocylindrical notation for the full hyperopic correction can be expressed as

       RE: +3.5 −1.5 × 180

       LE: +5.5 −1.0 × 180

    b. The child will have an induced 0.5Δ left hyperphoria looking 1 cm below the centers of
       spectacle lenses containing the full hyperopic correction.

    c. The child will have an induced 2Δ exophoria looking 1 cm to the right of the centers of
       spectacle lenses containing the full hyperopic correction.

    d. If the examiner decreases the working distance to 0.5 m after neutralizing the retino-
       scopic reflex, "with" motion will be seen in all meridians.

27. A 92-year-old patient with dry age-related macular degeneration (AMD) complains of deteriorating vision in 1 eye. Best-corrected visual acuity 12 months earlier was 20/30. With the same spectacle correction, it is now 20/100. Attempted refinement of the manifest refraction using ±0.25 D and ±0.50 D spherical lenses and a ±0.50 D Jackson cross cylinder elicits no change in the refraction. What is the next step?

    a. Perform a darkroom pinhole test.

    b. Repeat the manifest refraction using a ±0.75 D or ±1.00 D change in sphere and a ±0.75 D or ±1.00 D Jackson cross cylinder.

    c. Perform a slit-lamp examination for cataract or other media opacity.

    d. Dilate the pupil and examine for a choroidal neovascular membrane.

28. You fit a patient who has −3.50 D of myopia with an RGP contact lens that is flatter than K. If the patient's average K reading is 7.80 mm and you fit a lens with a base curve of 8.00 mm, what is the shape of the tear lens?

    a. plano

    b. teardrop

    c. concave

    d. convex

29. For the patient in question 28, what power RGP lens should you order?

    a. −3.50 D

    b. −4.00 D

    c. −2.00 D

    d. −2.50 D

30. You fit a toric soft contact lens on a patient with a refractive error of −2.50 D −1.50 × 175. The trial lens centers well, but the lens mark at the 6 o'clock position appears to rest at the 4 o'clock position when the lens is placed on the patient's eye. What power contact lens should you order?

    a. −2.50 D −1.50 × 175

    b. −2.50 D −1.50 × 115

    c. −2.50 D −1.50 × 55

    d. −2.50 D −1.00 × 175

31. All of the following statements regarding irregular astigmatism are true *except*:

    a. Manifest refraction and automated refraction may be dissimilar if there is significant irregular astigmatism.

    b. Irregular astigmatism may cause a poor endpoint in clinical refraction.

    c. Irregular astigmatism may be induced by a decentered refractive surgical procedure, pellucid marginal degeneration, and keratoconus.

    d. Best-corrected visual acuity is usually better with spectacles than with rigid contact lenses in the setting of significant irregular astigmatism.

32. Compared with spectacles, contact lenses

    a. increase the accommodative requirements of myopic eyes

    b. increase the accommodative requirements of hyperopic eyes

c. increase the convergence demands of hyperopic eyes

d. decrease the convergence requirements of myopic eyes

33. Which of the following increases the risk of infection in a patient wearing extended-wear contact lenses?

a. swimming with the contact lenses

b. exposure to smoke

c. corneal neovascularization

d. all of the above

34. The power of an intraocular lens (IOL) should be increased

a. as the power of the cornea increases and the axial length increases

b. as the power of the cornea decreases and the axial length increases

c. as the power of the cornea increases and the axial length decreases

d. as the power of the cornea decreases and the axial length decreases

35. Multifocal IOLs

a. offer increased image clarity and contrast for both near and far viewing

b. are independent of pupil size if they are well centered

c. offer a trade-off between decreased image quality and increased depth of focus

d. are indicated for all patients

36. Which of the following statements about piggyback IOLs is true?

a. Piggyback IOLs modify the vergence of light entering the eye after it leaves the incorrectly powered primary IOL.

b. Piggyback IOLs can be used in a second operation only if the original IOL power was too low and additional dioptric strength is indicated.

c. A piggyback IOL may be useful after removal of an incorrectly powered IOL.

d. Piggyback IOLs may be less necessary as standard IOL power ranges increase.

37. Aiming for a slight residual myopia in IOL power selection may be desirable because

a. weaker lenses are thinner and are less likely to cause surgical or postoperative complications due to size, disruption of tissues, inflammation, and so on

b. the A constant is calculated for a slight degree of residual myopia

c. residual myopia is closer to emmetropia than residual hyperopia

d. an error in power calculation is less likely to produce a resultant hyperopia, which would result in blurry vision at all distances

38. A patient comes for refractive surgery with keratometry readings of 43.0 D/42.0 D and a manifest refraction of −9.5 D. If LASIK were performed, you would expect the postoperative average keratometry reading to be

a. 34.9 D

b. 36.3 D

c. 37.3 D

d. 34.0 D

39. The principle of the astronomical telescope is used for magnification in which of the following ophthalmic instruments?

    a. indirect ophthalmoscope

    b. direct ophthalmoscope

    c. retinal fundus camera

    d. a and c

40. When a binocular indirect ophthalmoscope is used on a patient with small pupils, binocular visualization can be improved by

    a. moving the ophthalmoscope's mirror closer to the observer

    b. narrowing the observer's effective interpupillary distance

    c. moving the ophthalmoscope's eyepieces farther apart

    d. increasing the distance between the observer's head and the patient

    e. all of the above

41. Which of the following is not true of how keratometers work?

    a. They measure the radius of curvature of the central cornea.

    b. They assume the cornea to be a convex mirror.

    c. They directly measure the refractive power of the cornea.

    d. They use a mathematical formula to convert radius of curvature to approximate refractive power.

42. Which of the following is not an optical component of the slit-lamp biomicroscope?

    a. field lens

    b. astronomical telescope

    c. inverting prism

    d. Galilean telescope

43. Which of the following is not a component of an optical coherence tomography (OCT) system?

    a. movable mirror

    b. beam splitter

    c. reference beam

    d. split prism

44. Proper distance visual acuity testing for a low vision patient includes all of the following *except:*

    a. a testing chart with an equal number of symbols on each line

    b. nonstandardized room illumination

    c. a Snellen visual acuity chart at 20 ft

    d. a test distance of 10 ft

45. A patient with moderately low vision (20/160 in each eye) wants a prescription to be able to read; the best choice would be a(n)

a. +8.00 D single-vision reading spectacle

b. +4.00 D half-glass reader with a total of 6Δ BI prism

c. +8.00 D half-glass reader with a total of 10Δ BI prism

d. +8.00 D half-glass reader with 10Δ BI prism per lens

e. 8.0× magnifier

46. Which of the following statements regarding a patient with a central scotoma is false?

a. Most patients will fixate using an eccentric retinal location, the *preferred retinal locus.*

b. The location, shape, and number of scotomata variably affect visual function.

c. Eccentric fixation and PRL training can sometimes help patients improve coordination, tracking, and scanning and thereby facilitate function.

d. Reading is usually not possible because central macular function is required to read.

e. The best device for mapping a central scotoma is a scanning laser ophthalmoscope.

47. Which of the following statements regarding the prescription of visual aids is false?

a. The Kestenbaum rule provides a starting point to determine the appropriate addition required to read 1-M size print.

b. Base-in prisms increase effective magnification for binocular patients using reading spectacles.

c. Illuminated stand magnifiers help overcome stability and lighting problems associated with higher-power magnification.

d. Optical magnification without contrast enhancement may be insufficient for patients with severely reduced contrast sensitivity function.

e. In some states it is legal to drive with bioptic telescopes even when visual acuity falls below the normally accepted cutoff limit.

48. Which of the following best characterizes a person with "low vision"?

a. a bitemporal hemianopia

b. best-corrected visual acuity of 20/70 or worse

c. myopia greater than −20 D

d. a disability related to visual dysfunction

49. All of the following typically cause peripheral visual field deficits *except:*

a. retinitis pigmentosa

b. age-related macular degeneration

c. retinal detachment

d. panretinal photocoagulation

50. All of the following conditions commonly cause glare *except:*

a. iritis

b. corneal scarring

c. posterior subcapsular cataract

d. albinism

Answers

1. **a.** *Temporal coherence* is the principle by which the Michelson interferometer works. Spatial coherence, on the other hand, is a measure of the ability of 2 separated portions of the same wave to interfere. It is the principle by which wavefront splitting interferometers work. Polarization, directionality, and intensity refer to other important properties of laser light.

2. **d.** Many lasers emit a polarized beam. However, medical applications do not currently use this specific laser property.

3. **e.** A diopter is the reciprocal of distance in meters. A prism diopter measures the deviation in centimeters at 1 m, or centimeters per meter. Refractive index is the ratio of speeds and, therefore, has no dimensions. Wavelength can be measured in any unit of length. For optical wavelengths, the nanometer is convenient. Frequency is measured in cycles per second or hertz (Hz). Spatial frequency is measured in cycles per degree.

4. **a.** The index of refraction *(n)* of a transparent medium is defined as the ratio of the speed of light in a vacuum to the speed of light in the given material. Each lens material has a unique index of refraction, determined by the velocity with which light travels through it. The more the transparent material slows down light, the higher its *n* value and the greater its ability to refract light, thereby allowing thinner spectacle lenses.

5. **c.** The Airy disk is the pattern of light and dark rings formed when light from a point source passes through an aperture and is affected by diffraction. The size of the Airy disk increases with smaller pupil size (especially smaller than 2.5 mm), longer wavelengths of light, and longer focal lengths. Retinal conditions such as macular degeneration have no effect on the size of the Airy disk.

6. **b.** Light scattering occurs when small particles interfere with the transmittance of light and cause photons to deviate from a straight path. Short wavelengths of light are scattered more strongly than longer wavelengths. Larger particles scatter light more intensely than do smaller particles. In the healthy cornea, the tightly arranged and regularly spaced collagen molecules minimize the effects of scattering. When the cornea becomes edematous, the excess fluid in the stroma disrupts the very regular collagen structure, resulting in light scattering.

7. **a.** *Candela* is the unit of measure of *luminous intensity*, which is defined as the light emitted per unit of solid angle. *Luminous flux* is the quantity of light leaving a source or passing through a region of space, and it is measured in *lumens*. *Illuminance* is the quantity of light per unit area incident on a surface or at an image, and it is measured in *lux*. *Luminance* is the light reflected or emitted by a surface per unit area and per unit solid angle, and it is measured in *apostilbs*.

8. **d.** Laser light is created when atoms of an active medium are exposed to a source of energy (the *pumping source*). This causes most of the active medium's electrons to rise to a higher energy state, a condition called *population inversion*. Some of these high-energy electrons undergo spontaneous emission, generating photons. If these photons first encounter low-energy electrons, they are merely absorbed. However, if they encounter other high-energy electrons, *stimulated emission* occurs. In order to maintain the chain reaction of stimulated emissions, mirrors are placed at each end of the cavity, an arrangement called an

optical feedback. One mirror reflects totally and the other partially. Most of the coherent light generated is reflected back into the cavity to produce more stimulated emissions. The relatively small amount of light that is allowed to pass through the partially reflecting mirror produces the actual laser beam.

9. **d.** Light from the object, which is 1 m in front of the first lens, has a vergence of −1 D as it enters the lens (see the following figure). Vergence (diopters) = n/distance (meters) = −1/1 = −1 D. The lens adds an additional −1 D of vergence. Light leaving the lens, therefore, has a vergence of −2 D. Light rays with a vergence of −2 D appear to be coming from a point 0.5 m in front of the lens.

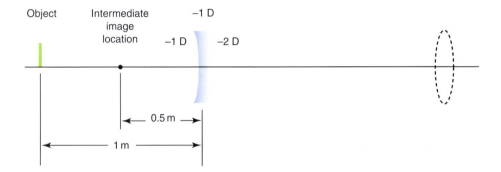

10. **d.** A −1 D lens has an anterior focal point, F_a, 1 m behind the lens and a posterior focal point, F_p, 1 m in front of the lens (see the following figure). A light ray from the tip of the object that enters the lens heading toward F_a will exit the lens parallel to the optical axis. A light ray that enters the lens parallel to the optical axis will exit the lens divergent, as if it had come from F_p. A ray traversing the nodal point of the lens, which corresponds to the optical center of the lens, will exit the lens undeviated. Back tracing the 3 rays as they leave the lens produces an upright virtual image at the location determined previously. The image is virtual because it is on the same side of the lens as the object. If a screen were placed at this location, no image would form. The ray-tracing diagram shows that the image is minified.

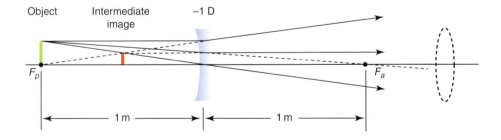

11. **c.** By similar triangles, the height of the intermediate image is one-half the height of the object (see the following figure). The transverse magnification is 0.5.

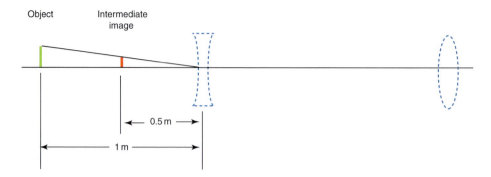

12. **b.** To answer questions 12–14, one makes the intermediate image the new object and forgets the first lens (see the following figure). The intermediate image is 2 m in front of the second lens. The vergence of light entering the second lens is, therefore, −0.5 D. The lens adds +1.5 D of vergence. The light exiting the lens, therefore, has a vergence of +1.0 D. Light rays with a vergence of +1.0 D come to a focus 1 m behind the second lens.

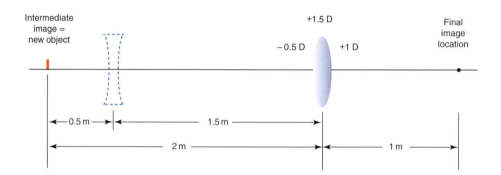

13. **d.** The +1.5 D spherical lens has an anterior focal point, F_a, 67 cm (2/3 m) in front of the lens and a posterior focal point, F_p, 67 cm behind the lens (see the following figure). A light ray from the tip of the object that enters the lens after going through F_a will exit the lens parallel to the optical axis. A light ray that enters the lens parallel to the optical axis will exit the lens and travel through F_p. A ray traversing the nodal point of the lens, which corresponds to the optical center of the lens, will exit the lens undeviated. All 3 rays intersect at the final image location determined previously. The image is real because it is on the opposite side of the lens as the object. A screen placed at this location would form a real image. The ray-tracing diagram shows that the image is inverted and minified.

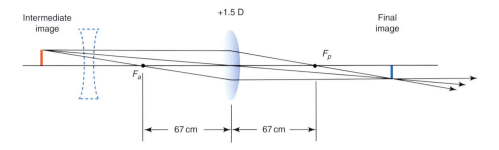

14. **b.** By similar triangles, the height of the final image is one-half the height of the intermediate image (see the following figure). Because the intermediate image is one-half the height of the object, the final image is one-fourth the height of the object. The transverse magnification is −0.25.

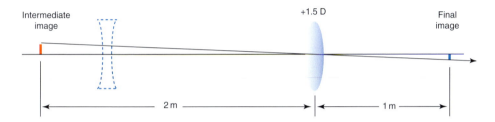

15. **a.** Light from the object has a vergence of −4 D when it strikes the mirror. The mirror adds +1 D, so light exiting the mirror has a vergence of −3 D. Because the mirror reverses image space, the image appears 0.33 m to the right of the mirror. The image can be drawn by tracing rays, as shown in part A of the figure. The image is upright. Image height can be determined by similar triangles, as shown in part B. The transverse magnification is 1.33/0.75 = 1.77. A negative transverse magnification would indicate an inverted image.

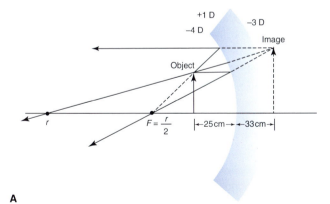

A

(continued)

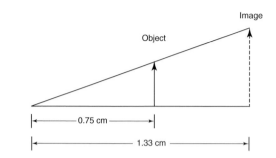

B

(continued from previous page)

16. **b.** Because red rays focus behind blue rays, the eye must make an accommodative effort to focus on red print after looking at blue print. It must relax accommodation to focus on blue print after looking at red print. The brain therefore perceives that the red print is in front of the blue print when both are displayed against the same background.

17. **a.** The far point of the eye and the fovea are always corresponding points when accommodation is relaxed. All the other statements are false.

18. **e.** The nonaccommodated hyperopic eye has a far point behind the eye. A virtual image of the retina forms at this location. As the eye begins to accommodate, the point of focus recedes to minus infinity. Minus infinity and plus infinity are essentially the same optically. As the eye continues to accommodate through optical infinity, the point of focus moves in front of the eye to a point between plus infinity and the cornea. The near point of the eye, in diopters, is equal to the far point location, in diopters, plus the amplitude of accommodation. Because we are told neither the amount of hyperopia nor the amplitude of accommodation, we cannot determine the location of the near point.

19. **e.** The Snellen fraction (eg, 20/20), the minimum angle of resolution (eg, 1.0), logMAR (eg, 0.0), and the 4-m standard (eg, 4/4) are all measures of visual acuity.

20. **a.** In mixed astigmatism, 1 focal line forms in front of the retina and the other line forms behind the retina. In compound myopic astigmatism, both focal lines fall in front of the retina. In compound hyperopic astigmatism, both focal lines fall behind the retina. In simple myopic astigmatism, 1 line forms on the retina and the other falls in front of it. In simple hyperopic astigmatism, 1 line forms on the retina and the other falls behind it.

21. **d.** The optical system's nodal point is the point through which light rays entering or leaving the system are undeviated. In the reduced schematic eye, the nodal point is located 5.6 mm posterior to the corneal surface. Since all light rays passing through this point are undeviated, a light ray that leaves the tip of an object will pass through the nodal point and strike the retina undeviated. Retinal image size can be calculated by similar triangles.

22. **b.** The best reading add for a low vision patient can easily be obtained from the visual acuity by using the Kestenbaum rule. The VA is expressed as a fraction $1/x$. The *dioptric* power of the add is simply x. In this example, x is determined to be 3.50. Note that a 3.5× magnifier is equivalent to a +14.0 D lens.

23. **a.** As the eyes look down to read through the add segment, there will be an abrupt upward image jump at the top edge of the segment. This jump is due to the prismatic effect of the plus lens (the add segment). Based on the Prentice rule, the amount of jump will depend on the power of the segment and on the distance from the top of the segment to the optical center of the segment.

24. **d.** As a rule of thumb, the number of prism diopters (Δ) is approximately twice the angle in degrees. However, this works only for small angles (<20°). An angle of 45° means that at 1 m, a beam is deviated by 1 m (100 cm). Thus, 45° corresponds to 100Δ. An angle of 90° is infinity in prism diopters.

25. **c.** In general, patients perceive image jump as more of a problem than image displacement. Flat-top segments minimize image jump because the optical center is near the top. In patients with myopia, flat tops also reduce prism displacement because the base-down effect of the distance portion is reduced by the base-up effect of the segment.

26. **b.** The power cross for this retinoscopy, before subtraction of the effect of the working distance, is shown in the figure. In plus cylinder terms, the corresponding spherocylinder refraction is

RE: +3.50 +1.50 × 090
LE: +6.00 +1.00 × 090

Subtracting 1.50 D to compensate for the effect of the working distance produces a spherocylinder refraction of

RE: +2.00 +1.50 × 090
LE: +4.50 +1.00 × 090

This result can be expressed in minus cylinder terms. Referring again to the power cross, note the 2.5 D difference between the eyes acting in the vertical meridian. This anisometropia produces a net 2.5Δ base-up prism effect in front of the left eye, creating a 2.5Δ left hyperphoria. There is a 2 D difference between the eyes in the horizontal meridian. This meridional anisometropia produces a net 2Δ base-in prism effect before the left eye, resulting in a 2Δ exophoria. Once a retinoscopic reflex has been neutralized at the peephole of a retinoscope, the far point of the eye is at 0.67 m. Moving closer produces "with" motion, and moving away produces "against" motion.

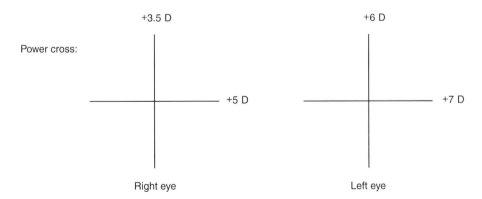

Power cross:

+3.5 D   +5 D   Right eye

+6 D   +7 D   Left eye

27. **b.** Changes of ±0.25 D and ±0.50 D in sphere and cylinder are likely to be below the "just noticeable" threshold for a patient with 20/100 visual acuity. Because the first thing to rule out when vision changes is a change in refraction, an additional attempt should be made to refine the refraction using larger-step changes in sphere and cylinder. The darkroom pinhole test is a test of potential vision. It should be performed after the refraction has been maximized.

28. **c.** The tear lens is formed by the posterior surface of the contact lens and the anterior surface of the cornea. If these 2 curvatures are the same, as with a soft lens, the tear lens is plano. If they are different (as is typical of RGP lenses), a + or − tear lens will be formed. In this case, the contact lens is flatter than K, so the tear lens is negative, or concave, in shape.

29. **d.** Use the rule of thumb that for every 0.05-mm radius of curvature difference between the base curve and K, the induced power of the tear film is 0.25 D. The power of the concave tear lens in this case is −1.00 D. The power of the RGP contact lens you should order is −3.50 D − (−1.00 D) = −2.50 D. An easy way to remember this is to use the following rule: *SAM = steeper add minus* and *FAP = flatter add plus*.

30. **b.** The amount and direction of rotation should be noted. In this case, they are, respectively, 2 clock-hours and rotation to the right. Each clock-hour represents 30° (360°/12 = 30°), so the adjustment needs to be 60°. Because the rotation is to the right, you should order a contact lens with axis 115 instead of 175—that is, −2.50 D −1.50 × 115. An easy rule to remember is *LARS = left add, right subtract*.

31. **d.** *Irregular astigmatism* is a catchall phrase for higher-order monochromatic aberrations. Most irregular astigmatism arises at the anterior surface of the cornea. RGP contact lenses create a smooth air–lens interface when they sit on the surface of an irregular cornea. Soft contact lenses cannot do this; rather, they mold to the surface of the cornea. If glasses could be manufactured to compensate for higher-order aberrations, they would work in 1 gaze direction only. For this reason, RGP contact lenses provide the best acuity for patients with irregular corneas and irregular astigmatism.

32. **a.** Contact lenses eliminate the accommodative advantage enjoyed by those with spectacle-corrected myopia and the disadvantage experienced by those with spectacle-corrected hyperopia. Compared with that of spectacle lenses, contact lens correction of myopia increases the accommodative and convergence demands of focusing on near objects proportional to the size of the refractive error. The reverse is true in hyperopia.

33. **d.** There are many risk factors associated with even the latest extended-wear contact lenses, including swimming with the lenses, previous history of eye infection, any exposure to smoke, abnormal lid function, severe dry eye, and corneal neovascularization.

34. **d.** A certain vergence of light is necessary to focus incoming light on the retina. As the power of the cornea decreases, a corresponding amount of vergence power (corrected for the different location of the refractive element) must be added. Similarly, as the eye becomes shorter, more vergence power is needed to bring the light into focus on the now-less-distant retina.

35. **c.** Multifocal IOLs present both near and distant foci to the retina at the same time. This leads to an unavoidable decrease in image quality and contrast sensitivity, particularly at low levels of illumination. Pupil size may be a factor, particularly with certain types of multifocal IOLs. (Smaller pupil size results in increased depth of focus regardless!)

36. **d.** Piggyback IOLs have been used to reach a total dioptric power that was unavailable in a single lens. As IOLs are becoming available in a wider range of powers, it is less likely that a piggyback IOL will be needed to reach an unusually high or low power. Piggyback IOLs are placed anterior to the primary lens and thus modify the light vergence *before* it reaches the primary IOL. These IOLs may be used to correct inaccurate primary IOLs in a second operation if the original IOL power was too low *or* too high. They are not used after removal of an incorrectly powered IOL—"piggyback" implies that a second IOL is in the eye.

37. **d.** No IOL power formula is 100% accurate. Aiming for a small degree of myopia increases the chances that the patient will have good uncorrected vision at some useful distance. There is no significant increase in surgical risks or complications related to different lens thicknesses due to different dioptric powers for a given IOL model. The *A* constant of the SRK formulas is related to the IOL type and is unaffected by the choice of refractive endpoint.

38. **a.** The formula is keratometry change = 0.8 × refractive change. Here, the keratometry change = 0.8 × 9.5 D = 7.6 D, so the calculated final postoperative average is K = (43.0 D + 42.0 D)/2 − 7.6 D = 34.9 D.

39. **d.** Both the indirect ophthalmoscope and the retinal fundus camera use the principle of the astronomical telescope, thereby producing magnified, real, and inverted images of the retina. The direct ophthalmoscope, however, applies the principle of a simple magnifier, using the refractive power of the patient's eye to produce magnified, virtual, upright images of the retina.

40. **e.** When looking through a small pupil, the observer can improve visualization by narrowing his or her effective interpupillary distance. This can be accomplished by several means. Moving the ophthalmoscope's mirror closer to the observer (the "small-pupil feature" available on some ophthalmoscopes) decreases the distance between the light paths to the observer's left and right eyes, effectively narrowing the observer's interpupillary distance. Moving the ophthalmoscope's eyepieces farther apart also decreases the distance between the light paths to the observer's eyes, similarly narrowing the observer's effective interpupillary distance. Increasing the distance between the observer and the patient decreases the angle formed by the observer's 2 eyes and the patient's eye, thereby allowing the light paths from the observer's eyes to "squeeze through" a smaller pupil.

41. **c.** Keratometers approximate the refractive power of the cornea by measuring the radius of curvature of the central cornea and assuming the cornea to be a convex mirror. The formula $r = 2u(I/O)$ is then used to convert this radius of curvature into an approximate refractive power, where r is the radius of curvature of the reflective cornea, u is the distance from the object to the cornea, I is the size of the image, and O is the size of the object.

42. **a.** A slit-lamp biomicroscope is a high-power binocular microscope with a slit-shaped illumination source. Most of the microscope's magnifying power is produced by an astronomical telescope, while additional magnifying power is produced by a Galilean telescope. The resulting magnified image is inverted, so an inverting prism is used to create an upright image. An objective lens, which moves the working distance from infinity to a distance close enough to focus on the eye, is the last component of the slit-lamp biomicroscope. A field lens, which is often used in a lensmeter, is not a component of the slit-lamp biomicroscope.

43. **d.** Optical coherence tomography (OCT) is used to create cross-sectional images of the living retina at extremely high resolutions. Rays from a light source (usually a superluminescent diode) are split by a beam splitter into a reference beam, which is directed to a movable mirror, and an object beam, which is directed to the retina. The 2 reflected beams are then superimposed by the same beam splitter and transmitted together to a light detector. By correlating the resulting interference patterns with the position of the movable mirror, information about the reflectivity of the internal structure of the retina can then be constructed.

44. **c.** For low vision patients, distance acuity testing is best done at a distance of 10 ft; standard projection charts, such as the Snellen chart, are not ideal for obtaining accurate visual acuity measurements for these patients. The ETDRS chart has a geometric progression of optotypes, with letter sizes from 10 to 200 and with each line having the same number of letters. In contrast to a Snellen-type chart, the ETDRS chart has a 160 line and a 125 line between the 100 and 200 lines. Performance on visual function tests often varies depending on room illumination, which should be adjusted to obtain the patient's best response.

45. **d.** A patient with 20/160 vision should still be able to maintain binocularity with reading despite requiring a reading add of +8.00 D (see the Kestenbaum rule). This will require adding to each lens a base-in prism that is 2.0Δ more than the dioptric strength of the lens. A half-glass reader is the most convenient spectacle form for this type of lens because the lens bulk and weight are minimized.

46. **d.** Patients with central scotomata can still read by using eccentric fixation, along with appropriate magnification and enhanced contrast, if necessary. Reading speed is usually decreased, but reading ability can often be improved with training and practice.

47. **b.** Base-in prisms should be incorporated into high-power reading spectacles to assist accommodative convergence in patients who have similar visual function binocularly. They do not affect magnification.

48. **d.** A person is considered to have "low vision" when a visual deficit significantly affects his or her activities. Visual disability is related to the interaction of a number of factors, including the complexity of the task, the skill of the person, the individual's response to reduced vision, and other aspects of visual function, including contrast sensitivity. A visual field deficit (such as bitemporal hemianopia) or a specific level of visual acuity (such as less than 20/70) does not in and of itself qualify as low vision if it does not significantly affect that person's particular activities or if he or she is able to adequately compensate. Conversely, a patient who performs relatively well on a Snellen test may be considered to have low vision if he or she is not able to perform necessary tasks because of visual loss.

49. **b.** Loss of peripheral visual field makes it difficult to navigate unfamiliar territory and may cause the patient to bump into objects or people. Retinitis pigmentosa, panretinal photocoagulation, and retinal detachment typically affect the peripheral visual field, whereas age-related macular degeneration typically affects central acuity.

50. **a.** Glare occurs when light is scattered by an optical medium, resulting in a reduction of contrast. This scattering of light can be caused by corneal scars and cataracts (especially posterior subcapsular cataracts). In albinism, the unpigmented iris allows too much light to pass, and light is scattered by the peripheral lens and zonules. In iritis, patients are often photophobic, but the photophobia is due to spasm of the ciliary body; it is not the result of glare.

Index

(*f* = figure; *t* = table)